ANNALS OF THE NEW YORK ACADEMY

VOLUME 164, ART. 2 PAGES 307–634

October 14, 1969

SECOND CONFERENCE ON PSYCHOPHYSIOLOGICAL ASPECTS OF CANCER*

Conference Chairman and Consulting Editor

CLAUS BAHNE BAHNSON

CONTENTS

Photograph of DAVID M. KISSEN .... Frontispiece

Scroll ....

Dedication. In Memory of DR. DAVID M. KISSEN: His Work and His Thinking. *By* CLAUS BAHNE BAHNSON 313

Part I. The Psychophysiological Problems in Cancer

Psychophysiological Complementarity in Malignancies: Past Work and Future Vistas. *By* CLAUS BAHNE BAHNSON 319

Emotion, Stress, the Central Nervous System, and Immunity. *By* GEORGE F. SOLOMON 335

Tumor-Specific Transplantation Antigens. *By* EVA KLEIN 344

Psychic and Cellular Aspects of Isolation and Identity Impairment in Cancer: A Dialectic of Alienation. *By* GRAHAM BENNETTE 352

Immunological Paradoxes: Theoretical Considerations in the Rejection or Retention of Grafts, Tumors, and Normal Tissue. *By* JONAS SALK 365

Part II. Early Experience, Psychopathology, and Cancer

Psychosocial Factors Modifying Host Resistance to Experimental Infections. *By* STANFORD B. FRIEDMAN, LOWELL A. GLASGOW, AND ROBERT ADER 381

Psychological and Somatic Variables Associated with the Development and Course of Monozygotic Twins Discordant for Leukemia. *By* WILLIAM A. GREENE AND SCOTT N. SWISHER 394

A Speculative Mathematical Model of the Psychophysiologic System. *By* ROBERT H. RIFFENBURGH 409

Discussion. *By* LAWRENCE LESHAN 425

* This series of papers is the result of a conference entitled Second Conference on Psychophysiological Aspects of Cancer, held by the New York Academy of Sciences on May 20, 21, and 22, 1968. The conference was supported in part by grants from the National Institutes of Health and the Damon Runyon Medical Foundation for Cancer Research.

Discussion. *By* DAVID W. WEISS ... 427
Comment. *By* CLAUS BAHNE BAHNSON ... 430

Part III. Emotion, Immunology, and Cancer

Immunological Parameters of the Host-Parasite Relationship in Neoplasia. *By* DAVID W. WEISS ... 431
The Relationship of Immunology to Carcinogenesis. *By* RICHMOND T. PREHN ... 449
Emotions and Immunity. *By* A. F. RASMUSSEN, JR. ... 458
Remarks on Dr. Korneva's Work. *By* GEORGE F. SOLOMON ... 463
The Hypothalamus and Immune Process. *By* MARVIN STEIN, RAUL C. SCHIAVI, AND THOMAS J. LUPARELLO ... 464
Discussion. Emotions, Immunology, and Cancer: How Might the Psyche Influence Neoplasia? *By* CHESTER M. SOUTHAM ... 473

Part IV. The Nervous System, Hormones, and Cancer

Steroid Excretion Patterns and Personality in Lung Cancer. *By* DAVID M. KISSEN AND L. G. S. RAO ... 476
Pretreatment Urinary Hormone Patterns and Survival in Patients with Breast Cancer, Prostate Cancer, or Lung Cancer. *By* JESSIE MARMORSTON, PAUL J. GELLER, AND JOHN M. WEINER ... 483
Neuroendocrine Factors in Experimental Carcinogenesis. *By* ELIZABETH STERN, MAX R. MICKEY, AND ROGER A. GORSKI ... 494
Psychoendocrine Considerations in Cancer of the Breast. *By* JACK KATZ, THOMAS GALLAGHER, LEON HELLMAN, EDWARD SACHAR, AND HERBERT WEINER ... 509
Induced Carcinogenesis under Various Influences on the Hypothalamus. *By* R. E. KAVETSKY, N. M. TURKEVICH, R. N. AKIMOVA, I. K. KHAYETSKY, AND Y. D. MATVEICHUK ... 517
Some Electrophysiological Peculiarities of the Nervous System in Malignant Growth. *By* K. P. BALITSKY, A. P. KAPSHUK, AND V. F. TSAPENKO ... 520
Discussion. Physiologic Responses to Avoidable and Unavoidable Psychologic Stress in Relation to Genetic Differences. *By* SAMUEL A. CORSON ... 526

Part V. Psychodynamic Process and Cancer

A Further Report on Personality and Psychosocial Factors in Lung Cancer. *By* DAVID M. KISSEN, R. I. F. BROWN, AND MARGARET KISSEN ... 535
Ego Defenses in Cancer Patients. *By* MARJORIE BROOKS BAHNSON AND CLAUS BAHNE BAHNSON ... 546
Regression as an Intervening Mechanism: A System-Theoretical Approach. *By* ÁRPAD MEZEI AND GYÖRGY NÉMETH ... 560
General and Organ-Specific Object Relationships in Cancer. *By* GOTTHARD BOOTH ... 568
Integration, Discipline, and the Concept of Shape. *By* HARLEY C. SHANDS ... 578

Part VI. Theoretical Psychophysiological Considerations

General Discussion. CLAUS BAHNE BAHNSON, *Moderator* ... 590

Part VII. Integration and Evaluation of Current Psychophysiological Approaches to Cancer

Panel Discussion 1: The Neuroendocrinologic Approach. SYDNEY MARGOLIN, *Moderator* 611
Panel Discussion 2: The Immunologic Approach. JONAS SALK, *Moderator* ... 620
Panel Discussion 3: The Psychological Approach. CLAUS BAHNE BAHNSON, *Moderator* ... 628

Dedicated to

DAVID M. KISSEN

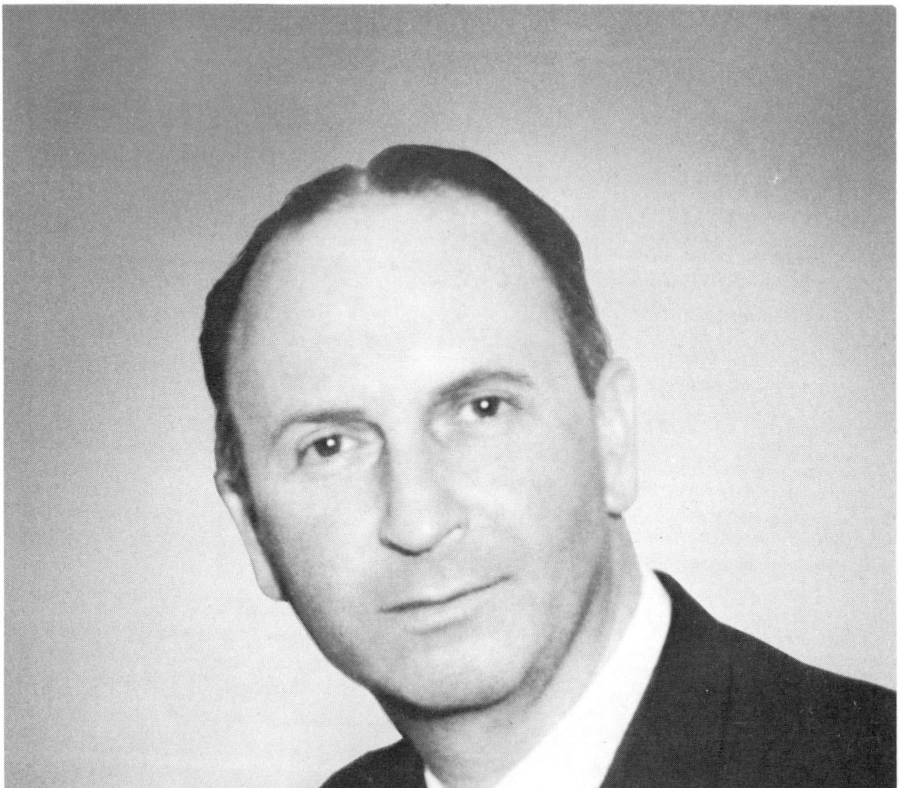

DAVID M. KISSEN

1916–1968

The New York Academy of Sciences, and the organization committee and participants of the second conference on psychophysiological aspects of cancer, express their deep appreciation and recognition of the initiative and vision which

David M. Kissen, B.Sc., M.D.

Director of the Psychosomatic Research Unit
Department of Psychological Medicine
University of Glasgow

showed in his pioneering psychosomatic research and in his origination of and contributions to the NYAS conferences on psychophysiological aspects of cancer.

Dr. Kissen studied psychophysiological relationships in several somatic diseases and contributed particularly to current research on personality correlates of lung cancer.

Dr. Kissen's work integrated theoretical boldness with empirical clarity and precision. He founded and directed the Psychosomatic Research Unit of the Department of Psychological Medicine, and with the assistance of his staff created a research unit which surely will continue to play a leading role in the further search for psychosomatic relationships.

Dr. Kissen also was an international promoter in the area of psychosomatic research in cancer, and, as the president of the International Psychosomatic Cancer Study Group, he inspired other researchers to study personality factors in relation to cancer.

For all this we, his colleagues, shall ever hold him in high esteem.

DEDICATION

IN MEMORY OF DR. DAVID M. KISSEN: HIS WORK AND HIS THINKING

Claus Bahne Bahnson

We shall all miss David M. Kissen, who so suddenly and prematurely passed away only several weeks prior to the conference on which this monograph is based. Dr. Kissen had looked forward to participating in it with particular expectations because he had been so very much disappointed at not being able to attend the first conference because of the sudden illness that presaged his recent death, although it was his vision to originate and initiate the arrangement for that first conference. Fortunately, the two studies Dr. Kissen worked on with his group in Glasgow were sufficiently well developed before his death to make it possible for his co-workers to complete the analyses and present the results in two papers at this conference.

In order to bring added perspective to this new work, which Dr. Kissen's co-workers will present, a review of some of the main trends in his research and in that of the Psychosomatic Research Unit, which he founded and directed in Glasgow, may be helpful.

David M. Kissen began his earliest studies in the psychosomatic field as a chest physician, and was particularly attracted to the study of emotional factors in pulmonary tuberculosis. The paper "The Patient's Personality" (1958) reflects the sensitivity and sophistication with which he approached complex psychosomatic problems from the very beginning of his work in this field. However, David Kissen soon turned his main interests to the study of personality in lung cancer, and he initiated this research, which he was to continue for a decade, in the best possible and most thorough fashion: he carried out intensive psychological interviews in several chest departments with a variety of chest patients whose diagnoses were unknown to him and to themselves at the time of the interview. About half of these 900 patients subsequently were found to suffer from lung cancer, and could be compared with the remainder of the patients serving as controls. On the basis of this essentially clinical procedure, he first characterized lung cancer patients, as opposed to noncancer pulmonary patients, as having "poor outlets for emotional discharge." By this, he meant that they have a facility for absorbing and containing emotional conflict, at an unconscious level, which results in an absence of apparent response. The basic clinical observation of "poor outlets for emotional discharge" in lung cancer patients was made quite independently of similar observations by other workers at approximately the same time, although phrased in a different terminology. This theoretical formulation of his observations was to become one of the main conceptual strains in his research, to be cross-validated on other subject groups and with different techniques of evaluation in several of the studies that followed.

David Kissen, however, was not satisfied with just carrying out empirical research without coming to grips with basic conceptual and methodological problems raised by the scientific approach to psychosomatic research. His paper "A Scientific Approach to Clinical Research in Psychosomatic Medicine" (1960a) reflects his critical and analytical interest in research methodology.

Evaluating the methodology of psychoanalytic studies in psychosomatic conditions, Dr. Kissen emphasized (in addition to the usual critique that psychoanalytic studies frequently use small numbers and have no controls) that they are characterized by an inherent danger of assigning to temporally concomitant attributes and dynamics not necessarily related to the disease at all, the causal role for the psychosomatic disease in these patients. Although this is a basic and logical point applicable to all research involving multiple variables, the fact that Dr. Kissen mentions this point in relation to psychoanalytic, or depth, studies indicates his concern for not becoming lost in the clinical jungle, but for attempting to circumscribe research to more clearly defined and "objective" measurements. Dr. Kissen writes, "What is important is that too many deep studies, involving too few patients, and without controls or objectivity, are used as the basis of too many profound conclusions." However, Dr. Kissen also writes in the same paper about psychoanalytic methods that "they are an important and possibly a principal means of exploration of unchartered territory–as in the past–and may point the way to more definite investigation" (1960a).

Concerning the definition of what constitutes a psychosomatic disorder, and concerning the popular concepts of proof of such conditions, David Kissen also had much to say. Often referring to Halliday's sevenfold criteria for psychosomatic afflictions, he took great pains to differentiate exactly what he did and did not mean by a psychosomatic condition. Defining, with Halliday, a psychosomatic condition as one that requires an investigation of emotional and psychological disturbances in addition to the somatic processes, he turned sharply against such naïve concepts as those expressed in the expectancy that when a psychological stress is removed, the psychosomatic disturbance will disappear. "The fact that organic change is only, or more effectively, reversible by physical means does not imply that it cannot be due to stress" (1960a).

In his quest for an impeccable methodology, David Kissen did not compromise on any of the criteria he deemed important. He insisted on carefully selected controls, on "objective" methods of measurement, and on sound statistical methods of analysis. Not only in his writings but also in his own work did he honor these rigid criteria for scientific research. David Kissen often was impatient with colleagues who would generalize expansively on the basis of meager data. He was critical of research that used a handful of patients without control subjects for the investigation of psychodynamic characteristics, and in which random or arbitrary results from these few subjects then would be generalized to pertain to the illness category as a whole. He always was most scientific and cautious in the presentation of his own data, and made it a point to oppose any enthusiastic follower who would broaden or generalize from these findings beyond the very precise limits of his own definition of his sample. This scientific modesty and commitment to careful investigation of facts earmarked all his scientific work, and makes it extremely valuable as a source of information, because one can be quite assured that what is stated is absolutely correct and indisputable, and that all generalizations that might have tempted others have been omitted. Thus, in spite of his enthusiasm for the psychosomatic approach, he restrained himself remarkably, and paid homage to critical fact, rather than to colorful theory.

The rigor of theoretical and empirical position did not inhibit the scope of David Kissen's production. On the basis of his clinical investigation of lung cancer and tuberculosis patients, he set out to investigate by more precise and objective methods the hypotheses he had formulated during his first study phase. Characteristically, the first thing he did was to investigate all factors *other* than the emotional ones that could be related to the differentiation between lung cancer and noncancer patients in his pulmonary population. He reviewed social class, income, intelligence, several aspects of smoking, and reasons given by subjects for starting to smoke, somatotypes, heredity, and other variables that might possibly be related to the cancer/noncancer differentiation, before entering into a discussion of personality features, emotionally stressful situations, and psychoanalytic variables (1960b).

Having convinced himself that there was something to the "poor emotional outlet" hypothesis, Dr. Kissen wrote several papers reporting on carefully designed studies of the subject matter. In a study on the "Relationship between Primary Lung Cancer and Peptic Ulcer in Males" (1962b), in which he controlled by social class and age within two subject groups, one group consisting of men found to have nonmalignant pulmonary conditions and another group of men admitted for treatment of a variety of psychosomatic conditions such as bronchial asthma, angina pectoris, hypertension, dermatitis, and pulmonary tuberculosis, he concluded that significant differences between lung cancer patients and controls were confined to those subjects in the age group of 45–64 years. In this group he found that 1) peptic ulcer is more common in lung cancer patients, 2) more lung cancer patients have histories of psychosomatic disorders other than peptic ulcer, 3) rheumatism, dermatitis, and neuroses are more common in lung cancer patients, 4) there is an association between cigarette smoking and lung cancer and also between cigarette smoking and peptic ulcer, whereas there is no association between cigarette smoking and history of past psychosomatic disorders other than peptic ulcer, and 5) adenocarcinomas, on the whole, tend to be associated with a greater proportion of peptic ulcer and other psychosomatic disorders than do the other histological types of lung cancer.

During his work with a variety of psychosomatic syndromes, Dr. Kissen arrived at the conviction that a psychosomatic disorder group exists, that it includes several psychosomatic conditions, and that it is characterized by syndrome shifts from one disease to another in the same patients (1963d). This point of view was founded on clinical history studies carried out on more than 700 adult males.

David Kissen needed some objective and quantifiable personality measures to substantiate his clinical conclusions. He found such a measure in the Maudsley Personality Inventory (MPI), developed by Eysenck.* Controlling for smoking history, which suddenly had become the uncritically accepted sole etiological variable in lung cancer, Dr. Kissen set to work, evaluating sample after sample, and teasing out exact interrelationships between different sets of scores on the MPI and different, exactly defined smoking-behavior classes. After premature conclusions had been drawn by other researchers, Kissen wrote, "The evidence . . . . suggests that both cigarette smoking and a characteristic personality appear to be involved in the development of lung cancer." (1964e) Relating the "neuroticism scores" on the MPI to smoking, Dr. Kissen concluded that "the poorer the outlet for emotional discharge the less the exposure to cigarette smoke required to induce lung cancer," thus proposing a two-factor theory of prediction. The "neuroticism scale" of the MPI measures an individual's emotional instability and his emotional over-responsiveness and liability to neurotic breakdown under emotional stress. Thus, low scores on this scale suggest lack of emotional discharge and were interpreted by Dr. Kissen to reflect that aspect

* Eysenck, H. J. 1959. The differentiation between normal and various neurotic groups on Maudsley Personality Inventory. Brit. J. Psychol. **50:** 176–177.

of the lung cancer patient's personality which he previously had identified clinically as "lack of outlet for emotional discharge." Other studies, using similar methodologies, cross-validated these test findings (1963b, 1963c, 1964b, 1964c, 1965b, 1966b, 1966c, 1966d). These MPI studies also revealed that lung cancer patients have a trend toward extraversion, as compared with controls, a finding that corroborates the social and "reality" orientation of cancer patients observed by other workers.

David Kissen also evaluated neuroticism and extraversion scores for smokers, irrespective of lung cancer status, and found that smokers in general score high on extraversion and fairly average on neuroticism. On this basis, he concluded that lung cancer patients do not appear to be a random sample but a special group of cigarette smokers, and that the lung cancer group consisting of nonsmokers also appears to be a special subgroup of these nonsmokers. In other words, his studies indicated that the relationship between smoking and lung cancer is an intricate and complex one.

David Kissen was concerned about the concepts of unconscious denial or inhibition, and in one of his studies (1963b, 1963c) set out to investigate whether lung cancer patients tended to conceal or "bottle up" consciously, rather than as an unconscious defense mechanism. He did that by questioning his subjects directly, asking each patient whether he tended to conceal or "bottle up" his emotional difficulties or tended to talk them over with someone. He found that, also on this conscious level, lung cancer patients tend to conceal their emotional difficulties significantly more often than do control patients. However, there were no suggestive correlations between conscious concealment and the extraversion or neuroticism scores on the MPI, suggesting that this conscious concealment factor may operate independently of the other personality factors he demonstrated in his samples.

David Kissen searched for other correlates of the tendency to "poor outlets for emotional discharge," and among these correlates reported a low degree of childhood behavior disorders among these "poor outletters" and low neuroticism scores on the newer Eysenck Personality Inventory, which replaced the MPI in his methodology (1963b, 1963c).

After having demonstrated clearly the relationships between smoking, emotional inhibition, and lung cancer, Dr. Kissen turned his attention to the study of autonomic activity and the awareness of such activity in lung cancer patients. He constructed a scale consisting of 11 items, each referring to a different system associated with autonomic activity, and found that lung cancer patients, according to their own reporting, operate on lower levels of autonomic activity on all 11 items (1968b).

David Kissen also broadened his interest in the psychosocial aspects of the study of lung cancer patients and reported that although lung cancer patients do not show an emotional response to adverse life situations by a rise in neuroticism scores, as do noncancer patients, they nonetheless do report significantly more adverse life situations than do controls, both in childhood and in adult life. Kissen suggested that this too is consistent with unconscious repression and denial of emotional difficulties.

Lung cancer patients reported, for their childhood, death of either parent, unhappy home, and other adverse life situations significantly more often than did control patients. In adult life, the adverse events relate to work and interpersonal difficulties, particularly marital strife of long standing (1967b).

Not only autonomic activity, but also hormonal activity entered into the research repertoire of Dr. Kissen's unit not too long ago, and some of the results he obtained are reported in this monograph. This biochemical work indicated that adrenal function is altered in cancer patients, compared with controls, since control patients respond to hospital admission with increased excretion of steroids followed by a gradual decrease over a period of seven days, whereas cancer patients do not show such a marked response to admission but maintain fluctuating and higher levels than controls. Thus, lung cancer patients respond differently to the stress of hospitalization than do controls, who apparently reflect the "fight-flight" reaction one would presume exists under such circumstances. Whether this is a correlate of the psychobiological inhibition also expressed in the several measures of "poor emotional outlet" is a question to which David Kissen directed his attention shortly before his untimely death, and to which his colleagues are addressing themselves at this time, by correlating steroid-excretion values with measurements of personality by means of the Eysenck Personality Inventory.

During the last few years, David Kissen also turned his interest toward the area of prevention, prophylaxis, and early detection of cancer, and because he was able to discriminate between cancer and noncancer patients on the basis of a combination of variables that he had isolated and cross-validated, he felt that these predictive measures should be applied in a prevention and early-detection program. He emphasized the "significance of carefully ascertained personality and psychosocial factors, together with physical factors, as means of identifying cancer-prone individuals. In this way preventive measures could be concentrated on the cancer-prone minority, for whom the hazards are most real, with greater likelihood of success than existing propaganda techniques which make no distinction between individual susceptibilities" (1965b). In his opening paper to the first New York Academy of Sciences conference on Psychophysiological Aspects of Cancer (1966b), Kissen also emphasized the prophylactic potential of personality and psychosocial data. "Would it not be of immense value if simple techniques were available to identify the susceptibles on whom specific preventive measures, psychological, and other, could be concentrated? Personality and other psychological characteristics, as well as physical and constitutional features, conducive to the development of these diseases, could be utilized to help identify readily high-risk individuals."

Dr. Kissen's co-workers in Glasgow now continue the promising research that he initiated with so much imagination and scientific rigor. We all hope that they may be able to complete the crucial psychophysiological research program he staked out.

Beyond the influence that David Kissen had in his own research group, he also influenced his contemporary and junior research colleagues deeply with his persistent and clear questions, and he most certainly was one of those few contemporary students of psychobiological conditions who actively set the stage for future interdisciplinary research into the difficult area of the mind-body relationships that still remain puzzling to us. For this initiative and leadership we will continue to be indebted to Dr. David M. Kissen for a long time to come.

Selected Bibliography

KISSEN, D. M. 1958. The patient's personality. *In* Transactions of the NAPT Commonwealth Chest Conference : 164–166. London, England.

KISSEN, D. M. 1960a. A scientific approach to clinical research in psychosomatic medicine. Psychosom. Med. **22:** 118–126.

KISSEN, D. M. 1960b. Psycho-social factors in cigarette smoking motivation: A review. Medical Officer **104:** 365–372.

KISSEN, D. M. & H. J. EYSENCK. 1962a. Personality in male lung cancer patients. J. Psychosom. Res. **6**: 123–127.
KISSEN, D. M. 1962b. Relationship between primary lung cancer and peptic ulcer in males. Psychosom. Med. **14**: 133–147.
KISSEN, D. M. 1963a. A propos de quelques concepts psychosomatiques et de leurs corollaires practiques. Rev. Med. Psychosom. (Paris) **5**: 15–26.
KISSEN, D. M. 1963b. Aspects of personality of men with lung cancer. Acta Psychother. (Basel) **11**: 200–210.
KISSEN, D. M. 1963c. Personality characteristics in males conducive to lung cancer. Brit. J. Med. Psychol. **36**: 27–36.
KISSEN, D. M. 1963d. The significance of syndrome shift and late syndrome association in psychosomatic medicine. J. Nerv. Ment. Dis. **136**: 34–41.
KISSEN, D. M. & T. FREEMAN. 1964a. General practitioner training in psychosomatic medicine and psychotherapy by group discussions. Revue de Med. Psychosom. (Paris) **6**(4).
KISSEN, D. M. 1964b. Lung cancer, inhalation, and personality. *In* Psychosomatic Aspects of Neoplastic Disease. D. M. Kissen & L. L. LeShan, Eds. : 3–11. Pitman. London, England.
KISSEN, D. M. & L. L. LESHAN, Eds. 1964c. Psychosomatic Aspects of Neoplastic Disease. Pitman. London, England.
KISSEN, D. M. 1964d. Quelques considerations psychosomatiques dans le maniement du patient souffrant d'une maladie chronique. *In* Psychosomatique et Chronicite. P. Aboulker, L. Chertok & N. Sapir, Eds. : 249–255. Librairie Maloine, S.A. Paris, France.
KISSEN, D. M. 1964e. Relationship between lung cancer, cigarette smoking, inhalation and personality. Brit. J. Med. Psychol. **37**: 203–216.
KISSEN, D. M. 1964f. Syndrome shift and personality traits. *In* Role of Psychosomatic Disorders in Adult Life. J. O. Wisdom & H. H. Wolff, Eds. Pergamon Press. London, England.
KISSEN, D. M. 1964g. The influence of some environmental factors on personality inventory scores in psychosomatic research. J. Psychosom. Res. **8**: 145–149.
KISSEN, D. M. 1964h. The use of questionnaires in personality measurement in psychosomatic research. J. Psychosom. Res. **8**: 293–296.
KISSEN, D. M. 1965a. Methodologie de la Recherche Psychosomatique. Medecine et Hygiene **23**: 633–634.
KISSEN, D. M. 1965b. Possible contribution of the psychosomatic approach to prevention of lung cancer. Medical Officer **114**: 343–345.
KISSEN, D. M. 1966a. Mind and preventive medicine. Surgo (Glasgow Univ. Med. J.) **33**: 2–13.
KISSEN, D. M. 1966b. Psychosocial factors, personality and prevention in lung cancer: A report on men aged 55–64. Medical Officer **116**: 135–138.
KISSEN, D. M. 1966c. Psychosomatic histories in the relatives of male hospital chest unit patients with special reference to lung cancer. Int. J. Soc. Psychiat. **12**: 199–208.
KISSEN, D. M. 1966d. The significance of personality in lung cancer in men. Ann. N. Y. Acad. Sci. **125**(3): 820–826.
KISSEN, D. M. 1966e. The value of a psychosomatic approach to cancer. Ann. N. Y. Acad. Sci. **125**(3): 777–779.
KISSEN, D. M. 1967a. Problems and possibilities in the psychosomatic approach to prevention with special reference to lung cancer. *In* Trans. Int. Chest and Heart Conference. Eastbourne, England. The British Chest and Heart Association.
KISSEN, D. M. 1967b. Psychosocial factors, personality and lung cancer in men aged 55–64. Brit. J. Med. Psychol. **40**: 29–43.
KISSEN, D. M. 1967c. Some psychosomatic aspects of disease prevention. Medecine et Hygiene.
KISSEN, D. M., R. I. F. BROWN & M. KISSEN. 1968a. A further report on personality and psychosocial factors in lung cancer. This monograph.
KISSEN, D. M. 1968b. Personal communication.
KISSEN, D. M. & L. G. S. RAO. 1968c. Steroid-excretion patterns and personality in lung cancer. This monograph.

PART I. THE PSYCHOPHYSIOLOGICAL PROBLEMS IN CANCER

PSYCHOPHYSIOLOGICAL COMPLEMENTARITY IN MALIGNANCIES: PAST WORK AND FUTURE VISTAS

Claus Bahne Bahnson*

Department of Psychiatry, Jefferson Medical College
Philadelphia, Pa.

INTRODUCTION

The present monograph on psychophysiological aspects of cancer follows three years after the previous, and first, monograph on this topic, and in many ways serves as its continuation. The first conference succeeded in bringing together evidence from many quarters demonstrating unequivocally that malignant processes are related to certain psychosocial conditions and psychodynamic states. However, the physiological processes mediating among experiential, affective, and coping processes on the one hand, and the physiological, biochemical, and immunological processes related to the malignant development, on the other, were not clearly elucidated. In brief, the first work demonstrated that an empirical relationship does exist between psychological states and malignancies, but did not investigate how these relationships are mediated. That is the task of the present conference. Here, we wish to initiate a careful mapping of the physiological, biochemical, hormonal, immunological, and other processes that may mediate the psychological states that have been observed to antecede onset of clinical cancer.

The search for cross-relationships between different levels of investigation inevitably raises basic theoretical questions. One of these questions is whether it is possible to conceptualize somatic and psychological phenomena within one model, relating them to each other in a meaningful way. Although the mind-body problem is as old as science itself, and would require several conferences just to be properly presented, it was obvious at the end of our first conference that the participants were able to work with somatic and psychological concepts within a single theoretical construct without feeling too uncomfortable. There was a reasonable amount of agreement that the old-fashioned dualistic, or multifactorial, interactive concepts were too narrow and rigid for our purpose, and that in general, a monistic approach such as Grinker's field theory would be required as an effective working model. Grinker himself expressed it thusly: "We have, I hope, abandoned the convenient but restricted and artificial two-foci correlations linking single factors in causality of disease processes. Hence, we need no longer argue whether a disease is *caused* by heredity, constitution, disordered chemistry or physiology, infection, trauma or repressed pathogenic emotions. We are no longer concerned with such either-or single-factor polarities but currently attempt to map out the widest possible ranges of conditions, all of which in some way and at some time, seem to be implicated in a dynamic chain of causes and effects." (1966a, p. 876) Other participants in the first conference (1966), such as Reiser, Margolin, Rakoff, and I, also addressed ourselves to basic psychosomatic issues, and introduced encompassing working models that will allow for heuristic psychosomatic formulations. Now I shall

* Present address: Eastern Pennsylvania Psychiatric Institute, Institute of Pennsylvania Hospital, Philadelphia, Pa., and University of Connecticut, Storrs, Conn.

endeavor to formulate briefly our own model of psychosomatic complementarity, which presents one possible working scheme integrating physiological and psychological observations, and I shall also refer to the work of other participants in this effort.

This paper will be structured as follows: First, a brief survey will be made of the status of work presented at the previous conference, then our own theoretical formulation and a few pertinent research results will be discussed. Finally, current work on central nervous system (CNS), endocrinological, immune, and other processes relevant both to psychological observation and malignant development, will be surveyed.

Main Theoretical Trends in Psychosomatic Cancer Studies

Loss-Depression Theories

Several workers have observed that object-loss, despair, depression, and hopelessness often are precursors to clinical cancer. Dr. Greene, who is a pioneer in this field of research, observed that leukemias and lymphomas often occur in a setting in which the patient deals with loss or separation, with concomitant feelings of sadness, anxiety, helplessness, and hopelessness. Greene also has suggested that psychological decompensation is a characteristic precursor to clinical cancer. Lymphomas and leukemias may develop when the patient, in his words, is "running out of psychological resources engendering shame and hopelessness" (Greene, 1966). To this worker, this formulation is reminiscent of some of the key concepts in the immunological approach to be discussed in this monograph, in which defensive incompetence seems to be a factor.

LeShan and his colleagues (LeShan & Worthington, 1956a, 1956b; LeShan & Reznikoff, 1960; Le Shan, 1966) have interviewed and carried out psychotherapy with nearly 500 patients, and suggest that cancer patients have a particular life of desertion, loneliness, and often guilt and self-condemnation. Although their patients are in "utter despair of being themselves" (Kierkegaard's phrase), they continue to carry out their activities and routines, although without achieving satisfaction, and deplete themselves by giving more to others than they themselves receive. Notice that, also in LeShan's formulation, the depletion-of-energy theme has been raised. Schmale (1958) and Schmale and Iker (1964, 1966), studying women with uterine cervical cancer, have reported similar findings. In a group of 51 essentially healthy and asymptomatic women, but predisposed to cervical cancer (Class III Papanicolau cells), he was able to predict correctly cancer versus noncancer in 36 out of 51 cases on the basis of psychological characteristics alone, yielding a two-tailed probability of $<.02$. His predictions of cancer were based on a recent life history indicating that these women had responded to a life event with feelings of hopelessness within the last six months prior to the first positive smear. Hagnell (1966), in a longitudinal population study in Sweden, found that women with "substable" personality characteristics, according to Sjöbring's personality types (1963), showed significantly higher cancer rates than did women with super- or mediostable personality characteristics. Sjöbring's substable type is characterized by depression, inertia, and inhibition, as well as concreteness, extraversion, and industriousness. Thus, his category encompasses both depressive and repressive personality aspects.

Our own clinical investigations of 80 cancer patients (1965a, 1965b, 1967) resulted in an extension of the loss-depression hypothesis in an attempt to detail why a loss should be more traumatic and crucial to cancer patients than to other people. Most people experience loss and separation, and many experience depressive episodes, but most often without the concomitant development of a malignancy. In cancer patients the traumatic loss of separation during adulthood gains its particularly devastating effect on the basis of early despair experienced by the child in relationship to its parents. Retrospectively, it appears that cancer patients had a primitive, but unsatisfying, relationship to their parents, particularly to the mother, of a pregenital and most often oral character, with ample ambivalence and rage. Only with the greatest effort could these children maintain an uncertain relationship to the significant parent, and the adolescent separation from the parents was painful and perceived as a severe deprivation against which they struggled in their adult years by attempting to establish an emotional relationship with a mate or spouse, or through substitute investments in creativity or work. Often, this was a difficult task because the child's mistrust and hostility were transferred to the adulthood partners. When this precariously established relationship or investment in adulthood breaks down, the original despair and hopelessness of the deprived and longing child reemerges, throwing the individual back to his own resources in the face of a renewed insult received from the environment, leaving him with little hope that any warmth or solace can be obtained from others. It is based on this idiosyncratic interpretation of loss that the cancer patient turns toward himself, and gives up efforts to interact emotionally with other people. Psychodynamically, this reexperience of depletion and hopelessness sets the stage for intensive regression to modes of discharge of drive that are self-contained and may reflect a wish for self-propagation. As we have expressed it elsewhere (1964b), the cancer patient, probably due to the many years of rehearsal with tolerating ungratifying reality, does maintain impeccable and realistic relationships to the society around him, and does not seem to show any behavioral regression in the face of stress other than the emotional turning toward himself (affective autism). Stated more simply, the cancer patient regresses somatically, but not behaviorally.

In addition to clinical and projective studies of these relationships, we have carried out a more "objective" investigation of how cancer patients perceive their parents, compared with patients with myocardial infarction and a normal, age-matched control sample.† We used the Roe-Siegelman Parent Child Relationship Questionnaire (Roe and Siegelman, 1964), which investigates patients' perception of their parents in retrospect, and found that cancer patients indeed perceive their parents as more neglecting and cold than do other patients and normal control subjects. (TABLES 1 & 2). These results lend support to the contention that the loss that has been observed to precede exacerbation or clinical manifestation of cancer must be understood as a special variety of loss experience, based on a history of childhood affective deprivation, before this loss may be considered predictive for a malignant development. These considerations are in agreement with those of Booth (1964), and have an affinity with those of Spitz (1945, 1946, 1949), Harlow and Harlow (1962a, 1962b), and Ader and Friedman (1964, 1965), with regard to the importance of early conditions of nurturance in animals: body contact, early handling, et cetera, for effective coping with later stresses.

Considering the coping mechanisms and their antecedents rather than the external events triggering the depressive reaction, we shall now review some of the studies of ego defenses.

† Some of these data are drawn from the Southeastern Connecticut (SECON) Heart Study, supported in part by grant no. HE–07522, The National Institutes of Health: W. I. Wardwell and C. B. Bahnson, principal investigators.

TABLE 1

CHI SQUARES AND PROBABILITY LEVELS FROM CONTINGENCY TABLES FOR PARENT-CHILD RELATIONSHIP SCORES (ROE-SIEGELMAN) FOR CANCER PATIENTS, MYOCARDIAL INFARCTION PATIENTS, HEMOPHILIC PATIENTS, AND WELL CONTROL SUBJECTS

			Mother					
				Summary of Results from Tables*				
Variable	x^2	df	total p	CA	p	MI	HE	p
1. Protective	16.2	6	.02	—	.05	=	+	.02
2. Punishment, symbolic love	16.8	9	.06	—	.06	+	+	
3. Rejecting	18.4	12	.11	—	.03	=	=	
4. Casual	19.9	9	.02	—	.01	=/—	—	
5. Reward, symbolic love	21.0	9	.02	—	.04	=	—	
6. Demanding	4.7	9	—	=/—	n.s.	=	=/—	
7. Punishment, direct object	5.5	6	—	—	n.s.	=/—	=	
8. Loving	30.3	12	.005	—	.005	=	—	
9. Neglecting	18.5	9	.04	+/—	n.s.	+/—	=	
10. Reward, direct object	10.0	9	.04	—	n.s.	=/—	+	

Total N for contingency tables total 114 in 9 instances; 113 in 1 instance.

CA = Cancer; MI = Myocardial Infarction; HE = Hemophilia; + indicates higher scores than well comparison group; — indicates lower scores than well comparison group; = indicates scores similar to well comparison group.

* Comparison of the three sick groups with the well normal subjects.

Ego Defense Theories

Whereas the loss-depression hypothesis deals with life-history parameters and content of conflicts, the ego-defense hypothesis turns the focus on coping patterns and structure of personality, albeit with the understanding that these parameters also have their ultimate precursors in the dynamics of early experience. Greene and co-workers (1956) noted that women with lymphomas and leukemias reacted to separation and loss with identification and introjection of the lost object, and with denial of affect and dependency needs. Later, however, Greene (1966) pondered whether the denial he had observed previously might be a function of the doctor's rather than the patient's defense. Kissen, to whom we dedicate this monograph, and who worked intensely with lung cancer patients for several years, concluded from all of his studies, (Kissen *et al.,* 1962; Kissen, 1963, 1964, 1965, 1966a, 1966b, 1966c) that lung cancer patients show a typical trend to suppress emotional problems and conflicts and, in his words, have a "diminished outlet for emotional discharge." He based this conclusion on precise and careful empirical work, making use of the Maudsley Personality Inventory devised by Eysenck, and of other "objective" methods. Our own studies (1964a, 1964b, 1965b, 1966a) have dealt specifically with the operational assessment of ego defenses in cancer patients, making use of a new method by which to assess affect and defense against affect. Another paper, later in this monograph, will report on our latest findings, which continue to support our previous results, indicating that cancer patients indeed do repress and deny unpleasant affect such as anxiety,

TABLE 2

CHI SQUARES AND PROBABILITY LEVELS FROM CONTINGENCY TABLE FOR PARENT-CHILD RELATIONSHIP SCORES (ROE-SIEGELMAN) FOR CANCER PATIENTS, MYOCARDIAL INFARCTION PATIENTS, HEMOPHILIC PATIENTS, AND WELL CONTROL SUBJECTS

Father								
				Summary of Results from Tables*				
Variable	x^2	df	total p	CA	p	MI	HE	p
1. Protective	48.1	9	.001	−	.001	+/−	+	.001
2. Punishment, symbolic love	5.6	6	n.s.	+	n.s.	+	+	
3. Rejecting	7.8	9	n.s.	−	n.s.	=	=/+	
4. Casual	26.6	9	.005	−	.01	=/−	=/−	
5. Reward, symbolic love	17.6	9	.05	+	.03	=	−	
6. Demanding	17.1	9	.05	−	.02	=	+	
7. Punishment, direct object	9.5	9	n.s.	−	n.s.	=	=	
8. Loving	7.0	9	n.s.	=	n.s.	+	−	
9. Neglecting	13.2	6	.05	−	n.s.	=/−	+/−	
10. Reward, direct object	8.8	9	n.s.	=/−	n.s.	=	+	
Total N for all contingency tables total 112.								

CA = Cancer; MI = Myocardial Infarction; HE = Hemophilia; + indicates higher scores than well comparison group; − indicates lower scores than well comparison group; = indicates scores similar to well comparison group.

* Comparison of the three sick groups with the well normal subjects.

hostility, or guilt to a higher degree than do matched normal control subjects. Henderson (1966) showed how conspicuous denial of malignancies were in both physicians and patients, resulting in dangerous or fatal delay in the institution of treatment, and Cobb (1952) showed that denial in cancer patients is extreme and remarkable. Grinker (1966b), evaluating the role of personality in cancer, stated: "It is more likely that a composite of drives, defenses, displacements and regressions are related to physiological regressions." To sum up, the concentration of studies in the area of ego defenses implicates the concept of regression of adaptation, which remains a key concept in psychophysiological cancer research.

PSYCHOPHYSIOLOGICAL COMPLEMENTARITY

Encompassing psychosomatic models in cancer have been sparse. However, a few attempts are on record, among them Jonas' formulation in our first monograph (1966), suggesting that cancer may represent an archaic asexual propagation mechanism useful to invertebrates, but useless or damaging in higher animals. He theorized that a malignancy may result from an autoamputative reflex in the CNS aimed at eliminating tissue once it has become the source of supranormal irritation, for physiological or symbolic reasons. Obviously, Jonas's concept is one of phylogenetic regression in a psychobiological organism under stress. Stevenson (1963) introduced similar concepts when he stated that "the neuro-biogenesis of neoplasia may be explained in patterns of defensive organization from remote evolution," and, independently of Jonas, also introduced the concepts of autoamputation and regeneration. Bennette (1965) introduces the concepts of impairment of self-identity and recognitional control in cancer, and continues to develop this hypothesis in his paper to follow today, including somatic, psychic, and psychosocial conditions within a basic framework of the concepts of alienation and self-recognition.

In order to communicate the axiomatic basis on which our research group operates, allow me to present very briefly a few primary thoughts and models related to complementarity of regression. One aspect of psychophysiological complementarity is the conceptual similarity between the manifestations of behavioral and physiological regression under stress. Whereas psychological behavioral regression results in elimination of self-object differentiation and facilitates the ego-defense projection, in physiological regression the self-object barrier is maintained and social behavior remains functional at a late developmental level, leaving the physiological medium as the only arena for archaic expression of drive potentials closely guided by the multileveled "symbolics" of body parts and functions. When this is the case, those parts of ego functions that relate to perception and control of the social environment are left intact, whereas ego function related to maintenance of inner psychobiological processes crumble and regress. Fenichel (1945), Deutsch (1953), Alexander (1950), Fisher and Cleveland (1956), Booth (1965), and several others have written about different aspects of this process. The basic hypothesis is simple: we postulate that the psychobiological organism disposes over two main channels of discharge of drive, need, or tension continuously generated within itself, sometimes in proaction with environmental stimulation. One way is to act on the environment, either in fantasy or actuality; the other is to disassociate the drive representation from thought, conscious feeling, and action, discharging it within the biological medium without involving later phylogenetic levels of interpersonal (social) expression (FIGURE 1). Our hypothesis specifies that the "choice" of behavioral versus somatic regression is associated with the type of ego defense utilized by the individual. Projective defenses, involving interpersonal discharge, predisposes to psychological regression under stress, whereas repressing and denying defenses, serving to maintain an effective external adaptation, result in internal somatic discharge and regression. Obviously, the severity of regression also is a function of the intensity of the conflictual drives or impulses. A hypothetical arrangement of behavioral and somatic regressive patterns are depicted in FIGURE 2, arranged along axes of increasing regression, one in terms of psychological behavioral manifestations, the other in terms of somatic dysfunction. The somatic and psychological conditions are arranged symmetrically, roughly according to the severity of the regressive levels of the symptoms. These models allow us to conceptualize psychological and somatic diseases as alternative, or complementary, results of conflict and regression. Note that both malignancies on the somatic side and deteriorated psychoses on the experiential-behavioral side represent the most extreme degrees of disorganization and self-alienation, although usually we do not perceive the similarity between these psychobiological conditions.

We operate here with a model within the framework of which reductionism, or arbitrary causal assignment to one observational level (e.g. physiological, biochemical, immunological, or psychological) is automatically rejected, since manifestations on different levels of observation by definition represent only multiple and arbitrary manifestations of a total psychobiological process. The selected manifestations are arbitrary and depend on the theoretical biases and methodologies put to use. In spite of this statement, I probably risk being mis-

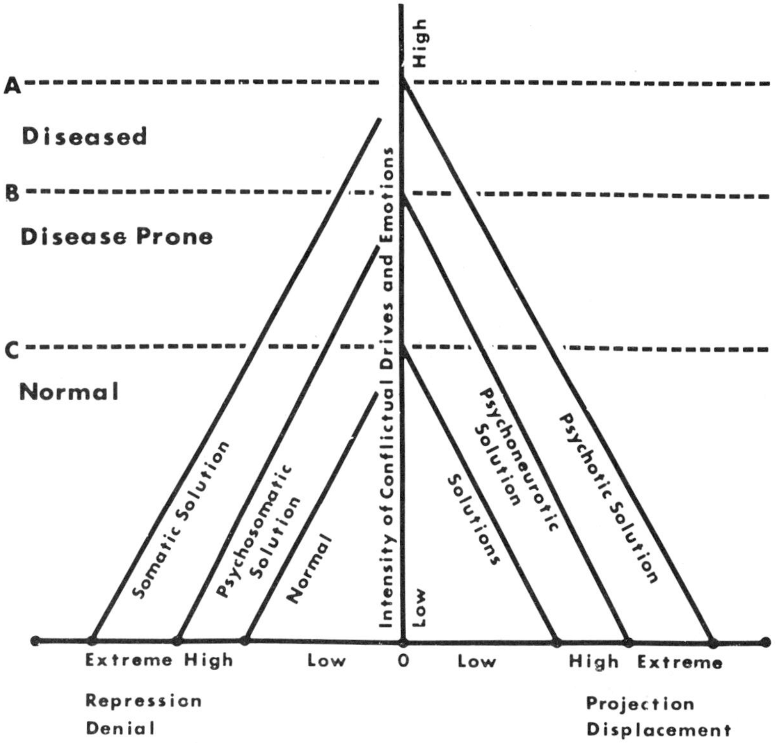

FIGURE 1. Relation between ego defenses, level of conflict, and symptom formation.

understood when presenting the following diagram of psychophysiological interaction, which specifies a possible "path" from environmental stress, through psychological experience and physiological reactions, to malignant development. Each sequence is hypothesized to have its equivalents on all observational levels, although here are specified only the most obvious and most readily observable aspects (FIGURE 3). The individual interacts with the environment in which a change such as loss of object occurs. A phenomenological experience ensues. The perceived strain is represented by CNS changes (hypothalamus) and stimulation of the hippocampus, and possibly may be associated with a reduced psychobiological defense. Cortical changes are associated with pituitary, ANS, and biochemical reactions, which, again, involve endocrine glands and hormones. Both neural and endocrine changes are associated with changes of both circulating and cellular immune reactions and possibly changes in the CNA coding transmitted. DNA and immune reactions interact with the present viral organisms and may produce the malignant development.

In the balance of this paper I will attempt to survey very briefly research results and conclusions relevant to the sequences of psychobiological carcinogenesis just outlined.

Loss and Depression in Cancer

Following the sequence of our etiological schema, some of the most important studies detailing the relationship between environmental trauma and cancer

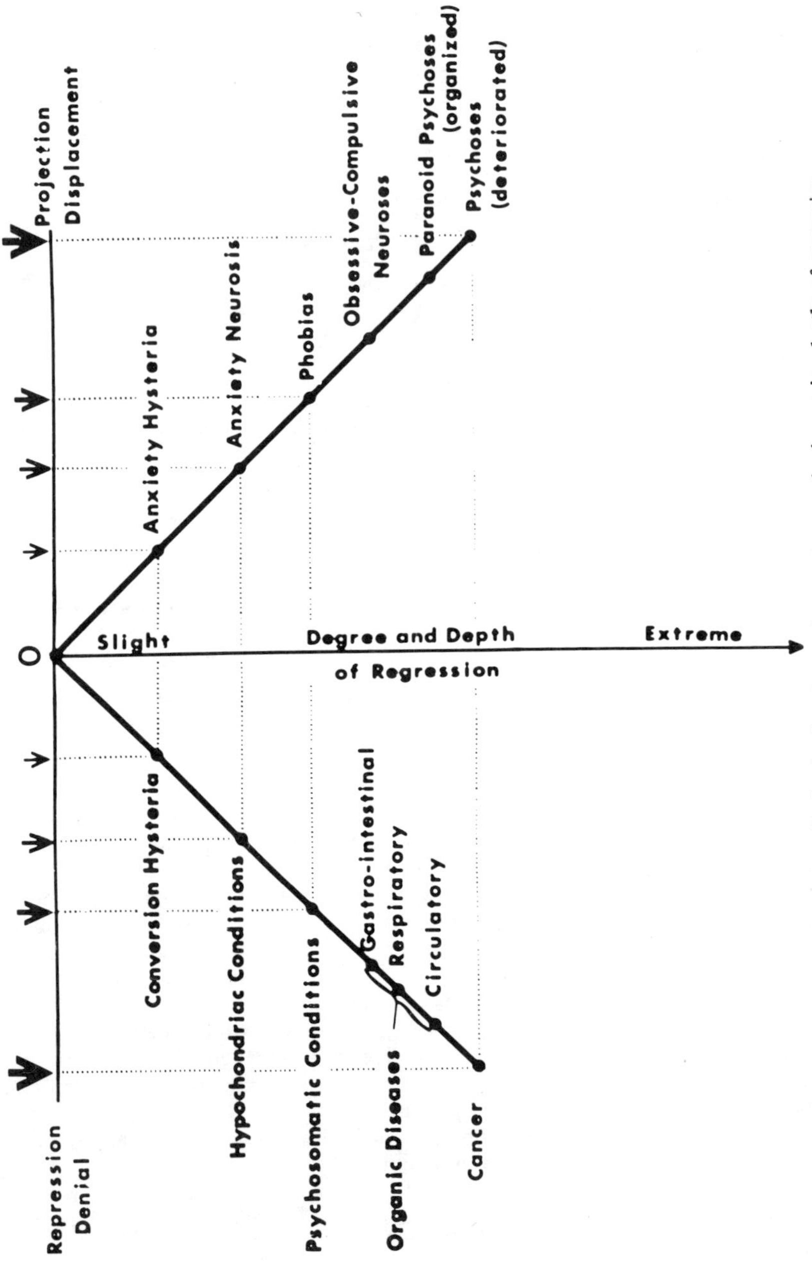

FIGURE 2. Complementarity of behavioral and somatic symptoms under increasing depths of regression.

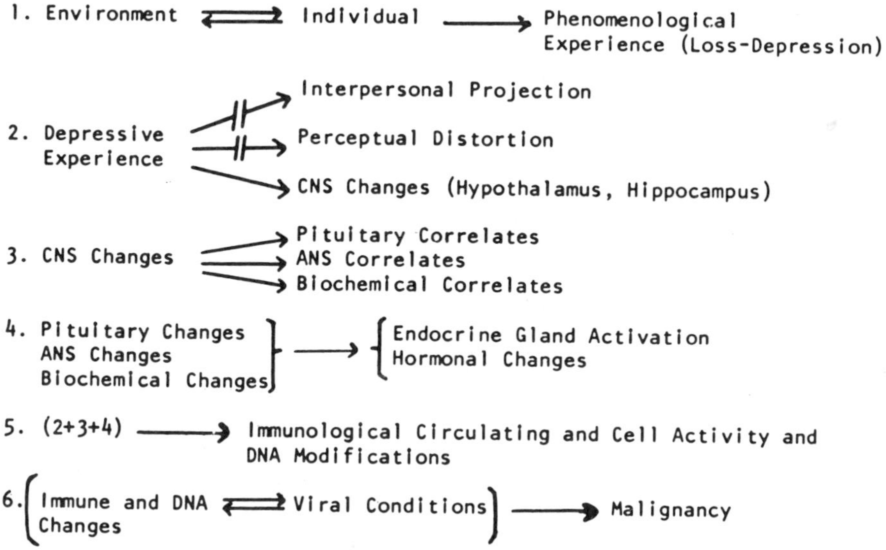

already have been discussed in the first part of this paper. The studies of Greene, LeShan, Schmale, Majorie Bahnson and myself have demonstrated that a correlation between loss and depression and the clinical development of cancer does exist. However, although LeShan was able to show a statistical relationship between objective loss and cancer morbidity, it seems crucial to point out about this first stage of the etiological chain that the phenomenological experience of loss, despair, and strain is the significant variable, since individuals react quite differently to conditions of "external" stress. The phenomenological depressive experience, of course, depends on the total Gestalt of the individual's past and present, and particularly on the solution of key interpersonal relations early in life. Most individuals, when perceiving severe loss and depression, live through a process of mourning, as described by Freud (1917) and manifested by temporary withdrawal and internalization of behavioral characteristics of the lost person in their efforts to maintain the lost relationship on a symbolic level. This mourning process involves interpersonal behavioral changes and, often, also transient perceptual distortion. Characteristically, cancer patients fail to show the reality-distorting aspects of the mourning process, and maintain their life routines unaltered during this mourning process. Several researchers have commented on this fact (e.g. LeShan, Cutler, and Bahnson). Following the model of complementarity, we hypothesize that at this point the phenomenological depressive state is denied access to consciousness and is expressed instead in CNS changes, possibly involving the hypothalamus and hippocampus as integrating stations for affective experience. Studies, particularly by the Russian experimentalists Kavetsky, Balitsky, and their co-workers (1966, 1968) have addressed themselves to the relationship between CNS changes and malignancies. Some of their latest findings will be reported here later. Kavetsky has shown that lesions of the paraventricular and dorsomedial nuclei of the hypothalamus lead to regression of adenomatosis in thyroid tumors. Balitsky, studying changes in bioelectric activity of the cerebral cortex in animals with grafted tumors, observed that bioelectrical activities in the cortex changed, and that the frequency of afferent impulsation of involved nerves declined. Here, then, are hardnosed empirical data pertinent to our broader schema. Rakoff (1962, 1963, 1966a, 1966b) has emphasized the important role of the hypothalamic-pituitary system in carcinogenesis. FIGURE 4, borrowed from Rakoff (1966b), depicts two alternate pathways of transmittal from the hypothalamus to target tissues. One leads via the endocrine glands and the other directly via biochemical changes to possible malignant changes.

Various workers have emphasized different aspects of the transmittal from the CNS to the target tissues. Kissen and Rao (1968) find that cancer patients, compared with control patients, show less initial adrenergic response at the time of admission to the hospital, but otherwise retain higher and more fluctuating levels. Cardon and Müller (1966) concluded that the elevated FFA levels in cancer patients may be related to adrenergic preponderance. Corson (1966) suggested on the basis of his experimental research that "unstable" animals with preponderance of adrenergic factors may be more prone to develop tumors. Seymour Levine (1961), who studied the effects of early handling of rats, concluded that one of the reasons that handled rats resist implanted tumors better than nonhandled rats was that their adrenal cortical response was more vigorous, although briefer. This finding, of course, dovetails with Kissen's and Rao's observations. These data may be interpreted as a defensive incompetence in the cancer-prone individuals, at least as measured by firm adrenal response followed by fading.

The work of Stein and co-workers (1968), which will be described in detail in this conference, is of particular importance because it relates hypothalamic changes (lesions) to the modification of circulating antibodies as well as to neuroendocrine and ANS reactions. Thus, Stein's work addresses itself to a broad span of the suggested etiological chain. Katz (1968), in an important study of corticoid and androgenic steroids in women with breast cancer, found that the corticoid-androgenic ratio foresaw the prognosis of cancer of the breast, with high corticoid outputs related to poor prognosis, and low relative corticoid outputs predicting a good prognosis. His group also was able to obtain an impressive correlation (.56, $p<.01$) between breakdown of ego defenses and hydrocortisone production in these patients. These findings support those of the workers mentioned above, but raise an important question, since elevated rates in their study were associated with a breakdown of defenses, and low rates with hope, faith,

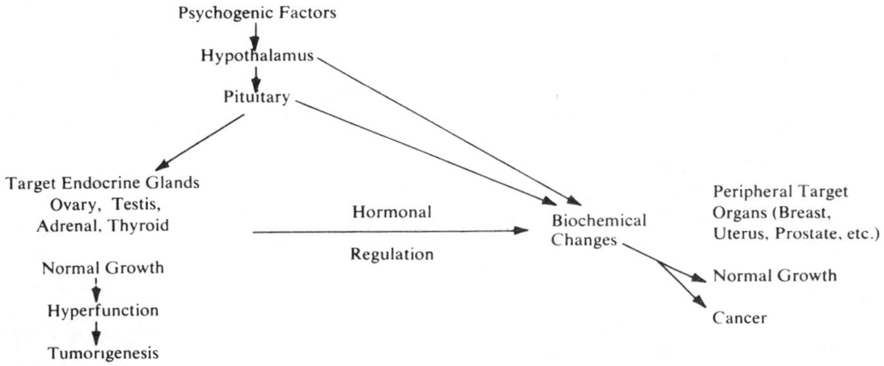

FIGURE 4. Some postulated mechanisms by which psychoendocrine factors may influence tumorigenesis. (By permission of A. E. Rakoff, 1966b.)

control, and denial. In order to relate these findings to the denial hypothesis, it will be imperative to define more clearly in future studies exactly what is meant by defensive failure. Defense cannot be considered an undifferentiated process, but the exact type of defensive mechanism must be outlined and measured.

Moore (1964) clearly demonstrated the importance of hormonal activity when showing that virus alone is hardly carcinogenic, whereas in combination with hormonal stimulation, it appears highly carcinogenic. Marmorston and colleagues (1966) compared hormone metabolites in malignant and nonmalignant tumors and found significant differences. Multivariate analyses of such hormones as estrone, 17-ketosteroids, Porter-Silber Chromogen, and the beta part of 17-ketosteroids, all discriminated significantly between the two tumor types. Marmorston and co-workers (1965a, 1965b, 1965c, 1966) showed that estrogen, androsterone, dehydroepiandrosterone, 17-ketogenic steroids, 17-hydroxycorticosteroids, and other hormone metabolites were diminished in cancer patients, when compared with nonmalignant and healthy control patients. They also showed that every cancer type has its own profile of changed hormone production, so that such a profile may serve as a predictor.

Turning now to the immune reactions, which will be considered so carefully in this monograph by some of the world's finest experts, I shall, as a non-immunologist, refer only to a few basic points. In our psychosomatic model of complementarity, emotional decompensation can well be likened to immunological failure, in the sense that both processes refer to diminished control, organization, and capacity for resistance and defense. The isomorphism between the concepts of psychologic and immunologic defense seems to me both fascinating and striking, and fits with the complementarity concept. Solomon (1966) and Solomon and Moos (1964), among the first workers to emphasize the psychophysiological importance of the immune reactions, have suggested that stress reduces the antibody response, and that adult immunological responsivity may be a function of early infantile experiences. These hypotheses are supported by the studies of Ader and Friedman (1964), showing that early life experiences and environmental manipulations of rats modify their responses to injected Walker-256 Carcino-Sarcoma, by Ader and Friedman's finding (1965) that rats prematurely separated from their mothers have greater mortality rates from implanted tumors, and Newton's results (1964) that rats handled and petted early in life resisted Walker Carcinoma 256 longer than rats raised in isolation, and without handling.

Weiss (1968) finds that native or acquired immunologic disability often precedes the onset of neoplasia and will describe some mechanisms by which psychogenic stimuli may affect host-tumor interactions via the immunological apparatus. Rasmussen (1968) directs himself to the intricate effects of stress on both immunological and anaphylactic responses, pointing out that stress may stimulate as well as deplete immunological defensive reactions, thus implicitly warning against premature and oversimplified concepts of reactions to stress, before the great variety of experiences included under this heading have been differentiated clearly from each other. Kidd (1961) and Sommers (1958) have approached the immune problem from a slightly different point of view, suggesting that latent cancer cells often are present within body tissues without developing further and that the sudden proliferation of such cancer cells may be a function of the breakdown of the immune resistance at a particular time. Southam and Siegel (1966), in their careful experiments, have gone far to show that immune reactions definitely influence the course of cancer, paying special attention to autoimmune processes. Bennette (1965), over and above his psychobiological theorizing and interest in immunological relationships, emphasizes the role of DNA as a carrier of information, and suggests that immunological reactions may interfere, or interact, with the distribution of the information code carried along by the DNA molecules for the purpose of identification.

This brief survey of recent and current studies has carried us from the level of broad and abstract psychosocial thinking all the way through hypothesized intervening media to the aberrant development of neoplastic cells. Although much too brief, and sometimes superficial, this hurried travel may alert us to what is to come, both now and during the coming years of intensified research.

FUTURE CONSIDERATIONS

The psychological and immunological considerations related to cancer reveal certain conceptual similarities. They both have to do with relationships to self, on the psychological or somatic levels; with the handling of psychobiological stress matrices, and with exhaustion and breakdown of defensive systems; and, probably, with dual-control systems governing each area. There is a peculiar isomorphism between the psychological process of self-alienation and self-estrangement (Bahnson and Bahnson, 1965a) and the biological failure of discriminating between alien and familiar configurations expressed in the impairment of immune reactions, which should allow for a theoretical reformulation on a higher level of abstraction, including both levels of psychobiological processing. Early life experience, self-relationships and self-image, affective reactions, autoimmune processes, and the mechanisms of RNA communication—all must be considered within a single global theory as multifaceted expressions of the total psychobiological process. Although we are not this far as yet, there seems to be no doubt that such a theoretical development is the next necessary step, which will enable us to conceive of, and not only describe, the malignant process as a total life development, encompassing data which today still are understood as reflecting independent, and at most, interactive, phenomena. This monistic construct implies a leap away from the disciplinary segregation characterizing cancer research today, but will be worthwhile, since it will allow for integration and the mutual stimulation of all participating disciplines.

REFERENCES

ADER, R. & S. B. FRIEDMAN. 1964. Social factors affecting emotionality and resistance to disease in animals. IV. Differential housing, emotionality, and Walker-256 carcinosarcoma in the rat. Psychol. Rep. **15:** 535–541.

ADER, R. & S. B. FRIEDMAN. 1965. Social factors affecting emotionality and resistance to disease in animals. V. Early separation from the mother and response to a transplanted tumor in the rat. Psychosom. Med. **27:** 119–122.

ALEXANDER, F. 1950. Psychosomatic Medicine. W. W. Norton, New York, N. Y.

BAHNSON, C. B. 1966a. Panel discussion: Retrospects and prospects. Ann. N. Y. Acad. Sci. **125**(3): 1028–1055.

BAHNSON, C. B. 1966b. Gegenwärtige Strömungen in der psychosomatischen Forschung und Skizzierung eines komplementären theoretischen Modells. *In* Therapie uber das Nervensystem **6:** 11–45. Hippokrates Verlag. Wiesbaden, Germany.

BAHNSON, C. B. 1967. Psychological aspects of cancer. Presented at the International Congress for Psychosomatic Medicine and Hypnosis. Kyoto, Japan. (Paper available in mimeograph form.)

BAHNSON, C. B. & M. B. BAHNSON. 1964a. Cancer as an alternative to psychosis: A theoretical model of somatic and psychological regression. *In* Psychosomatic Aspects of Neoplastic disease. D. M. Kissen & L. L. LeShan, Eds. : 184–202. Pitman. London, England.

BAHNSON, C. B. & M. B. BAHNSON. 1964b. Denial and repression of primitive impulses and of disturbing emotions in patients with malignant neoplasms. *In* Psychosomatic Aspects of Neoplastic Disease. D. M. Kissen & L. L. LeShan, Eds. : 42–62. Pitman. London, England.

BAHNSON, C. B. & M. B. BAHNSON. 1965a. Psychodynamics of cancer. Presented at Fourth International Conference on Psychosomatic Aspects of Neoplastic Disease. Turin, Italy. (Paper available in mimeograph form.)

BAHNSON, C. B. & M. B. BAHNSON. 1965b. Ego defensive functioning in cancer patients: The utilization of denial and projection as measured by self attributed and projected mood and emotion. Presented at Fourth International Conference on Psychosomatic Aspects of Neoplastic Disease. Turin, Italy. (Paper available in mimeograph form.)

BAHNSON, C. B. & M. B. BAHNSON. 1966. Role of the ego defenses: Denial and repression in the etiology of malignant neoplasm. Ann. N. Y. Acad. Sci. **125**(3): 827–845.

BENNETTE, J. G. 1965. Immunological mechanisms in possible mediators of psychosomatic competence in relation to chemical, viral and physical carcinogenic changes. Presented at the Fourth International Conference on Psychosomatic Aspects of Neoplastic Disease. Turin, Italy.

BOOTH, G. 1964. Cancer and humanism: Psychosomatic aspects of evolution. *In* Psychosomatic Aspects of Neoplastic Disease. D. M. Kissen & L. L. LeShan, Eds. : 159–169. Pitman. London, England.

BOOTH, G. 1965. Irrational complications of the cancer problem. Amer. J. Psychoanal. **25:** 41–60.

CARDON, P. V., JR. & P. S. MÜLLER. 1966. A possible mechanism: Psychogenic fat mobilization. Ann. N. Y. Acad. Sci. **125**(3): 924–927.

COBB, B. 1952. A socio-psychological study of the cancer patient. Unpublished doctoral dissertation. University of Texas. Austin, Texas.

CORSON, S. A. 1966. Neuroendocrine and behavioral response patterns to psychologic stress and the problem of the target tissue in cerebrovisceral pathology. Ann. N. Y. Acad. Sci. **125**(3): 890–915.

CUTLER, M. 1954. Behavioral characteristics of 40 women with cancer of the breast. *In* The Psychological Variables in Human Cancer. J. A. Gengerelli & F. I. Kirkner, Eds. Univ. California Press. Berkeley, Calif.

DEUTSCH, F. 1953. The psychosomatic concept in psychoanalysis. Monograph Series of the Boston Psychoanalytic Society and Institute. International Universities Press. New York, N. Y.

FENICHEL, O. 1945. The Psychoanalytic Theory of Neurosis. W. W. Norton & Co., Inc. New York, N. Y.

FISHER, S. & S. E. CLEVELAND. 1956. Relationship of body image to site of cancer. Psychosom. Med. **18:** 304–309.

FREUD, S. 1917. Mourning and melancholia. *In* Collected Papers, **4:** 152–170. Hogarth. London, England.

GREENE, W. A. 1966. The psychosocial setting of the development of leukemia and lymphoma. Ann. N. Y. Acad. Sci. **125**(3): 794–801.

GREENE, W., L. E. YOUNG & S. N. SWISHER. 1956. Psychological factors and reticuloendothelial disease. II. Observations on a group of women with lymphomas and leukemias. Psychosom. Med. **18:** 284–303.

GRINKER, R. 1966a. Psychosomatic aspects of the cancer problem. Ann. N. Y. Acad. Sci. **125**(3): 876–882.

GRINKER, R. 1966b. Discussion of the papers. Ann. N. Y. Acad. Sci. **125**(3): 874–875.

HAGNELL, O. 1966. The premorbid personality of persons who develop cancer in a total population investigated in 1947 and 1957. Ann. N. Y. Acad. Sci. **125**(3): 846–855.

HARLOW, H. F. & M. K. HARLOW. 1962a. The effect of rearing conditions on behavior. Bull. Menninger Clin. **26:** 213–224.

HARLOW, H. F. & M. K. HARLOW. 1962b. Social deprivation in monkeys. Sci. Amer. **207:** 136–146.

HENDERSON, J. G. 1966. Denial and repression as factors in the delay of patients with cancer presenting themselves to the physician. Ann. N. Y. Acad. Sci. **125**(3): 856–864.

JONAS, A. D. 1966. Theoretical considerations concerning the influence of the central nervous system on cancerous growth. Ann. N. Y. Acad. Sci. **125**(3): 946–951.

KATZ, J. L., T. GALLAGHER, L. HELLMAN, E. J. SACHAR & H. WEINER. 1968. Psychoendocrine considerations in cancer of the breast. This monograph.

KAVETSKY, R. E., N. M. TURKEVICH, R. M. AKIMOVA, I. K. KHAYETSKY & Y. D. MATVEICHUK. 1968. Induced cancerogenesis under various influences on the hypothalamus. This monograph.

KAVETSKY, R. E., N. M. TURKEVICH & K. P. BALITSKY. 1966. On the psychophysiological mechanism of the organism's resistance to tumor growth. Ann. N. Y. Acad. Sci. **125**(3): 933–945.

KIDD, J. G. 1961. Does the host react against his own cancer cells? Cancer Res. **21**: 1170.

KISSEN, D. M. 1963. Personality characteristics in males conducive to lung cancer. Brit. J. Med. Psychol. **36**: 27–36.

KISSEN, D. M. 1964. Lung cancer, inhalation, and personality. *In* Psychosomatic Aspects of Neoplastic Disease. D. M. Kissen & L. L. LeShan, Eds. : 3–11. Pitman. London, England.

KISSEN, D. M. & H. J. EYSENCK. 1962. Personality in male lung cancer patients. J. Psychosom. Res. **6**: 123.

KISSEN, D. M. 1965. Possible contribution of the psychosomatic approach to prevention of lung cancer. Medical Officer **114**: 343–345.

KISSEN, D. M. 1966a. The significance of personality in lung cancer in men. Ann. N. Y. Acad. Sci. **125**(3): 820–826.

KISSEN, D. M. 1966b. The value of a psychosomatic approach to cancer. Ann. New York Acad. Sci. **125**(3): 777–779.

KISSEN, D. M. 1966c. Psychosocial factors, personality and prevention in lung cancer. Medical Officer **116**: 135–138.

KISSEN, D. M. & L. G. S. RAO. 1968. Steroid excretion patterns and personality in lung cancer. This monograph.

LESHAN, L. L. 1966. An emotional life-history pattern associated with neoplastic disease. Ann. N. Y. Acad. of Sci. **125**(3): 780–793.

LESHAN, L. L. & R. E. WORTHINGTON. 1956a. Some recurrent life history patterns observed in patients with malignant disease. J. Nerv. Ment. Dis. **124**: 460–465.

LESHAN, L. L. & R. E. WORTHINGTON. 1956b. Personality as a factor in the pathogenesis of cancer. Brit. J. Med. Psychol. **29**: 49–56.

LESHAN, L. L. & M. REZNIKOFF. 1960. A phychological factor apparently associated with neoplastic disease. J. Abnorm. Soc. Psychol. **60**: 439–440.

LEVINE, S. 1961. Plasma-free corticosteroid response to electric shock in rats stimulated in infancy. Science **135**: 795–796.

MARGOLIN. 1966. Panel discussion: Retrospects and prospects. Ann. N. Y. Acad. Sci. **125**(3): 1028–1055.

MARMORSTON, J., L. G. CROWLEY, S. M. MYERS, E. STERN & C. E. HOPKINS. 1965a. Urinary excretion of neutral 17-ketosteroids and pregnanediol by patients with breast cancer and benign breast disease. Amer. J. Obstet. Gynec. **92**: 447–459.

MARMORSTON, J., H. W. GIERSON, S. M. MYERS & E. STERN. 1965b. Urinary excretion of neutral 17-ketosteroids and pregnanediol by patients with lung cancer and emphysema. Amer. Rev. Resp. Dis. **92**: 404–416.

MARMORSTON, J., L. J. LOMBARDO, S. M. MYERS, H. W. GIERSON & E. STERN. 1965c. Urinary excretion of neutral 17-ketosteroids and pregnanediol by patients with prostatic cancer and benign prostatic hypertrophy. J. Urol. **93**: 276–286.

MARMORSTON, J., J. M. WEINER, E. STERN & C. E. HOPKINS. 1966. Urinary hormone metabolite levels in patients with cancer of the breast, prostate and lung. Ann. N. Y. Acad. Sci. **125**(3): 959–973.

MOORE, D. H. 1964. The role of viruses in breast cancer causation. Presented at the Fifth National Cancer Conference. Philadelphia, Pa.

NEWTON, G. 1964. Early experience and resistance to tumor growth. *In* Psychosomatic Aspects of Neoplastic Disease. D. M. Kissen & L. L. LeShan, Eds. : 71–79. Pitman. London, England.

RAKOFF, A. E. 1962. Psychogenic factors in anovulatory women: Part I. Hormonal patterns in women with ovarian dysfunctions of psychogenic origin. Fertil. Steril. **13**: 1.

RAKOFF, A. E. 1963. Hormonal patterns in psychogenic amenorrhea and anovulation. Adv. Neuroendocrinol. **14**: 460–510.

RAKOFF, A. E. 1966a. Discussion of the papers. Ann. N. Y. Acad. Sci. **125**(3): 817–820.

RAKOFF, A. E. 1966b. In panel: Retrospects and prospects. Ann. N. Y. Acad. Sci. **125**(3): 1029–1031.

RASMUSSEN, A. J., JR. 1968. Emotions and immunity. This monograph.

REISER, M. 1966. Panel discussion: Retrospects and prospects. Ann. N. Y. Acad. Sci. **125**(3): 1028–1055.

ROE, S. & M. SIEGELMAN. 1964. The Origin of Interests. American Personnel and Guidance Association. Washington, D. C.

SCHMALE, A. H., JR. 1958. Relation of separation and depression to disease. I. A report on a hospitalized medical population. Psychosom. Med. **20**: 259–277.

SCHMALE, A. H., JR. & H. P. IKER. 1964. The affect of hopelessness in the development of cancer. I. The prediction of uterine cervical cancer in women with atypical cytology. Psychosom. Med. **26:** 634–635.

SCHMALE, A. H., JR. & H. P. IKER. 1966. The psychological setting of uterine cervical cancer. Ann. N. Y. Acad. Sci. **125**(3): 807–813.

SJOBRING, H. 1963. La Personalité, Structure et Developpement. Doin. Paris, France.

SOLOMON, G. 1966. Panel discussion: Retrospects and prospects. Ann. N. Y. Acad. Sci. **125**(3): 1028–1055.

SOLOMON, G. & R. H. MOOS. 1964. Emotions, immunity and disease. Arch. Gen. Psychiat. **2:** 657–674.

SOMMERS, S. C. 1958. Host factors in fatal human lung cancer. Arch Path. (Chicago) **65:** 104–111.

SOUTHAM, C. & A. H. SIEGEL. 1966. Serum levels of second component of complement in cancer patients. J. Immunol. **97:** 3.

SPITZ, R. A. 1945. Hospitalism: An inquiry into the genesis of psychiatric conditions in early childhood. *In* The Psychoanalytic Study of the Child. Vol. I. International Universities Press. New York, N. Y.

SPITZ, R. A. 1946. The smiling response: A contribution to the ontogenesis of social relations. Genet. Psychol. Monogr. **34:** 57–125.

SPITZ, R. A. 1949. The role of ecological factors in emotional development. Child Develop. **20:** 145–165.

STEIN, M., R. SCHIAVI & T. J. LUPARELLO. 1968. The hypothalamus and immune processes. This monograph.

STEVENSON, D. 1963. Evolution and the neurobiogenesis of neoplasia. *In* Psychosomatic Aspects of Neoplastic Disease. D. M. Kissen & L. L. LeShan, Eds. : 152–169. Pitman. London, England.

WEISS, D. W. 1968. Immunological parameters of the host-parasite relationship in neoplasia. This monograph.

DISCUSSION OF THE PAPER

DR. GREENE: I should like to make one comment. You kindly referred to some of my work. At one point in your presentation you mentioned my reference some years ago to the women who developed leukemia manifesting psychological decompensation and then you went on to say that this was reminiscent of key immunological concepts that are developing today. I think it is important to point out that this is your association; this is not my association.

What I should like to emphasize is that, I think, there is a tendency to lend what I should call physiological luster to psychological processes. There is also a tendency to lend emotional luster to physiological and immunological processes, which I think is intellectually enticing, but I'm not sure how helpful it is. I also think that the use of the word "complementarity" lends very far-reaching fundamental scientific luster to psychophysiologic processes, but I'm not sure that these manifestations need this, if you will. In terms of modeling–we all like to model, and at the conference three years ago I pointed out that it is difficult for any of us to consider psychophysiologic processes as operating in neoplasia without there being a relating mechanism. I think it may be possible to conceptualize in terms of psychological processes and physiological processes and immunological processes without having to come to any kind of modeled, integrating closure. The real problem in getting a model, I think, is to find the model of a man or of a medical team, if you will, than can work with both the immunological dysfunction, perhaps therapeutically, and the psychological dysfunction, perhaps therapeutically.

DR. BAHNSON: I will be very brief, Dr. Greene, in my answer to your remarks. Of course, it is anybody's privilege to operate within the system of his own theoretical preference and to choose whether he wishes to decentralize observations in terms of many pell-mell plots or independent systems, or whether he prefers to be more "continental" or "spinozean" and think in terms of integrated systems.

There is no proof for or against any of these approaches, and we all understand that theory represents an arbitrary, or, perhaps, personally motivated choice. Theory is for somehow bringing system to our limited minds out of a number of different, observed phenomena. When we study psychophysiological aspects of malignancies, it seems to me to be reasonable to search for theoretical formulations that may integrate rather than segregate phenomena that we usually perceive at different conceptual levels; and for this reason I have preferred to use a monistic model, which, of course, is a completely arbitrary choice, just as all other models combining observations represent such choices.

In terms of luster, I must say that it seems to be helpful to introduce a bit of luster into our theoretical discussions, rather than the usual dullness, so I will accept this accusation.

EMOTIONS, STRESS, THE CENTRAL NERVOUS SYSTEM, AND IMMUNITY

George F. Solomon

Stanford University School of Medicine

and

Veterans Administration Hospital
Palo Alto, Calif.

Hypotheses

Stress and emotional distress may influence the function of the immunologic system via central nervous system and possibly endocrine mediation.[1] Thus, environmental and psychologic factors might in some circumstances be implicated as aspects of the pathogenesis of cancer, the resistance to which growing evidence finds immunologic in nature, and of infections as well as of autoimmune diseases, which seem to have an association with states of relative immunologic incompetence. There are considerable data to link personality factors, stress, and, particularly, failure of psychologic defenses or adaptations to the onset and course of cancer and of infectious and autoimmune diseases, particularly rheumatoid arthritis. We are concerned especially with physiologic mechanisms, nervous and humoral, by which emotions and stress may relate to the diseases associated with dysfunction and hypofunction of the immunologic system. One possible link is the effect of stress-responsive adrenal cortical steroid hormones, which may be immunosuppressive.

Stress effects on immunologic response might be expected to be observed under clinical conditions of gross failure of psychologic defenses, as generally occurs during acute mental illness. (However, in some forms of schizophrenic and depressive illnesses, the psychologic defenses may have "succeeded" in warding off psychic distress. Such patients do not show elevated adrenal cortical hormone levels.[2]) Abnormal central nervous system function in mental illness might be reflected immunologically; on the other hand, it is conceivable that abnormal immunologic factors may play a role in the pathogensis of mental illness, particularly schizophrenia, as suggested by Fessel[3,4] and by Heath and Krupp.[5] The possibility that at least some forms of schizophrenia might be related to autoimmunity is intriguing in view of evidence to be presented that autoimmunity itself has emotional and stress antecedents.

Infectious Diseases and Emotions

Clinicians have long been aware of the importance of host resistance in the etiology of infectious diseases. Osler is supposed to have commented on the importance of knowing what is going on in a man's head in order to predict the outcome of his tuberculosis. The British authority, Day, states, "To develop chronic active pulmonary tuberculosis a person needs some bacilli, some moderately inflammable lungs (not celluloid like the guinea pig's nor asbestos like the elephant's) and some internal or external factor which lowers the resistance to the disease," and he goes on to say that unhappiness is a cause of lowered resistance.[6] Elaborating on an appealing multifactorial approach to disease, Salk speculates illness may concern genetic, behavioral, social, and immune relationships.[7] In research studies, emotions, especially depression[8] and social factors,[9] have been linked to susceptibility to and recovery from infectious diseases. Families of ill children were found to have been more disorganized during the prior six-month period and to have exposed their children to a greater number of psychologic and social changes, which were threatening and had a disruptive impact, than was the case with a comparison group of healthy children.[9] Delayed recovery from infectious mononucleosis has been correlated with deficient ego strength[10] and prolonged convalescence from tuberculosis and influenza correlated with depression.[11,12] Experimentally, avoidance learning and restraint leads to increased susceptibility to herpes simplex virus in mice.[13] Though neither stress nor Coxsackie B virus alone is sufficient to produce disease in mice, the combination results in a loss of body weight.[14] Disappearance of vesicular stomatitis virus from the site of innoculation is retarded in stressed mice.[15] Under certain conditions, stress increases susceptibility to virus-induced tumors.[16]

Cancer and Emotions

Personality factors have been tied to the presence and the rapidity of dissemination of cancer in a large number of studies, rapid progression of cancer being associated with unsuccessful psychologic defenses and psychic distress. (Even Galen considered that melanchollý women suffer from cancer more frequently than sanguine women!) Four consistent factors are found in reports of personality studies on some patients with cancer: (1) the patient's loss of an important relationship prior to the development of a tumor, (2) the cancer patient's inability to express hostile feelings and emotion, (3) the cancer patient's unresolved tension concerning a parent figure, (4) sexual disturbance.[17] As will be seen, these are very similar to the factors that have been described in patients with autoimmune diseases. In a predictive study, Klopfer related long survival either to successful denial of reality or, more rarely, to a mature, calm acceptance of reality, and rapid death to ego defensiveness with a high degree of subjective distress.[18]

Cancer and Immunity

This is a great deal of growing evidence that resistance to cancer is immunologic in nature. Some event reducing immunologic competence at a critical time may allow a mutant cell (ordinarily rejected like a foreign graft) induced by virus, chemical carcinogen, radiation, or chance somatic mutation to thrive and multiply. There is evidence for tumor-specific antigens[19] and for lowered immunologic capacity in patients with cancer.[20] In regard to experimental tumors, Habel states, "Perhaps the only way in which the mouse, naturally infected as an adult or with a small amount of virus as a newborn, can develop polyoma tumor is by the chance occurrence of some event which temporarily reduces its immunologic competence at the proper time after virus transformation of normal cells to tumor cells."[21] Cancer is thus seen as analogous to infectious disease, with the balance between the inoculum of foreign pathogenic material and host resistance factors determining the emergence of disease.

Autoimmune Diseases and Immunologic Incompetence

Though the etiologic significance of autoantibodies themselves remains uncertain, relative immunologic incompetence may be related to the pathogenesis of autoimmune diseases such as rheumatoid arthritis, systemic lupus erythematosus, myastenia gravis, and acquired hemotlytic anemia.[22] These diseases occur with relative frequency in patients and experimental animals with immunologic deficiency states and with neoplastic diseases of immunologically competent cells. Dixon and associates relate autoimmune disease to the presence of circulating antigen-antibody complexes, which occur when antibody appears in an environment of antigen excess.[23] In rabbits injected daily with small amounts of purified serum proteins, only those animals with a poor antibody response, in contrast to those with an absent or with a vigorous antibody response develop chronic glomerulonephritis with deposits of antigen, host-globulin and host-complement in the glomerular basement membranes. Immunologic complexes can produce chronic degenerative tissue change, and the injured tissue needs no immunologic relationship to the antigen involved. Antigen-antibody complexes inactivate complement, release amines from mast cells, and may produce disseminated inflammatory lesions and also activate the proteolytic enzyme plasmin, which has been noted to be elevated in conditions of emotional stress.[24] It is conceivable that *in vivo* denaturation of body constituents by proteolytic activity might lead to autoimmunity. Weigle has shown that administration of proteins modified *in vitro* and given to animals tolerant to that protein breaks the tolerance for the original protein.[25] Also, antigen-antibody complexes themselves might act as new antigens for formation of new antibody. Rheumatoid factor is probably such an autoantibody.[26] Another hypothetical mechanism by which immunologic incompetence, perhaps based partly on genetic predisposition, might relate to autoimmunity is the failure to eliminate by rejection mechanisms abnormal clones of immunologically competent cells reactive against self.[22] Alternatively, a bacterium, virus, or mycoplasm ordinarily readily handled by the immune system may attack a specific tissue and alter it immunologically to induce autoimmunity.[22]

Emotions and Social Factors in the Onset and Course of Autoimmune Diseases

In view of evidence that relative immunologic incompetence, which may be stress-induced, may be important in the pathogenesis of autoimmune disease, our findings in regard to emotional factors in the autoimmune diseases seem pertinent. As we shall see, these factors are similar to those cited for infectious disease and cancer.

Moos' review of the literature of over 5,000 patients with rheumatoid arthritis found that investigators agreed that arthritics, when compared with various control groups, tend to be self-sacrificing, masochistic, conforming, self-conscious, shy, inhibited, perfectionistic, and interested in sports.[27] Moos and I found that female rheumatoid patients were nervous, tense, worried, moody, depressed, concerned with the rejection they perceived from their mothers and the strictness they perceived from their fathers, and showed denial and inhibition of the expression of anger in contrast to their healthy sisters.[28,29] Women with definite or classical rheumatoid arthritis scored higher than healthy female family members on Minnesota Multiphasic Personality Inventory scales reflecting inhibition of anger, anxiety, depression, compliance-subservience, conservatism, security-seeking, shyness, and introversion.[30] We related rapidity of progression of disease,[31] relatively high degrees of functional incapacity,[32] and lack of response to medical treatment in rheumatoid arthritis[33] to an inability to utilize previously successful ego adaptations. Arthritics who did poorly were more anxious and depressed, were more isolated, introverted, and alienated, and were more unable to maintain compulsive defenses and suppression of anger than were those with a more benign course. These findings are quite analogous to those already cited in the cases of infectious disease and cancer. We compared two groups of healthy female relatives of rheumatoid arthritic patients, one group having, and the other lacking rheumatoid factor in their sera, since there is some evidence that the presence of rheumatoid factor in the serum may predispose to arthritis.[34] Psychologic test results indicated that there was a greater incidence of emotional decompensation – anxiety, depression, low self-esteem, alienation, fear and worry, and lack of impulse control and ego mastery – in those relatives *lacking* rheumatoid factor. It seemed as if the occurrence of psychic disequilibrium in the presence of rheumatoid factor might lead to overt rheumatoid disease, so that physically healthy persons with rheumatoid factor, to remain so, need be psychologically healthy as well. Thus, emotional decompensation in the predisposed individual might result in a specific physical illness. Interestingly, the rheumatoid factor *positive* relatives were more similar to the arthritic patients in their *type* of character structure defense and adaptation, but were distinguished from the patients by the *success* of these adaptations.

It is of considerable interest that personality data similar to those we and others have reported for patients with rheumatoid arthritis have been published for patients with other autoimmune diseases. Engel, in his classical studies of ulcerative colitis, a disease often associated with anticolon antibodies, refers to obsessive-compulsive character traits of consciousness, neatness, indecision, conformity, overintellectualization, rigid morality, and worrying.[35] Engel's colitis patients, as arthritics have been described, could not directly express hostility and seemed basically immature and dependent. Colitis patients' mothers were controlling and had a propensity to assume the role of martyr, again as arthritics' mothers have been described. McClary and associates speak of the role of the mechanism of depression in patients with disseminated lupus erythematosus. They observed an unusual need for activity and independence, which they consider a denial of the guilt-provoking wish for maternal affection.[36] McClary, like Otto and Mackay,[37] found that onset of lupus frequently followed major life stress situations.

The Central Nervous System and Immunity

Several lines of evidence point to a direct role of the central nervous system in control of immunogenesis. Fessel demonstrated that mental stress produces a rise in 19S gamma globulin.[38] Fessel and Forsyth demonstrated alteration in gamma globulin levels by electrical stimulation of the lateral hypothalamus of rats.[39] Korneva and Khai reported that a destructive lesion of the portion of the dorsal hypothalamus leads to a complete suppression of the production of complement-fixing antibodies and to prolonged retention of antigen in the blood.[40] In a more recent report, Korneva claims that electrical stimulation of the same region enhances the antibody production.[41] Soviet workers in questionable work have for a long time claimed to be able to condition antibody response, to obtain anamnestic antibody increase by a conditioned stimulus without antigen.[42] Soviet workers also claim that denervation of the site of antigen deposition diminishes antibody response, and nervous stimulation in conjunction with antigen administration enhances antibody response.[43]

Immunologic Abnormalities and Mental Illness

A relationship among immunoproteins, stress, and central nervous system is suggested by the findings of various dysproteinemias and autoimmune agglutination reactions in conjunction with schizophrenic illnesses. Elevation of gamma globulin levels and of macroglobulin as well as qualitative disturbances in the electrophoretic patterns of gamma globulin have been reported in various groups of patients with functional psychoses.[44] An increased incidence of positive FII (rheumatoid factor) and nucleoprotein latex agglutination tests has been found in the sera of psychotic state hospital patients.[3] Using various agglutination techniques, antibrain antibody activity has been found in the sera of acutely and chronically ill mental patients.[4] Heath now claims that the substance "taraxein" derived from the serum of disturbed schizophrenic patients, which is reputedly capable of eliciting psychotic symptoms upon injection into normal voluteers and monkeys and of producing electroencephalographic spike activity in the septal region similar to that he finds in schizophrenic patients, is an Ig G autoantibody directed against oligodendroglia of a portion of the septal region (particularly of schizophrenic brain) as determined by immunofluorescence and ferritin-tagged globulin techniques.[5,54]

Our own work suggests a positive correlation between severity of general psychotic symptoms and 19S macroglobulin levels and a negative correlation of these symptoms with overall gamma globulin levels in schizophrenic patients.[45] Neither behavior nor serum protein levels were altered by the administration of small amounts of the immunosuppressant antimetabolite chlorambucil in a group of chronic schizophrenic patients with relatively elevated levels of gamma globulin and/or macroglobulin.[45] New data of ours suggest that psychiatric patients show significant elevation of Ig A and Ig M immunoglobulins without regard to diagnosis or other subcategory.[55]

There is disputed evidence that schizophrenic patients have a relatively poor antibody response to administered antigen.[46–48] However, Rubbo and I recently found no significant difference in secondary response to tetanus toxoid in schizophrenic patients as compared with hospitalized nonschizophrenic psychiatric patients and normal controls.[56] If present, such relative immunologic incompetence might relate to the higher incidence of autoantibodies in schizophrenic patients[3] and to the higher death rate observed in such patients.[49] The presence of abnormal globulins and of altered immunologic responsivity in schizophrenic patients may be related to the finding of abnormal lymphocytes in schizophrenics and in their family members reported by Fessel and Hirata-Hibi.[50,51]

Rheumatoid Factor and Stress

We have some evidence that rheumatoid factor, an antiglobulin autoantibody, appears or increases in titer in some healthy athletes under stress of a very hard-fought, emotionally charged, close football game and that this appearance or increase is more likely in the presence of prior psychic distress. (Stress has been reputed to affect the presence of thyroid autoantibody.[52])

Stress and Antibody Response

We have evidence that some forms of stress, especially overcrowding, significantly reduce primary and secondary antibody response to flagellin, a potent bacterial antigen that is novel to the rat.[57] Overcrowding virtually eliminated booster response. This finding may relate to natural epizootics following overpopulation.

Early Experience and Antibody Response

A clear finding is that early experience alters adult immunologic responsivity in the rat.[58] Fisher rats were handled from birth by being picked up and placed in a small box for three minutes and then returned to the nest. Handled rats responded more vigorously to primary challenge with flagellin at nine weeks, particularly in the 19S globulin, and also showed somewhat higher titers, which were sustained longer, after booster immunization four weeks following primary than did unhandled controls.

Antigen Clearance and Stress

Stress seems to accelerate initial elimination of circulating antigen by the reticuloendothelial system and to alter its distribution.

Interferon, Stress, and Adrenal Steroid Hormones

A project was carried out in conjunction with Thomas Merigan and Seymour Levine on the effects of stress and variations in levels of adrenal cortical steroid hormons within physiologic ranges on interferon production in mice.[53] (Interferon is a nonspecific protein elaborated in response to virus infection, one which is increasingly implicated in resistance to virus diseases including, perhaps, virus-induced tumors.) Both stress and pharmacologic levels of adrenal cortical hormones had been reported to suppress the synthesis of interferon. We measured interferon in mice six hours after intravenous injection of Newcastle disease virus and related interferon titers to plasma corticosterone levels. The stress of repeated random electric shocks preceded by a warning buzzer during interferon production did not alter the response from that of controls; such stress administered for five hours prior to virus inoculation significantly *enhanced* interferon production. Administration of ACTH did not alter interferon response. Corticosterone administration adequate to produce high circulating steroid levels just greater than maximal attainable physiologic levels also did not alter response. Adrenalectomized animals had relatively high interferon titers; however, neither prior stress nor partial corticosterone replacement therapy in any combination significantly altered interferon production in adrenalectomized mice. Administration of the virus itself produced an adrenal response as measured by plasma corticosterone level in intact animals not subjected to other exogenous stress as great as that in animals subjected to exogenous stress prior or subsequent to injection of virus. Thus, observed preinoculation stress-induced enhancement of interferon production may have been due to relative adrenal exhaustion, so that the viral challenge was not able to effect maximal adrenal response.

Summary

Stress and emotional distress may influence the function of the immunologic system. Thus, environmental and psychologic factors might in some circumstances be implicated in the pathogenesis of cancer, the resistance to which growing evidence finds immunologic in nature, as well as of infections and of autoimmune diseases, which seem to have an association with states of relative immunologic incompetence. There are considerable data to link personality factors, stress, and, particularly, failure of psychologic defenses to the onset and course of cancer and of infectious and autoimmune diseases. We are concerned with nervous and hormonal mechanisms by which emotions and stress may relate to specific dysfunctions of the immunologic system.

Clinical situations of emotional decompensation and mental illness may be associated with immunologic disturbances, which in turn might affect mental function.

We have experimental evidence that some forms of stress may reduce primary and secondary antibody response in rats and that adult immunologic responsivity may be altered by early infantile experience. In contrast, we found that stress prior to inoculation enhances interferon production, which may have implications in virus-induced tumors.

References

1. SOLOMON, G. F. & R. H. MOOS. 1964. Emotions, immunity and disease: a speculative theoretical integration. Arch. Gen. Psychiat. **11:** 657.
2. SACHAR, E. J. 1967. Corticosteroids in depressive illness. II. Longitudinal psychologic endocrine study. Arch. Gen. Psychiat. **17:** 554.
3. FESSEL, W. J. 1961. Disturbed serum proteins in chronic psychosis. Arch. Gen. Psychiat. **4:** 154.
4. FESSEL, W. J. 1963. "Antibrain" factors in psychiatric patients' sera. I. Further studies with hemagglutination technique. Arch. Gen. Psychiat. **8:** 614.
5. HEATH, R. G. & I. M. KRUPP. 1967. Schizophrenia as an immunologic disorder. Arch. Gen. Psychiat. **16:** 1.
6. DAY, G. 1951. The psychosomatic approach to pulmonary tuberculosis. Lancet (May 12): 6663.
7. SALK, J. 1962. Biological basis of disease and behavior. Perspect. Biol. Med. **5:** 198.
8. SCHMALE, A. H., JR. 1958. The relation of separation and depression to disease. Psychosom. Med. **20:** 259.
9. MUTTER, A. Z. & M. J. SCHLEIFER. 1966. The role of psychological and social factors in the onset of somatic illness in children. Psychosom. Med. **28:** 333.
10. GREENFIELD, N. S., R. ROESSLER & A. P. CROSLEY, JR. 1966. Ego strength and length of recovery from infectious mononucleosis. J. Nerv. Ment. Dis. **128:** 125.
11. IMBODEN, J. B., A. CARTER, E. C. LEIGHTON & R. W. TREVOR. 1959. Brucellosis III. Psychologic aspects of delayed convalescence. Arch. Intern. Med. **103:** 406.
12. IMBODEN, J. B., A. CARTER & E. C. LEIGHTON. 1961. Convalescence from influenza: a study of the psychological and clinical determinants. Arch. Intern. Med. **108:** 115.
13. RASMUSSEN, A. F., JR., E. S. SPENCER & J. T. MARSH. 1957. Increased susceptibility to herpes simplex in mice subjected to avoidance-learning stress or restraint. Proc. Soc. Exper. Biol. Med. **96:** 183.
14. FRIEDMAN, S. B., R. ADER & L. A. GLASGOW. 1965. Effects of psychological stress in adult mice inoculated with Coxsackie B viruses. Psychosom. Med. **27:** 361.
15. YAMADA, A., M. M. JENSEN & A. F. RASMUSSEN, JR. 1964. Stress and susceptibility to viral infections. III. Antibody response and viral retention during avoidance-learning stress. Proc. Soc. Exper. Biol. Med. **116:** 677.
16. RASMUSSEN, A. F., JR., W. H. HILDEMANN & M. SELLERS. 1963. Malignancy of polyoma virus infection in mice in relation to stress. J. Nat. Cancer Inst. **30:** 101.
17. LESHAN, L. L. & R. E. WORTHINGTON. 1956. Personality as factor in pathogenesis of cancer: review of literature. Brit. J. Med. Psychol. **29:** 49.
18. KLOPFER, B. 1957. Psychological variables in human cancer. J. Project Techn. **21:** 331.
19. PREHN, R. T. 1963. Role of immune mechanisms in biology of chemically and physically induced tumors. *In* Conceptual Advances in Immunology and Oncology. Hoeber. New York, N. Y.
20. SOUTHAM, C. M., A. E. MOORE & C. P. RHOADES. 1957. Homotransplantation of human cell lines. Science **125:** 158.
21. HABEL, K. 1963. Immunologic aspects of oncgenesis by polyoma virus. *In* Conceptual Advances in Immunology and Oncology. Hoeber. New York, N. Y.
22. FUDENBERG, H. H. 1968. Are autoimmune diseases immunologic deficiency states? Hosp. Prac. **3:** 43.
23. DIXON, F. J., J. FELDMAN & J. VASQUEZ. 1961. Experimental glomerulonephritis. J. Exp. Med. **113:** 899.
24. LATNER, A. I. 1947. Anxiety as a cause of fibrinolysis. Lancet **1:** 194.
25. WEIGLE, W. O. 1965. The antibody response in rabbits to previously tolerated antigens. Ann. N. Y. Acad. Sci. **124:** 133.
26. AHO, K. & K. SIMMONS. 1963. Studies of the nature of rheumatoid factor: reaction of rhumatoid factor with human specific precipitates and with native human gamma globulin. Arthritis Rheum. **6:** 676.
27. MOOS, R. H. 1964. Personality factors associated with rheumatoid arthritis: review. J. Chronic Dis. **17:** 41.
28. MOOS, R. H. & G. F. SOLOMON. 1965. Psychologic comparisons between women with rheumatoid arthritis and their non-arthritic sisters. I. Personality test and interview rating data. Psychosom. Med. **27:** 135.
29. MOOS, R. H. & G. F. SOLOMON. 1965. Psychologic comparisons between women with rheumatoid arthritis and their non-arthritic sisters. II. Content analysis of interviews. Psychosom. Med. **27:** 150.

30. Moos, R. H. & G. F. Solomon. 1964. Minnesota Multiphasic Personality Inventory response patterns in patients with rheumatoid arthritis. J. Psychosom. Res. **8:** 17.
31. Moos, R. H. & G. F. Solomon. 1964. Personality correlates of the rapidity of progression of rheumatoid arthritis. Ann. Rheum. Dis. **23:** 145.
32. Moos, R. H. & G. F. Solomon. 1965. Personality correlates of the degree of functional incapacity of patients with physical disease. J. Chronic Dis. **18:** 1019.
33. Solomon, G. F. & R. H. Moos. 1965. Psychologic aspects of response to treatment in rheumatoid arthritis. GP **32:** 113.
34. Solomon, G. F. & R. H. Moos. 1965. The relationship of personality to the presence of rheumatoid factor in asymptomatic relatives of patients with rheumatoid arthritis. Psychosom. Med. **27:** 350.
35. Engel, G. 1953. Studies of ulcerative colitis: III. Nature of the psychologic process. Amer. J. Med. **19:** 231.
36. McClary, A. R., E. Meyer & D. J. Weitzman. 1955. Observations on role of mechanism of depression in some patients with disseminated lupus erythematosus. Psychosom. Med. **17:** 311.
37. Otto, R. & I. Mackay. 1967. I. Psychosocial and emotional disturbance in systemic lupus erythematosus. Med. J. Aust. **2:** 488.
38. Fessel, W. J. 1962. Mental stress, blood proteins, hypothalamus: experimental results showing effect of mental stress upon 4S and 19S proteins; speculation that functional behavior disturbances may be expressions of general metabolic disorder. Arch. Gen. Psychiat. **7:** 427.
39. Fessel, W. J. & R. P. Forsyth. 1963. Hypothalamic role in control of gamma globulin levels. (abst.) Arthritis Rheum. **6:** 770.
40. Korneva, E. A. & L. M. Khai. 1963. Effect of destruction of hypothalamic areas on immunogenesis. Fiziol. Zh. SSSR. Sechenov. **49:** 42.
41. Korneva, E. A. 1967. The effect of stimulating different mesencephalic structures on protective immune response patterns. Fiziol. Zh. SSSR. Sechenov. **53:** 42.
42. Luk'yanenko, V. I. 1961. The problem of conditioned reflex regulation of immunobiological reactions. (In Russian). Vspekhi Sovremmenoy biologii. **51:** 170.
43. Gordienko, A. N. Control of immunogenesis by the nervous system. U.S. Dept. of Commerce Translation TT60–51069.
44. Fessel, W. J. & B. W. Grunbaum. 1961. Electrophoretic and analytical ultracentrifuge studies in sera of psychotic patients: elevation of gamma globulins and macroglobulins and splitting of alpha$_2$ globulins. Ann. Intern. Med. **54:** 1134.
45. Solomon, G. F., R. H. Moos, W. J. Fessel & E. E. Morgan. 1966. Globulins and behavior in schizophrenia. Int. J. Neuropsychiat. **2:** 20.
46. Vaughn, W. J., Jr., J. C. Sullivan & F. Elmadjian. 1949. Immunity and schizophrenia: survey of ability of schizophrenic patients to develop active immunity following injection of pertussis vaccine. Psychosom. Med. **11:** 327.
47. Kerbicov, O. V. 1960. Immunologic reactivity in schizophrenia as influenced by some modern drugs. *In* Pavlovian Conference on Higher Nervous Activity. Joint Meeting between N. Y. Academy of Sciences and Academy of Medical Sciences of USSR, New York, N. Y. Oct. 13–15.
48. Friedman, S. B., J. Cohen & H. Iker. 1967. Antibody response to cholera vaccine: differences between depressed, schizophrenic and normal subjects. Arch. Gen. Psychiat. **16:** 312.
49. Niswander, G. D., G. M. Heslerud & G. Mitchell. 1963. Differences in longevity of released and retained schizophrenic patients. Dis. Nerv. Syst. **24:** 348.
50. Fessel, W. J. & M. Hirata-Hibi. 1963. Abnormal leukocytes in schizophrenia. Arch. Gen. Psychiat. **9:** 601.
51. Fessel, W. J., M. Hirata-Hibi & I. M. Shapiro. 1965. Genetic and stress factors affecting the abnormal lymphocyte in schizophrenia. J. Psychiat. Res. **3:** 275.
52. Goodman, M. *et al.* 1963. Effect of age, sex and schizophrenia on autoantibody production. Arch. Gen. Psychiat. **8:** 518.
53. Solomon, G. F., T. Merigan & S. Levine. 1967. Variation in adrenal cortical hormones within physiologic ranges, stress and interferon production in mice. Proc. Soc. Exp. Biol. Med. **126:** 74.
54. Heath, R. G., A. Fitzjarrel & I. M. Krupp. 1968. Schizophrenic gamma G immunoglobulin at specific brain sites. (abst.) Scientific Proceedings, 124th Annual Meeting, Amer. Psychiat. Assn. Washington, D. C.
55. Solomon, G. F., M. Allansmith, B. McClellan & A. Amkraut. 1969. Immunoglobulins in psychiatric patients. Arch. Gen. Psychiat. **20:** 272.

56. SOLOMON, G. F., S. D. RUBBO & E. BATCHELDER. Secondary immune response to tetanus toxoid in psychiatric patients. J. Psychiat. Res. (In press.)
57. SOLOMON, G. F. 1969. Stress and antibody response in rats. Int. Arch. Allergy **35:** 97.
58. SOLOMON, G. F. 1968. Early experience and immunity. Nature **220:** 821.

DISCUSSION OF THE PAPER

MISS DENAH HARRIS (*New York, N. Y.*) What is it that creates stresses that may cause the distress that comes up in our life when we must face these problems? May I ask for discussion on that question?

DR. P. V. CARDON: I just wonder if Dr. Solomon would repeat the postulated way that the autoimmune business starts? As I got it, the idea is that there is not quite enough antibody there, when the external antigen reacts with it. Then something happens that leads to an autoimmune process. That went faster than I could understand it.

UNIDENTIFIED SPEAKER: With reference to various models that you talked about, Dr. Solomon, of carcinomas perhaps being like certain infectious diseases, I had the opportunity during the past three months to study for the first time a patient with leprosy, in which the biggest problem was both the immunologic investigator and the psychological investigator's anxiety about being in juxtaposition with the patient.

DR. SOLOMON: With regard to the question of stress and distress, it seems very important how the organism is perceiving the stimulus. Certainly, in our experimental work with stress, we found a very marked effect from overcrowding on immune response, no effect from what looked to us as very disturbing to the rats (namely, apprehension followed by an electric shock), and a moderate effect on having them remain on small platforms above a pan of water. Thus, there are differences among stresses even in animals.

In humans, it is an even more complicated issue, because what's going on within the individual is important. For me, jumping out of an airplane with a parachute might be very stressful, but for a psychopath, remaining seated in this meeting all day might be very stressful, and he would be gleeful about jumping out of airplanes. Whether there is some sort of means of coping or habituation is crucial to whether or not one is going to have a physiological response. One cannot just look at the events themselves and make assumptions about their "stressful" nature.

The question that was raised about the mechanism of autoimmunity reflects an extremely difficult and complicated problem. Clinically, there is a correlation between states of immunologic deficiency; for example, hypogammaglobulinemia, with autoimmunity. How this works has been speculated on by a number of people. Circulating antigen-antibody complexes are formed only when there is much antigen and a little bit of antibody. There is a great deal of work showing that these complexes are related to inflammatory processes and various sources of tissue damage. There are other possible mechanisms that I mentioned. One is failure to eliminate by immunologic means mutant immunologically competent cells that are reactive against self. I think these all remain speculative. It's rather fun for me to realize that immunologists, as hard scientists, sometimes get as speculative as behavioral scientists! Perhaps some of the immunologic experts who are here may have an opportunity later on to clarify some of these physiological mechanisms for us.

TUMOR-SPECIFIC TRANSPLANTATION ANTIGENS*

Eva Klein

Institute for Tumor Biology, Karolinska Institutet
Stockholm, Sweden

The occurrence of tumor-specific transplantation antigens in experimental systems is the rule rather than the exception.[1–3] If transplantation antigens have to be expressed on the cell surface, as there are good reasons to believe, their existence may imply a change in membrane structure. Growth-controlling instructions of the organism, whether they operate by long distance with humoral forces or by contactual local signals, must be transmitted to the effector cell organelles by receivers with a cell surface component. It may therefore be conjectured that a profound change in the normal surface, whether due to the appearance of new structural constituents imposed by virus-derived genetic information or to spontaneous or induced genetic changes, may lead to a deficient responsiveness to controlling forces. This concept has received experimental support recently by the work of Borek and Sachs,[4] who found a remarkable parallelism between the surface antigen and contact inhibition pattern of virus-transformed, chemically induced, and x-ray-transformed neoplastic cells.

The development of this field started when Foley[5] discovered that methylcholanthrene-induced sarcomas were antigenic in inbred mice: Isografted hosts were shown to be resistant to a second inoculation after their first tumor was made necrotic by ligation. Prehn and Main[6] confirmed Foley's experiment and also showed that tumor resistance could be elicited within critically skin-compatible donor-host combinations. Révész[7] found that isograft resistance against methylcholanthrene-induced sarcomas could be built up by treatment with heavily irradiated cells of the same tumor line. Klein and colleagues[8] demonstrated subsequently the induction of resistance in the primary autochthonous tumor host following operative removal of the tumor, three inoculations of irradiated tumor cells, and challenge with small numbers of viable cells.

Cross-reactivity tests between different tumors induced by the same chemical carcinogen revealed a remarkable antigenic individuality: Cross-immunization was rare or absent, even between tumors of similar morphology and induced in the same host genotype[6–8] or, in the cases where this has been tested, even between independently induced primary tumors in the same host[9,10]

Demonstration of individually distinct antigenic specificities has later been extended to other chemically induced tumors, including sarcomas induced by other aromatic hydrocarbons,[11] mammary carcinomas induced by methylcholanthrene,[12] and hepatomas induced by azo dyes.[13] Even sarcomas induced by the implantation of cellophane films or Millipore filter were antigenic, but only very weakly.[14,15] The strength of antigenicity is an operational concept and is judged by the maximum number of tumor cells rejected by preimmunized but accepted by untreated syngeneic hosts. Within tumor groups induced by the same chemical agent, there was a certain inverted relationship between antigenic strength and the length of the latency period preceding the appearance of the same tumor after

* Support for this investigation was received from the Swedish Cancer Society and Medical Research Council, the National Cancer Institute (Grants CA–04747 and CA–03700), the Damon Runyon Memorial Fund (ORG–598), the Jane Coffin Childs Memorial Fund for Medical Research, and the Knut and Alice Wallenbergs Foundation.

carcinogen administration in the primary host.[11,15] Prehn's interpretation was that tumors arising after prolonged periods of latency have been subjected to a more efficient immunoselection than those which appeared after a short period of time.

Another line of most important development started when virus-induced tumors were found to be antigenic in isograft tests. The first finding was [16,17] that polyoma virus-induced tumors contain a common, group-specific transplantation antigen capable of inducing rejection response in syngeneic hosts. The identity or extensive cross-reactivity (available transplantation methods cannot distinguish between these two possibilities) of the polyoma antigen in tumors of very different morphology and histogenesis is in sharp contrast to the individuality of the chemically induced tumors. The antigen was not present on the mature virion, since antiviral antibodies were neither necessary nor sufficient for the induction of transplantation resistance and the antigen was present on polyoma-induced tumor cells, whether they released virus or not.[2]

Group-specific transplantation antigens have now been shown to exist in all other virus-induced tumor systems that have been investigated and in leukemias. Among the latter tumors, no nonvirus-releasing lines exist; thus the relationship of the rejection-inducing antigen to the mature virus particles released by budding through the cell membrane cannot be decisively settled at present. Rejection responses could be built up by preimmunization with virus-containing materials or with the leukemic cells themselves, administered as homografts, subthreshold isografts, or heavily irradiated cells.[18] The "strength" of the antigenicity was different for the different systems. The Gross and the Moloney agents induce thymic lymphomas of closely similar or even identical morphology and clinical history, but their antigenic specificities are distinct.[18–20] The antigenicity of Gross-virus-induced leukemias is weaker than that of leukemias induced by the Moloney agent. The antigenic weakness of the Gross lymphomas, and the findings concerning the natural occurrence of the Gross virus and the specific cellular antigen (G) determined by it, have led to the suggestion[21] that the Gross agent may represent a leukemia virus occurring in nature, whereas this is not necessarily true for some of the other agents that have been isolated from serially propagated tumors in the laboratory and that induce more strongly antigenic neoplasms, less probable to occur under natural circumstances.

The immunological nature of tumor-isograft rejections is indicated by the following facts:

The threshold dose required for regular takes of a given tumor can be reduced by experimental manipulations known to inhibit immune responses, such as total body irradiation or treatment with antilymphocytic serum,[22,23] and it can be increased by specific preimmunization.[2] The resistance of preimmunized animals is not abolished by whole body x-irradiation, in agreement with the fact that established immune responses are less affected by x-rays than new primary responses. Neonatal thymectomy in mice or rats counteracts the tumor-isograft rejection response.[24]

Both cell- and antibody-mediated effector mechanisms could be demonstrated. Lymph node cells or macrophages from sensitized animals were found to inhibit the growth of the neoplastic target cells against which they have been immunized, both in tissue culture system and when mixed together *in vitro* and subsequently inoculated into suitable recipient animals.[10,25–27] The sensitized state of lymphocytes followed the same rules as in transplantation experiments in the case of chemical-carcinogen-induced tumors; their inhibitory effect was strictly confined to the particular tumor against which the donor animals were immunized. In some systems, humoral antibodies could also be demonstrated. They were easiest to detect if the target cells were derived from leukemias or lymphomas; cytotoxic[1,19,27] or membrane immunofluorescence[19,28] reactions were particularly useful. In the experimental systems studied, immunofluorescence was of broader applicability than the cytotoxicity, since the threshold effects of antigen concentration affecting cytotoxic sensitivity in an all-or-none fashion do not seem to play the same limiting role.[29,30] The absence of cytotoxic reactions in a given cell system cannot be interpreted to exclude humoral antibodies. Tumor-specific antibodies can be demonstrated sometimes by their paradoxical effect, immunological enhancement.[31–34] Presumably, the foreign antigenic sites of the cell surface become covered by humoral antibodies; in target cells resistant to cytotoxicity, this is believed to counteract both immunogenicity and sensitivity to host-cell-mediated destruction.

The properties of tumor-specific transplantation antigens resemble genetically determined weak transplantation antigens. It is not certain to what extent they can be exploited for tumor prevention. This obviously depends on a number of factors such as the cross-reactivity of the antigen; its potential immunogenicity in the presumptive tumor host in relation to genetic constitution, age, and previous immunological experience; and the feasibility of experimental interference to booster cells' rejection and avoidance of enhancement. The limited evidence now available for experimental tumors already indicates that the situation differs for different systems.

The immune status of the autochthonus host and particularly its "attitude" towards its tumor was found to vary between complete and apparently irreversible tolerance, reversible tolerance, and various degrees of sensitization. The amount of the antigenic load and the developmental stage when it is introduced appear to be of importance, together with genetic factors influencing reactivity characteristics of the host species or strain. In addition, immunosuppression by the oncogenic agent or by increasing age may also play a role.

Full tolerance was found to prevail only in systems where a viral oncogen is introduced into fetal or newborn hosts capable of supporting its proliferation and maturation, i.e., a full infectious cycle. All known cases of this type concern RNA viruses growing in their natural host and lacking any major pathogenic or cytocidal effect. The mouse mammary tumor agent, the vertically transmitted murine leukemia agent of Gross, or other mouse leukemia viruses introduced experimentally into susceptible newborn recipients can be mentioned as examples.[35–38] In all these cases, the agent is present throughout the lifetime of the animal and can be isolated from normal and neoplastic tissues as well. Electron microscopy indicated that virus growth is not restricted to the oncogenic target, but occurs in a variety of other cells as well. The immune system of the host is thus continuously exposed to virus-determined antigens.

This is probably the reason why there is no demonstrable tumor-specific graft rejection or production of anticellular and antiviral antibodies in such situations. If the same agents are introduced into host animals of the same genetic constitution at a later stage of development, however, they can react well, as a rule. Mammary tumors arising in mammary-tumor-virus-carrying strains can thus be rejected by syngeneic preimmunized mice of agent-free sublines; reintroduction of the agent to newborns prevents this reaction. The leukemia agents induce not only rejection but cytotoxic, membrane-reactive, and virus-neutralizing antibodies as well after inoculation into adults, but may fail to do so after neonatal infection. To some extent, newborn reactivity is a question of genetically determined maturity of the immune system; it is more difficult to induce tolerance to the Moloney virus in C57B1 mice than in a number of other strains. The same is true for tolerance induction against "ordinary" transplantation antigens.

The situation is more complicated, more diversified, and from the immunological point of view, more interesting in tumors induced by chemical carcinogens or by viruses that enter into a nonproductive interaction with their target cell. At the present time, the latter category includes all known oncogenic DNA viruses and the Scmidt-Ruppin variant of the Rous virus. The immune status of the susceptible animals cannot be described as either full tolerance or sensitization, but more as a state of relative immunological "inertia": The animals are potentially reactive. They seem to manage to eliminate a certain proportion, as shown by the increased tumor incidence in neonatally thymectomized recipients.[24, 39–43] By injecting a second dose of the same oncogenic virus or attenuated tumor cells originally induced by it during the latency period of carcinogenesis, the reactivity of the animals could be reinforced and tumor incidence reduced.[44–48] This indicates that the immunological capacity of the nonvaccinated animal is not fully utilized. The amount of antigen released by the developing neoplastic cells is probably insufficient to induce an adequate host response in time, capable of coping with their increasing numbers before they reach an irreversible colony size. The underlying host-tumor relationship is probably the most accessible one for immunological manipulations by specific or nonspecific means. In contrast, attempts to protect against methylcholanthrene-induced carcinogenesis by pretreatment with pools of methylcholanthrene-induced tumors was unsuccessful.[8,49] The number of individual antigenic alternatives is probably larger than that included in the pools used. Treatment with Bacilluse Calmette-Guérin did, on the other hand, delay the appearance of methylcholanthrene-induced sarcomas, presumably by increasing the recipients' capacity to react against their own antigenic, potentially neoplastic cells.[50]

In addition to the above-postulated interplay in timing between antigen release and possibility for mobilization of the host response after neonatal infection, other factors may also play a role in the outgrowth of potentially immunogenic tumor cells, as demonstrated in some of the analyzed cases. Nonspecific immunodepression was found to be induced by chemical carcinogens (and not by related noncarcinogenic hydrocarbons).[51] When mice were rechallenged both with their methylcholanthrene-induced autologous tumors and with another tumor induced in the same genotype (in crisscross experiments), they supported the growth of autologous cells better in 45% of the cases. In the remaining cases, the growth of the two tumor categories were identical.[52] This probably indicates the presence of a superimposed specific component akin to tolerance or paralysis as well, presumably as the combined result of immunodepression and constant antigen release. As a possibility, immunological enhancement has also to be kept in mind in this system, although its actual operation during the oncogenic process has not yet been demonstrated experimentally.

Little is known about the specific immune status of the human tumor patient. The work of Southam and Brunschwig[53] showing the rejection of surprisingly large numbers of autografted neoplastic cells in cancer patients indicates, however, that autosensitization may be a reality, at least against certain types of tumor.

The remarkable success of chemotherapy against choriocarcinomas of the female (a tumor of fetal, i.e., homograft-like, origin) is widely but not universally attributed to a synergistic interaction of an immunological reaction against paternally determined isoantigens and a direct cytostatic effect. The absence of similar therapeutic success in the rare cases of male choriocarcinomas is in line with this explanation. Direct evidence in favor of this intriguing explanation is still lacking, however.

Tumor-specific immune reactions have been recently postulated to explain the remarkably good results of chemotherapy obtained in a certain fraction (15–25%) of Burkitt lymphoma cases in Africa. Long-lasting regressions and probably cures were obtained after the use of a large variety of drugs in very different dosage schedules. In theory, a relatively strong new tumor-specific transplantation antigen would be in line with the postulated viral etiology of this tumor and horizontal transmission of the presumptive agent. Using the indirect (membrane) immunofluorescence method, we have recently obtained evidence[54] of the presence of antibodies in a certain number of Burkitt patients capable of reacting with the Burkitt lymphoma cells. Although the strict specificity of this reaction of the Burkitt lymphoma and its possible clinical and epidemiological significance remains to be elucidated, it strengthens the assumption that immune responses may contribute, if not to the immediate primary effects of therapy, at least to the decreased probability of tumor recurrence.

References

1. OLD, L. J. & E. A. BOYSE. 1964. Immunology of experimental tumors. Ann. Rev. Med. **15:** 167–186.
2. SJÖGREN, H. O. 1965. Transplantation methods as a tool for detection of tumor specific antigens. Progr. Exp. Tumor Res. **6:** 289–322.
3. KLEIN, G. 1966. Tumor antigens. Ann. Rev. Microbiol. **20:** 223–252.
4. BOREK, C. & L. SACHS. 1966. The difference in contact inhibition of cell replication between normal cells and cells transformed by different carcinogens. Proc. Nat. Acad. Sci. **56:** 1705–1711.
5. FOLEY, E. J. 1953. Antigenic properties of methylcholanthrene induced tumors in mice of the strain of origin. Cancer Res. **13:** 835–837.
6. PREHN, R. T. & J. M. MAIN. 1957. Immunity to methylcholanthrene-induced sarcomas. J. Nat. Cancer Inst. **18:** 769–778.
7. RÉVÉSZ, L. 1960. Detection of antigenic differences in isologous host-tumor systems by pretreatment with heavily irradiated tumor cells. Cancer Res. **20:** 443–451.
8. KLEIN, G., H. O. SJÖGREN, E. KLEIN & K. E. HELLSTRÖM. 1960. Demonstration of resistance against methylcholanthrene-induced sarcomas in the primary autochthonous host. Cancer Res. **20:** 1561–1572.
9. GLOBERSSON, A. & M. FELDMAN. 1964. Antigenic specificity of benzo(a)pyrene induced sarcomas. J. Nat. Cancer Inst. **32:** 1229–1243.
10. ROSENAU, W. & D. L. MORTON. 1966. Tumor-specific inhibition of growth of methylcholanthrene-induced sarcomas in vivo and in vitro by sensitized isologous lymphoid cells. J. Nat. Cancer Inst. **36:** 825–836.
11. PREHN, R. T. 1960. Tumor-specific immunity to transplanted dibenz(a,h)-anthracene-induced sarcomas. Cancer Res. **20:** 1614–1617.
12. PREHN, R. T. 1963. Tumor specific immunity to nonviral tumors. Canad. Cancer Conf. **5:** 387–395.
13. BALDWIN, R. W. & C. R. BARKER. 1967. Antigenic composition of transplanted rat hepatomas originally induced by 4-dimethylaminoazobenzene. Brit. J. Cancer **21:** 338–345.
14. KLEIN, G., H. O. SJÖGREN & E. KLEIN. 1963. Demonstration of host resistance against sarcomas induced by implantation of cellophane films in isologous recipients. Cancer Res. **23:** 84–92.
15. PREHN, R. T. 1963. The role of immune mechanisms in the biology of chemically and physically induced tumors. *In* Conceptual Advances in Immunology and Oncology. : 475–485. Sixteenth Ann. Symp. Fundamental Cancer Res. Hoeber. New York, N. Y.
16. SJÖGREN, H. O., I. HELLSTRÖM & G. KLEIN. 1961. Transplantation of polyoma virus induced tumors in mice. Cancer Res. **21:** 329–337.
17. HABEL, K. 1961. Resistance of polyoma virus immune animals to transplanted polyoma tumors. Proc. Soc. Exp. Biol. Med. **106:** 722–725.

18. KLEIN, G., H. O. SJÖGREN & E. KLEIN. 1962. Demonstration of host resistance against isotransplantation of lymphomas induced by the Gross agent. Cancer Res. **22:** 955–961.
19. KLEIN, E. & G. KLEIN. 1964. Antigenic properties of lymphomas induced by the Moloney agent. J. Nat. Cancer Inst. **32:** 547–568.
20. OLD, L. J., E. A. BOYSE & E. STOCKERT. 1964. Typing of mouse leukemias by serological methods. Nature (London) **201:** 777–779.
21. AOKI, T., E. A. BOYSE & L. J. OLD. 1966. Occurrence of natural antibody to the G (Gross) leukemia antigen in mice. Cancer Res. **26:** 1415–1419.
22. KLEIN, G. & E. KLEIN. 1963. Antigenic properties of other experimental tumors. Cold Spring Harbor Symp. Quant. Biol. **27:** 463–470.
23. BREMBERG, S., E. KLEIN & J. STJERNSWÄRD. 1967. Effect of heterologous antilymphoid cell serum on tumor isografts and viral leukemogenesis. Cancer Res. **27:** 2113–2118.
24. LAW, L. W. 1966. Studies on thymic function with emphasis on the role of the thymus in oncogenesis. Cancer Res. **26:** 551–574.
25. KLEIN, E. & H. O. SJÖGREN. 1960. Humoral and cellular factors in homograft and isograft immunity against sarcoma cells. Cancer Res. **20:** 452–461.
26. OLD, L. J., E. A. BOYSE, B. BENNET & F. LILLY. 1963. Peritoneal cells as an immune population in transplantation studies. *In* Cell bound antibodies. B. Amos & H. Koprowski, Eds. : 89–99. Wistar Inst. Press. Philadelphia, Pa.
27. SLETTENMARK, B. & E. KLEIN. 1962. Cytotoxic and neutralization tests with serum and lymph node cells of isologous mice with induced resistance against Gross lymphomas. Cancer Res. **22:** 947–954.
28. PASTERNAK, G. 1965. Serologic studies on cells of Graffi virus-induced myeloid leukemia in mice. J. Nat. Cancer Inst. **34:** 71–83.
29. KLEIN, G., E. KLEIN & G. HAUGHTON. 1966. Variation of antigenic characteristics between different mouse lymphomas induced by the Moloney virus. J. Nat. Cancer Inst. **36:** 607–621.
30. FENYÖ, E. M., E. KLEIN, G. KLEIN & K. SWIECH. 1968. Selection of an immunoresistant Moloney lymphoma sublime with decreased concentration of tumor specific surface antigens. J. Nat. Cancer Inst. **40:** 69–89.
31. MÖLLER, G. 1964. Effect on tumor growth in syngeneic recipients of antibodies against tumor specific antigens in methylcholanthrene-induced mouse sarcomas. Nature **204:** 846–847.
32. BUBENIK, J. & P. KOLDOVSKY. 1965. Factors influencing the induction of enhancement and resistance to methylcholanthrene-induced tumors in a syngeneic system. Folia Biol. **11:** 258.
33. WEISS, D. W., L. J. FAULKIN, JR. & K. B. DEOME. 1964. Acquisition of heightened resistance and susceptibility to spontaneous mouse mammary carcinomas in the original host. Cancer Res. **24:** 732.
34. GLYNN, J. P., A. R. BIANCO & A. GOLDIN. 1964. Studies on induced resistance against isotransplants of virus-induced leukemia. Cancer Res. **24:** 502–508.
35. AXELROD, A. A. 1963. Changes in resistance to the proliferation of insotransplanted Gross virus-induced lymphoma cells, as measured with a spleen colony assay. Nature **199:** 80–83.
36. ATTIA, A. M., K. B. DEOME & D. W. WEISS. 1965. Immunology of spontaneous mammary carcinomas in mice. II. Resistance to a rapidly and a slowly developing tumor. Cancer Res. **25:** 451–457.
37. KLEIN, E. & G. KLEIN. 1966. Immunological tolerance of neonatally infected mice to the Moloney leukemia virus. Nature **209:** 163–165.
38. PASTERNAK, G. & L. PASTERNAK. 1967. Demonstration of Graffi leukemia virus and virus-induced antigens in leukemic and non-leukemic tissues of mice. J. Nat. Inst. **38:** 157–168.
39. DEFENDI, V. & R. A. ROOSA. 1964. The role of the thymus in carcinogenesis. Wistar Inst. Monographs **2:** 121–136.
40. KIRSCHSTEIN, R. L., A. S. RABSON & E. A. PETERS. 1964. Oncogenic activity of adenovirus 12 in thymectomized BALB/c and C3H/HeN Mice. Proc. Soc. Exp. Biol. Med. **117:** 198–200.
41. GRANT, G. A. & J. F. A. P. MILLER. 1965. Effect of neonatal thymectomy on the induction of sarcomata in C75BL Mice. Nature **205:** 1124–1125.
42. NISHIZUKA, Y., K. NAKAKUKI & M. USUI. 1965. Enhancing effect of thymectomy on hepatotumorigenesis in Swiss mice following neonatal injection of 20-methylcholanthrene. Nature **205:** 1236–1238.
43. TING, R. C. & L. W. LAW. 1965. The role of thymus in transplantation resistance induced by polyoma virus. J. Nat. Cancer Inst. **34:** 521–527.

44. DEICHMANN, G. J. & T. E. KLUCHAREVA. 1964. Immunological determinants of oncogenesis in hamsters infected with SV40 virus. Virology **24:** 131–137.
45. EDDY, B. E., G. E. GRUBBS & R. D. YOUNG. 1964. Tumor immunity in hamster infected with adenovirus type 12 or simian virus 40. Proc. Soc. Exp. Biol. Med. **117:** 575–579.
46. GOLDNER, H., A. J. GIRARDI, V. M. LARSON & M. R. HILLEMAN. 1964. Interruption of SV40 virus tumorigenesis using irradiated homologous tumor antigen. Proc. Soc. Exp. Biol. Med. **117:** 851–860.
47. GIRARDI, A. J. 1965. Prevention of SV40 virus oncogenesis in hamsters. I. Tumor resistance induced by human cells transformed by SV40. Proc. Nat. Acad. Sci. **54:** 445–451.
48. EDDY, B. E., R. D. YLUNG & G. E. GRUBBS. 1966. Resistance to viral-induced tumors. *In* Viruses Inducing Cancer, Implications for Therapy. W. J. Burdette, Ed. : 403–414. Univ. of Utah Press. Salt Lake City, Utah.
49. PREHN, R. T. 1961. Failure of immunization against tumorigenesis. J. Nat. Cancer Inst. **26:** 223;227.
50. OLD, L. J., E. A. BOYSE, D. A. CLARKE & E. A. CARSWELL. 1962. Antigenic properties of chemically induced tumors. Ann. N. Y. Acad. Sci. **101:** 80–106.
51. STJERNSWÄRD, J. 1965. Immunodepressive effect of 3-methylcholanthrene. Antibody formation at the cellular level and reaction against weak antigenic homografts. J. Nat. Cancer Inst. **35:** 885–892.
52. STJERNSWÄRD, J. 1968. Immune status of the primary host toward its own methylcholanthrene-induced sarcomas. J. Nat. Cancer Inst. **40:** 13–22.
53. SOUTHAM, C. M. & A. BRUNSCHWIG. 1961. Quantitative studies of autotransplantation of human cancer. Cancer **14:** 971–978.
54. KLEIN, G., E. KLEIN & P. CLIFFORD. Search for host defenses in Burkitt lymphoma: membrane immunofluorescence test on biopsies and tissue culture lines. Cancer Res. In press.

DISCUSSION OF THE PAPER

DR. RASMUSSEN: Dr. Klein, do you have any experimental data, or if not experimental data, any ideas, as to the relative importance of different immune mechanisms that you outlined in the actual rejection or immunization against virus tumors? Is this an immune response to the infectious phase of the virus prior to transformation, or is this an immune response to the transformed cells, or both? If it is an immune response to cells, is it antibody or is it cell-related?

EVA KLEIN: The systems that deal with histocompatibility antigen first and then also with the tumor-specific antigen, function in a way suggesting that rejection perhaps is mainly mediated by the cellular response. Thus the cellular response is the most important. We know from the histocompatibility system that the presence of humoral antibodies might work in another way; it may enhance tumor development. Thus, for rejection, the cellular response is the most important.

The second question you asked, whether we know from the leukemia system whether the immunity is directed against the virus or against cellular antigens in the leukemia system, can be answered simply: we do not know. We cannot distinguish between the viral antigens and the antigens that the viruses impose on the cell. However, in the DNA virus system we seem to know that the antigens are not identical with viral antigens.

DR. MARGOLIN: This presentation is notable for a number of reasons. First of all, we have a series of isogenic preparations with well-established, quantifiable reactivity to the particular challenge. Second, such isogenic preparations can be used to investigate the various stress hypotheses that have been referred to today. In short, it seems that we have learned of a way of measuring the influence of these hypothetical stresses on the reactivity of these particular mice.

I am so grateful for the clarity and lucidity of this report that I cannot resist asking questions.

One question is related to the frequency distribution of takes. What was the cause of this? Why were there not 100% takes? Why were there 16 out of 30, 10 out of 20? Finally, why were not the animal groups larger and why were they so variable in the different experiments?

DR. KLEIN: I agree that the selection of an appropriate system to test your questions is a very important issue. I want to show that you should select various systems to test the various questions.

UNIDENTIFIED SPEAKER: In that last slide, you showed enhancement as a possible consequence or risk as consequence of vaccination. Does this mean that there is, in fact, an enhancement effect known in terms of antibody directed against the inducing virus? And, in connection with the same question, has anybody looked at the possible cause of enhancement's being the now widely studied effect of antibody on feedback suppression of the antibody response?

DR. KLEIN: There is not much work done on the enhancement phase in the tumor-specific system; however, we know from histocompatibility antigens that this risk exists, not against a virus, but against the cellular antigens. It has been demonstrated that the balance between humoral antibodies and cellular antibodies can be disturbed in certain ways that we cannot control, so that humoral antibodies may come in a moment when this leads to enhancement. This can happen, because you cannot control when the humoral antibodies should appear and when the cellular response should appear, and in all humoral situations the outcome of the interplay between these two responses are a little bit different.

We know, for instance, that the presence of humoral antibodies can coat the surface of the tumor cells. It will not kill the tumor cells but will coat the antigenic side, and then, even if we should, by some means provide the cellular response, the cellular response cannot reach this site. But in *in vivo* systems we just cannot control it. Therefore, we have to be aware of the fact that this enhancement risk exists.

PSYCHIC AND CELLULAR ASPECTS OF ISOLATION AND IDENTITY IMPAIRMENT IN CANCER: A DIALECTIC OF ALIENATION

Graham Bennette

Faculty of Medicine, University of London, Middlesex Hospital
London, England

Introduction

For the scientific "mechanists" who try to explain biochemical and biophysical happenings solely in terms of reproducible objective evidence, it is so difficult to imagine ways, that is, mechanisms, by which psychic impulses could alter the physical properties of cells that the whole idea is discounted as absurd. The so-called psychic impulses themselves have never been demonstrated "scientifically" –they have never been measured–and so their supposed interaction with autonomous biochemical processes seems to be doubly absurd. Of course, many scientists do not think of the cell merely as a complex time sequence of physicochemical events, but for them too there is a serious difficulty when it comes to accounting for the manner in which subjective reality impinges on the performance of living systems that do, in fact, operate through biochemical and biophysical mechanisms.

There are many problems about cancer incidence in different communities that make it difficult to the point of impossibility to interpret them solely in terms of genetic predisposition, dietary habits, exposure to specific carcinogenic risks, and so on–that is, in terms of material factors acting directly on normal tissues, causing their cells to change into cancer cells. But if the idea is accepted that abnormal cells in a state of abnormal organization are arising all the time and that they form invasive cancers only when morphostatic controls break down, we find that we are concentrating our attention on another, less specifically material level of organization. It is not so difficult, qualitatively at least, to imagine that psychological and cultural influences of a nonmaterial order of reality can affect the vigor of nervous, hormonal, and immunological control of the body. How it works is still, of course, a mystery, but whereas the idea that psychic factors might directly alter biochemical reactions is utterly baffling and probably absurd, the idea that they can modify the way in which control systems are mobilized is a good deal more acceptable.

This leads us to consider in what way the seriality of levels of organization might offer a "way in" to understanding how psychic factors can influence individual cells and cell clusters indirectly. The nucleus of a cell is part of the internal environment of that cell, and the rest of the cell forms the immediate external environment of the nucleus. Neither can pursue normal function without the other. The cell itself is part of the internal environment of a more complicated whole, the tissue in which it participates as a unit. The internal environment of the tissue forms the immediate external environment of the cell. The tissue in turn is part of the internal environment of the whole organism, which represents the immediate external milieu of the tissue or organ. There is a continuity, an overlapping between the internal and external environments in this sequence, each participating in the other. To go further takes us into the field of social relations and species relations, in which the individual organism forms part of the internal environment of the group. The participation of the individual in the greater whole, which is its immediate external biological environment, is a necessary factor for harmonious functioning at the social levels of organization.

At all these levels of organization there is interaction, and as the complexity advances from the molecular to the cellular and thence through the whole animal to the community, it becomes more and more difficult to define the controlling factors in physicochemical terms. Psyche becomes more and more a dominant influence. Each level has a quality of selfness in its organization, an identity that is controlled, and as the total organization increases in complexity, the psychic self aspect differentiates. Smithers[1] quotes Koestler, who has written about this seriality and interpenetration of levels of biological organization, concerning the relation of the part to the whole in establishing identity: "The part has to maintain its individuality, otherwise the organism would lose its articulation and revert to amorphous heterogeneity: at the same time, it has to behave as a *part* in the whole, that is, in functional subordination. Now the individuality of the part consists in its being itself an integrated whole of a lower order—a sub-whole composed of a sub-parts, which in themselves are sub-wholes, and so on. In this organic heirarchy the functional units of each level are all Janus-faced, as it were: they are wholes when facing downwards, parts when facing upwards." The sciences of biology and medicine face downwards in their analytical search for causal relationships between and within the various levels of organization. Anthropology and psychology are concerned with the upward relationships, while psychobiology has to embrace the Janus-faced and paradoxical situation of looking both ways at once.

We are all aware of the great importance of making our investigation of the psychobiological factors in cancer a scientific one, that is, one that is critically relevant and where possible supported by measurable and quantitatively verifiable data. But this is exactly where our difficulty lies, and before discussing the questions of isolation and identify impairment included in the title it will be helpful to explore this difficulty, to ask where it *is* possible to be strictly scientific and where it is not. It depends, of course, on our definition of what is scientific. If our idea of science is narrowly identified with questions of measurement, reproducibility, and objectivity, then this will not be a scientific paper. But I am afraid that I cannot apologize to those who may hold this narrow definition because I believe that a much broader definition must be accepted in any investigation that includes subjective information, which by its very nature is not measurable, reproducible, or accessible to objective, reductive analysis. The broader definition must include the side of research that has to do with the descriptive exploration of reality, including subjective reality, which may often appear to be paradoxical and which *may indeed actually be* paradoxical—that is, logically inexplicable. If the study of cancer in all its aspects teaches us anything, it is that it is full of paradoxes. The question is how to deal with them critically, in an intellectually acceptable and profitable way. We are dealing with the very fundamental paradoxes of subjective psychological events and their interactions with objective material systems, and our concern is, of course, always focused on the problem of cancer in man, the most paradoxical creature of them all.

Analytical Reasoning and the Solving of Problems

Let us look at this a bit more closely—this cancer "problem," as we so often call it. Certainly there are problems that can and will be solved, but there are also aspects of this immensely complex situation that cannot be treated as problems at all. There is an anecdote about the philosopher, Ludwig Wittgenstein. One of his students is supposed to have said, "Professor Wittgenstein, my problem is that I don't feel at home in the universe," to which the professor replied, "You have my sympathy, but that is not a problem, it is a difficulty."

Problems suggest the sort of puzzles that can be solved by analyzing them logically, but difficulties are rather different. You either have to live through them or take evasive action (if you can), but you cannot exactly analyze yourself out of the dilemmas that may arise by falling in love or falling ill. Paradoxes, which are logical difficulties and not problematic puzzles, cannot be resolved by the sort of reductive reasoning that tries to break down the complexity into smaller and smaller bits for closer and closer study. This is the familiar method of technical science, and it works extremely well when the observer is in the position of standing outside the *thing* he is studying–the thing being an object or an objective system in the outer world. But when man is the *subject* of study, the observer is unable to detach himself to the same degree, and in a very real sense he is part of the experiment. Scientific, reductive analytical study, in the narrow sense, is no longer entirely satisfactory unless he *insists* on detaching himself and treating the subjects, human beings, as if they were objects, or as an abstraction, Man, considered as an object. If science is equated with objectivity, which seems to be increasingly the case, the social, medical, and anthropological scientists can be strictly scientific, narrowly scientific, only to the extent to which they objectify the subject of their study.

Laing[2] uses a quotation from Sartre in one of his books: "I am not fond of the word psychological. There is no such thing as the psychological. Let us say that one can improve the biography of a person." He is right, there is no such *thing,* and here Sartre seems to be pointing a questioning finger at the "logical" part of the word "psychological." There is no such thing as "the cancer problem" either. The study of the moving and evolving biographies of people, including the biographical episodes of illness, is concerned with issues that are certainly not primarily issues of logic. The application of logical reductive analysis has its place, but if we are to help patients as people as well as treat them as cases, we must be aware of the dangers of treating subjective information objectively and analytically.

The word "analysis" derives from Greek roots meaning "to unloose," "to disperse," or "to set free,"[3] but in scientific and general use it has come to mean "to break down into component parts," a reductive process following the rules of logic. Laing[4] has written, "One has to avoid any schema that falsely fragments the reality one is attempting to describe, without losing sight of the distinction between fragmentation that does violence to specifically personal facts, and a legitimate analysis of one aspect of the situation at a time . . . it is immensely difficult not to subject quite unwittingly our human reality to such conceptual mutilation that the original is quite lost in the process." He emphasizes the need for the descriptive approach, and it is clear from his other work that his use of the word "analysis" is in its "exploratory, unloosing" sense and not in the "fragmenting, reductive" sense. Elsewhere[5] he has written, "Language has developed within obvious limits imposed by the degree of self-consciousness which man has attained. The analytic-instrumental approach to the world and to oneself entails a language which expresses the results of the analytical process, but the language then expresses an analytically *reduced* reality."

Dialectical Reasoning and Paradox

If the analytical-logical process involves the danger of distorting inquiries into human affairs, giving us an analytically reduced picture, we need to balance this by another, complementary, intellectual approach that may reveal a picture which, though less precisely defined, is more expansive. This opposite process of synthesis, in which logic is not the primary element, involves a bringing together and evolution of concepts that include both the concrete facts and the subjective facts of the situation. It is the process of dialectic, the nature and characteristics of which have been particularly studied by Sartre.[6,7] It is a process rather than a method, and it consists of a never-ending dialogue in which the subject being studied is "analyzed" in the sense of being unloosed in order to examine it and to build a new concept of its nature in relation to other components that have been teased out of the tangle. Here the analysis is a destructuring process rather than a destructive, fragmenting one. Sartre calls it a conceptual process of detotalization and retotalization of the concrete and subjective factors contributing to the complex whole. The unloosing that is needed is an exploratory sorting-out that is not determined by the need to be logically coherent at each step. It is the imposition of rigid rules that Sartre believes to be the factor in logical analysis that leads to reductive or even destructive fragmentation of the whole. The process of detotalizing does not have to follow a strictly logical sequence but may include, and *does* include in any relevant imaginative exercise, the nonlogical dimension of intuition. The crucial point is that while the dialectic process is not itself logically restricted and may contain nonrational experiential information, the new synthesis of concepts that results from its application may contain new ideas that *can* be subjected to critical experimental verification. Dialectic is a process of questioning that provides no direct answers, but it can tell us more clearly which are the really relevant questions to ask and may suggest thereby new experimental approaches.

All this may seem to be very obvious because it is what we all do in any relevant discussion. It is interesting that the word "discussion" has supplanted the older word "discourse"–a comment on the way that the reductive analytical tradition has modified language. "Discussion" comes from the Latin, *discutere,* meaning "to dash to pieces, disperse, or dispel," while "discourse" derives from *discurrere*, meaning "to run to and fro."[3] Although we may all use dialectic reasoning in any profitable discussion, its use is often unconscious and uncritical. It is critical relevance we really need. Someone once said that every laboratory should have the motto above the door, "A research project that is not worth doing is not worth doing well." Medawar,[8] in a broadcast talk entitled "Is the scientific paper a fraud?" concluded that it usually is in its traditional format, because it embodies "a totally mistaken conception, even a travesty, of the nature of scientific thought." Again, it is relevance we need and not merely the appearance of a specious objectivity. Although the power of dialectic has been recognized since the time of Socrates, and although the modern exponents have not invented anything new, Sartre in particular is doing an incalculable service in his study and characterization of the process. It is immensely relieving, in the face of what Laing calls our traditional fascination with logic, to find that the investigation of systems that include subjective information can be capable of critical intellectual refinement.

Continuous detotalizations and retotalizations by what Sartre calls the progressive-regressive method produce an ever-changing conceptual synthesis. The new synthesis overtakes the previous one–Sartre's word is "dépassement"–so that the new interpretations partially invalidate the old, but much of the old is nevertheless restructured into the new picture. There is never a *totality* arrived at, never any final solutions, but only a series of new totalizations. An evolutionary synthesis of ideas is in progress that can be called a process of "intellectual becoming."

Although it is a process and not a method imposing a set of inflexible rules, its application requires a critical and disciplined habit of mind. Sartre's present work is concerned with the critique of dialectical reasoning. This has been described as an internal dialectic that is aimed to discover the relevance of the information to be assimilated and the ways in which meaningful totalizations can be built up. He is also trying to establish relationships between dialectic and the other dimension of analytical reasoning in order to clarify the limits of application of each mode. Dialectic obviously does not threaten to replace the logical mode of reasoning, but in human affairs it must take its place in the inquiry if the specifically human contents are to be understood without subjecting them to the violence of objectification. The biography of every illness is a psychosomatic and psychosocial evolution, and with the advent of a critical dialectical way of assessing the shifting emphasis of meaning we can look forward to being released from the position of apologists when we insist on the relevance of studying the psychic setting of so-called physical diseases in the face of the scepticism of some medical scientists who contemptuously dismiss personal facts as merely anecdotal.

A Psychobiological Dialectic of Alienation

How can we find a way to open a psychobiological dialectic towards a greater understanding of the cancer process? In bringing together facts from the laboratory and the psychological findings of various observers it is not my intention to try to establish correlations that could be used to construct a testable hypothesis. There is certainly a need for such hypotheses from which to deduce and predict, and to subject to experimental verification. I am suggesting that in addition, dialectic comparisons may be fruitful in confirming relevance and creating new possible experimental situations.

First it must be said that there are several dialectic movements already in full swing in cancer research. Perhaps the most exciting one is the dialogue among clinicians, epidemiologists, pathologists, immunologists, virologists, and several other specialists, which is showing the great power of this approach in the recent studies of Burkitt's tumor. Even though the participants in this dialectic share the same technical language, it is difficult enough. It is much more difficult, but at the same time more within the scope of dialectic, when the dialogue has to include the psychic dimension of reality. It is more within the scope of dialectic precisely because we are here confronted by the paradoxes of psychic and somatic interactions, and paradox is the business of dialectic. If there is no common language, then we will have to invent one. Let us start by looking for a common existential parameter. The first one that comes to mind, because it has come to so many other minds, is alienation. We could try to define what it means, but definition is itself logically restrictive. Let us look instead at what it might mean or could mean, and then see whether there is evidence from the laboratory and from the psychiatrists (the alienists, by the way) that might justify the conclusion that it is relevant. In the process we will hope to go some way towards evolving a meaning, which is as much as to say, inventing language.

Alienation, originally derived from words meaning "without a bond," can have a number of meanings attributed to it, including qualities of both injury and isolation, loss and meaninglessness. It is the opposite or the denial of participation and communication. The alienated is apart from the community, the stranger lacking some of the aspects of communal identification. Smithers[1,9] believes that injury and isolation are central biological factors in the induction of the disorganization that leads to invasive cancer. His books are filled with direct and indirect evidence for this contention from a wide field of biological study. From the laboratory we see that the cancer cell is certainly out of touch and cut off from the society of other cells, wandering about without normal cohesion and separated from the controls that integrate the structures and functions of the tissues in their participation in the corporate whole.

Evidence of Alienation from the Laboratory

Examples of spontaneous malignant transformation of cells of many different types when isolated in tissue culture and separated from homeostatic control by serial cultivation have been documented by Harris.[10] This work started with the experiments of Sanford, Earle, and their collaborators,[11] who found that malignant changes can occur in cultured cells that have received no specific treatment. Apparently it is in some way the result of isolation in the tissue-culture situation. It was argued that the tissue-culture fluids or the processes of handling long-term serial cultures might result in malignant change, but the work of Shelton and her colleagues[12] showed that untreated normal cells can undergo malignant conversion even in a completely isologous biological environment. They demonstrated malignant transformation of normal cells in the situation of isolation within semi-permeable capsules implanted into the peritoneal cavities of animals on the donor strain. These sealed chambers of Millipore filter material allowed the passage of body fluids but not of cells, so that the contained normal cells were isolated from contact with other cells but were otherwise environmentally situated, with access to humoral homeostatic influences. The experiments strongly suggest that the loss of cell contact is an essential quality of the alienation. Haddow[13] quotes a colleague, Dr. Delorme, who said that cells know a great deal more about each other than we know about them, implying that cells in contact can exchange chemical information. Recent studies of the phenomena of contact inhibition, allogeneic inhibition, contact adherence, and the transmission of drug resistance clearly show that cells do exchange information, and this is also plainly underlined by the phenomena of immunological recognition. The philosophical implications of this in the control of biological meaning and of cell and tissue identity are too wide to be entered into here.

An example of the failure of flow of information between cells in contact in the induction of cancer is found in that rather neglected area of experimental carcinogenesis, the induction of tumors by the implantation of impermeable sheets of various materials. This field of work has been reviewed by Clayson.[14] He quotes evidence that the material itself, whether it be plastics of various kinds, cellophane, metals, glass, or some other material, is not responsible for producing a specifically chemical effect. Goldhaber[15] showed that it is the physical barrier that constitutes the carcinogenic influence by measuring the effect of pore size on the incidence of tumors following the implantation of Millipore filter material. If the perforations in the sheet are big enough, cell contacts can be made and tumors do not arise. Clayson[14] quotes many examples of work in which the experimenters seemed to be bent upon proving that the phenomenon is chemical in nature. Following an imaginative paper by Alexander and Horning at a Ciba Symposium some years ago,[16] there was a discussion. Kaplan is quoted as saying, "I wonder if it is not appropriate to approach this phenomenon from a rather simple-minded viewpoint, namely that if there is anything that connective tissue knows how to do it is to connect, and in order to connect it must somehow get a signal to tell it whether it is connected or not. If one imposes an impermeable barrier, is this not simply a way to tell the connective tissue cells that they are disconnected?" Perhaps it would be fair comment to say that the strength of his approach depends on the simplicity and freedom of a flexible dialectical way of thinking. It is depressing that so little work has been done in this field since 1961. Notable exceptions are the studies of Klein and his colleagues,[17] who studied the immunogenicity of plastic film tumors, and Bates and Prehn,[18] who made the very interesting observation that homograft reactivity is impaired in the skin overlying the plastic film, again indicating a barrier effect to the passage of information between cells.

The immunological system in all its diversity and flexibility of appropriate response embodies the principles of recognition, learning, memory, and the transmission of meaningful information. These words are the best we can find until we can invent a language to describe biological purposiveness appropriately. All these words, with their strong psychic overtones, attempt to describe the function of the immune system in discriminating between self and not-self and in mediating an appropriate response to maintain the integrity of the self against the incursion of not-self, random elements. It has often been suggested that the immune system also exercises a positive surveillance in morphostatic control beyond that of merely eliminating the foci of abnormal cells and foreign substances that threaten the integrity of the self.

It is now generally agreed that the cancer cell has a changed identity. The evidence that malignancy is accompanied by alterations to the self patterns of cells is well documented in a recent book by Green and others.[19] The change in the surface protein patterns of cancer cells may entail the addition of new components, or loss or reorientation of existing components, or both. Antigenic loss, simplification, or deletion implies that some sort of replacement must occur, and whether the new pattern is formed by addition, reorientation, or deletion, it must acquire a changed identity in the process. Although something of the nature of the change may be detectable in the laboratory, it does not necessarily follow, as Sela pointed out,[20] that the new pattern will be recognized as such by the immunocytes, unless it is assumed either that these lymphoid cells have infinite recognitional capacities or that by recognizing characteristic self paterns, everything else is identified as not-self. But there is yet another possibility–that the changed pattern is not recognized at all, that it becomes relatively or completely anonymous. This could account for the fact that most spontaneous tumors evoke poor immunological reactivity by the host.

We have now touched on a number of the possible meanings of the word "alienation" at the cellular level, with examples of loss of meaningful communication of the information that is indispensable for organizational control. We have also looked at some of the associated changes of identity that may involve the isolation of foreignness or of anonymity in the context of what might be called the social biography at the cellular level.

Before turning our attention to alienation at the psychic and psychosocial levels in man, some reference must be made to important animal experiments. Andervont[21] showed that the gregarious C3H mouse develops spontaneous mammary tumors significantly earlier if the animals are raised in isolation. Newton[22] found that regular human handling of infant rats enhances their resistance to the growth of an experimental tumor, significantly delaying mortality in the gentled as compared to the nongentled group.

Evidence from Psychological and Philosophical Studies

In psychological investigations, the use of psychometric methods to look for specific conscious personality characteristics in cancer patients can be very misleading. Just as it may lead down false trails to make quantitative analytical studies of situations of artefact in the laboratory, a distorted and reduced picture of existential reality may result from psychometric studies, unless a deep awareness exists of the sources of possible confusion. The kind of psychological approach that reveals data about the easily accessible levels of conscious psychic functioning can be very confusing for the reason that much of the way the biography goes is determined in the unconscious. The use of dialectic is especially important in attempting to interpret the symbolic information that reaches consciousness. Hints of impending defeat and regression that break surface into consciousness may be revealed directly, but may often be so frightening that consciousness remains aware only of the products of defensive responses or attitudes of denial. On the other hand, beneath a consciously experienced despair there may be a mobilization of unconscious creative force, while again, a conscious attitude of optimism superficially motivating a lot of activity that *looks* creative may defensively cover a deeper self-destructive hopelessness and apathy. To penetrate the biography is the difficulty, and for this, feeling and intuitional awareness has to be included in the dialectic.

Although the biographical idea of an evolving psychobiological process as an interpretation of illness has a dialectic value and also a value as a basic attitude to counteract the tendency to make facile psychological or physicochemical theories, relevant experimental approaches are, of course, possible. The paradox of conscious and unconscious functioning calls for a great deal of discrimination in the choice of methods for studying psychological responses and in their assessment. It is not surprising that conflicting results are sometimes reported. The dialectic point can be made that they may both be right, in the sense that they may both be relevant aspects of a paradox. Bahnson,[25] Kissen,[23] and the others whose work is briefly referred to here have all been aware of the need to penetrate the defenses and to look for deeper meanings that may contradict the conscious attitudes.

Kissen's work[23] deserves special mention, because it combined imaginative experimental design with a meticulous statistical approach. We all very much regret the loss of this man who had such a gift for contributing insight, feeling, and experimental precision. His major finding, which was repeatedly confirmed–that men with lung cancer show impairment of discharge of affect and inadequate outlets for instinctive drive–is central to the point of this paper. Here we see containment and blockage of the communication of psychosocial feeling information, a potent cause of experiential alienation. Booth,[24] in comparisons of personality between patients with tuberculosis and those with cancer, based on Rorschach testing, concludes that the cancer patient is typically emotionally isolated and autistic. Bahnson and Bahnson[25] have found attitudes of denial and excessive ego defense in cancer patients as compared to other groups. They believe that these attitudes are associated with deep-seated guilt, leading to a division of the identity into "a conscious self that is socially adequate but empty and meaningless, and an unconscious self that is explosive, tragic and tormented." They have noted the same unfulfilled need for love and the same pathological dependency, coupled with an impoverishment of creative relationships with others that have been reported by LeShan and Worthington.[26] Here we see meaninglessness associated with an intense need to communicate, and a perversion of the normal relationship between the ego and the self aspects of identity due to injury and psychic invalidation associated with guilt. The interpretation of the findings of negativity, defeat, and affects of hopelessness in cancer patients by LeShan,[27] Green,[28] Schmale and Iker,[29] and others may well include the despair of unrelatedness. Laing[4] has studied the sickness of unrelatedness at a psychic level arising from the invalidation of feeling exchange between parent and child. To use the language of Buber,[30] this feeling exchange for the child is the I-Thou experience from which a secure, deep, Self identity is normally established. Later, the demands of the thinking function result in the development of a logical, analytical appraisal of the world, establishing the I-It relationships of subject to objects and building up the ego identity. It is no new idea that impoverishment of the deeper identity of the Self leads to hypertrophy of the ego function. In Kierkegaard's analysis of the inner state of relatedness to the Self,[31] it is exactly the hypertrophy of the ego at the expense of the deeper identity that is seen to lead to despair and meaninglessness. Guilt is related to meaninglessness through Kierkegaard's equation of sin, despair, and alienation—the "sickness unto death." It is not virtue, he says, but faith that is the opposite of sin, and we might guess that the eroson of the will to live towards a creative future will be accompanied by and augmented by the will to die, either to escape the anguish of unresolved guilt or to expiate it. The guilt of alienation is the failure of love, returning us to Kissen's work,[23] which defined the blockage of flow of feeling. LeShan[32] has stressed that there is a need to love as well as to be loved, emphasizing the blockage of affective release and surrender to the flow of feeling in interpersonal contacts. He quotes Freud: "In the last analysis, we must love in order not to fall ill, and must fall ill when, in consequence of neurosis, we cannot love."[33]

To this must be added the need to hate. The conflict of this particular paradox, love and hate, is especially relevant to the difficulty of inadequate affective discharge. The suppression of release of the aggressive instinctive forces because these impulses are seen to be destructive and bad is confirmed and encouraged by both the religious and the social codes, which strengthen the denial of hate impulses by authorizing the underlying feelings of guilt. The benign tumor used to be called innocent, and by inference the cancer is guilty. There are countless references to support the idea that internalized violence is a powerful component of self-destruction in somatic and psychic diseases. The obstruction of communication with the unconscious, the source of instinctive energy, deprives consciousness of emotional meaning. Habitual ego denial of unconscious vitality, because of the fear and pain of guilt, isolates the deep self center, further blocking communication with the unconscious. As the Bahnsons[25] put it, "the inhibited psychic drive is discharged along primitive and regressive physiological channels and the person kills himself."

The pathological dependency that arises in this situation can be seen as a search for outer meanings to compensate for the loss of the inner meanings that results from denial of the value of the deep identity. This compensation may be temporarily adequate, providing an opening that allows at least some degree of flow from the unconscious. But the loss of the dependent relationship may precipitate the physical illness. Mitchell,[34] Muslin and his colleagues,[35] Schmale,[36] and others have noted that separation experiences from life-saving dependent relationships frequently antedate the appearance of invasive cancer or its recurrence many years after the apparently successful eradication of the primary disease. The separation experience may be due to bereavement, a broken marriage, or other personal crises involving the loss of subject relationships as well as object relationships such as occur on retirement from work that was the only adequate source of emotional fulfillment and release.

Thus at the psychic level we have found evidence of meaninglessness, separation from the deep self center of identity, and suggestions of failure of internal communication between the conscious and unconscious psyche of the individual. There is also the implication of a poverty of feeling rapport between the individual and the community, indicating failures of emotional communication not only within the individual psyche but also in the outer sphere of psychic interaction.

Psychobiological Balances in the Biographical Manifestation of Illness

In the regression that leads to invasive cancer, two main contributory factors can be considered as the physical level: first, that increasing disorganization due to exposure to specific carcinogenic and mutational injuries to cellular identity strains the normal mechanisms of homeostatic control beyond their capacity; and second, that the competence of the controls themselves becomes impaired.

A similar situation may exist at the psychic level. Here I am distinguishing between the two levels for the sake of clarity, although this is unsatisfactory. The expression of psychobiological events is not, I think, a simple resultant of a balance between events occurring at the physical and the psychological levels, but until we have invented a new language from the application of dialectic, there may be no choice but to use the traditional idea of psyche and soma.

If isolational injury of the deep center of the self is a central factor in the induction of regressive illness, and if this center is vulnerable to both psychic and physical injury, we can speculate that the biographical manifestation of disease, whether primarily a psychotic or primarily a malignant randomness, is determined by the relative state of integrity and balance of the psychic and somatic controls as well as by the type and intensity of the trauma. Using a more holistic language, we could say that it depends on the internal balance set up within the total psychobiological homeostatic system of integration. From this we could develop the idea that invasive cancer results from an internalization of disturbances of identity and communication that cannot find psychic expression because of the strength of well-differentiated psychic controlling functions, that is, a strongly developed or hypertrophied ego, coupled with inadequate bodily homeostatic control. On the other hand, where the ego and other psychic controls are poorly developed, but there is a competent bodily homeostasis, a similar disturbance of deep identity would lead to psychotic regression. On this basis, malignant diseases and regressive psychoses could be seen as alternative biographical expressions of illness proneness, in the sense that they are comparable but differently balanced modes of evolution of the same underlying pathology, a pathology of alienation.

The complexity of such a system would lead us to expect a great variety of individual types of disease, and it would not be surprising that some cancer patients show profound psychological disturbances. But the idea that cancer is an alternative to psychosis is not meant to imply that one would necessarily expect a very low incidence of cancer among psychotics nor a low incidence of psychosis in cancer patients. This *may* be the case, but Bahnson and Bahnson,[37] who first proposed that the two disease states be seen as alternatives, meant rather to suggest, I believe, that they represent together a psychobiological complex. In this complex, the "psychic element" in cancer may be very dominant or it may be minimal. Increasing exposure to carcinogenic influences, an increased rate of natural genetic mutation, and loss of precision of homeostatic control with advancing age may result in cancer without the intervention of any notable psychological disorder. As Doll[38] put it when explaining the difficulties of assessing the smoking risk "The longer you smoke, the older you get." It is cancer in the young and early middle-aged, when death is inappropriate and tragic, that deserves study with a particular emphasis on the psychic factors in the psychobiological dialectic. Here it may be possible to improve the biography of the person in a way that is scarcely possible for the old. Cancer in childhood can be seen as a disastrous perversion of developing identity, but one that is also interpretable in psychobiological terms with an emphasis on alienation, invalidation, and possibly unconscious projection, as well as an emphasis on genetically determined proneness and possible exposure to specific carcinogens.

Summary

In conclusion–though no conclusions are ever possible in a dialectic approach to understanding–let us see how the cancer process can be described in terms of the dialectic of alienation.

Invasive cancer is seen as an evolving pathological condition allowed to proceed through failures of psychobiological control. The failure may be temporary and acute or chronic and slowly progressive, or it may fluctuate. It may be reversible, or by reason of long-standing abnormalities, it may be effectively irreversible or only partly reversible. It is associated with a perversion of the information that normally directs the balances of control of growth and differentiation, that is, a change or loss of appropriate meaning occurs through injury or disfigurement of identity at some level of organization. The systems involved may be subject to a deterioration of control because of a genetically determined weakness or incompetence in the face of challenge. A challenge becomes a threat when the appropriate responses cannot be mobilized. The systems deprived of informational control become isolated, and indeed the original injury may take the form of isolation. There is a loss or blockage of communication between systems that are interdependent in total psychobiological homeostasis. *Dynamic* aspects of identity, that is, the processes of identification and mutual recognition between the affected systems, deteriorate as a result of the impairment of communication. In so far as the integrity of *structural* identity depends on dynamic interactions of identification, there follows an actual loss or change of typical character, towards anonymity or foreignness. The unique patterning of the original identity is replaced in part by random patterns that are without specific meaning for the total functional organization. When identity deteriorates into relative anonymity, there is an overall impairment of self-recognition, and the local abnormality is not recognized as such by the control systems concerned with maintaining the self identity as a whole. The competence of the control systems themselves becomes impaired, so that even when the abnormality of identity assumes a foreign character, this is not recognized and eliminated, as would normally be the case. In other words, the false-self elements are tolerated as a result of defects in the control systems, which may themselves also reflect a pathology based on injury and isolation. The local and then more general breakdown of control leads to degrees of autonomy, with the subsequent invasion of the organized self by the random, disorganized false-self elements.

This generalized and nonspecific way of describing the cancer process has been chosen deliberately to emphasize the possibilities of making dialectical, descriptive comparisons between disease processes conventionally described as psychic or somatic. The last paragraph could be read as an interpretation of some of the basic aspects of the schizophrenic process, within the individual and within the psychosocial setting.

References

1. Smithers, D. W. 1960. A Clinical Prospect of the Cancer Problem. Introductory volume of monograph, Neoplastic Disease at Various Sites. Livingstone. London, England.
2. Laing, R. D. 1959. The Divided Self. Tavistock Publications. London, England.
3. Onions, C. T., Ed. 1966. The Oxford Dictionary of English Etymology, Clarendon Press. Oxford, England.
4. Laing, R. D. 1961. The Self and Others. Tavistock Publications. London, England.
5. Laing, R. D. & D. G. Cooper. 1964. Reason and Violence. Tavistock Publications. London, England.
6. Sartre, J-P. 1960. The Problem of Method. H. E. Barnes, Transl. Methuen & Co., Ltd. London, England.
7. Sartre, J-P. 1960. Critique de la Raison Dialectique. 1. Librairie Gallimard. Paris, France.
8. Medawar, P. B. 1963. Listener (London) **70:** 377.
9. Smithers, D. W. 1964. The Weild Lecture. *In* On the Nature of Neoplasia in Man. Livingstone. London, England .
10. Harris, M. 1964. Cell Culture and Somatic Variation. Holt, Rinehart & Winston, Inc. New York, N. Y.
11. Sanford, K. K., W. R. Earle, E. Shelton, E. L. Schilling, E. M. Duchesne, G. D. Likely & M. M. Becker. 1950. J. Nat. Cancer Inst. **11:** 351.
12. Shelton, E., V. J. Evans & G. A. Parker. 1963. J. Nat. Cancer Inst. **30:** 377.
13. Haddow, A. 1965. Brit. Med. Bull. **21:** 133.
14. Clayson, D. B. 1962. Chemical Carcinogenesis. Churchill. London, England.
15. Goldhaber, P. 1961. Proc. Amer. Ass. Cancer Res. **3:** 228.
16. Alexander, P. & E. S. Horning. 1959. *In* Carcinogenesis: Mechanisms of Action. Ciba Symposium. G. E. W. Wolstenholme, Ed. Churchill. London, England.
17. Klein, G., H. O. Sjögren & E. Klein. 1963. Cancer Res. **23:** 84.
18. Bates, R. R. & R. T. Prehn. 1965. Nature (London) **205:** 303.
19. Green, H. N., H. M. Anthony, R. W. Baldwin & J. W. Westrop. 1967. An Immunological Approach to Cancer. Butterworth & Co. (Publishers), Ltd. London, England.
20. Sela, M. 1964. *In* New Perspectives in Biology. M. Sela, Ed. Elsevier. Amsterdam, The Netherlands.
21. Andervont, H. B. 1944. J. Nat. Cancer Inst. **4:** 579.
22. Newton, G. 1964. *In* Psychosomatic Aspects of Neoplastic Disease. Pitman Medical Publishing Co. London, England.
23. Kissen, D. M. 1966. The significance of personality in lung cancer in men. Ann. N. Y. Acad. Sci. **125:** 820.
24. Booth, G. 1964. *In* Psychosomatic Aspects of Neoplastic Disease. Pitman Medical Publishing Co. London, England .
25. Bahnson, C. B. & M. B. Bahnson. 1966. Role of the ego defenses: Denial and repression in the etiology of malignant neoplasm. Ann. N. Y. Acad. Sci. **125:** 827.
26. LeShan, L. L. & R. E. Worthington. 1965. J. Nerv. Ment. Dis. **124:** 460.
27. LeShan, L. L. 1961. Psychiat. Quart. **35:** 314.
28. Greene, W. A. 1966. The psychosocial setting of the development of leukemia and lymphoma. Ann. N. Y. Acad. Sci. **125:** 794.
29. Schmale, A. H., Jr. & H. P. Iker. 1966. Psychosom. Med. **28:** 714.
30. Buber, M. 1923. I and Thou. 2nd Edit. R. G. Smith, Transl. Clark. Edinburgh, Scotland.
31. Kierkegaard, S. 1849. The Sickness unto Death. W. Lowrie, Transl. Princeton University Press (1954). Princeton, N. J.
32. LeShan, L. L. 1964. *In* Psychosomatic Aspects of Neoplastic Disease. Pitman Medical Publishing Co. London, England.
33. Freud, S. 1946. On Narcissism. Coll. Papers. **4**. Hogarth Press. London, England.
34. Mitchell, J. S. 1960. Studies in Radiotherapeutics. Blackwell. Oxford, England.
35. Muslin, H. L., K. Gyarfas & W. J. Pieper. 1966. Separation experience and cancer of the breast. Ann. N. Y. Acad. Sci. **125:** 802.
36. Schmale, A. H., Jr. 1958. Psychosom. Med. **10:** 259.
37. Bahnson, C. B. & M. B. Bahnson. 1966. *In* Psychosomatic Aspects of Neoplastic Disease. Pitman Medical Publishing Co. London, England.
38. Doll, R. 1965. *In* 15th Jaarboek van Kankeronderzoek en Kankerbestrijding in Nederland. De Bussy. Amsterdam, The Netherlands.

DISCUSSION OF THE PAPER

DR. WEISS: I wish to make one brief comment on a point raised by Dr. Bennette; namely, that spontaneous tumors are either nonantigenic or less antigenic than artificially induced ones. I think that the term "spontaneous" requires a moment's reflection. We very often encounter a concept that a spontaneous neoplasm, or a spontaneous event in biology in general reflects something more mysterious, more random, than a specifically induced event; in this case, a specifically induced neoplasm. I think this must be qualified, because when we speak of a spontaneous tumor, we merely mean a tumor that has arisen as part and parcel of the life history of an animal without the intentional manipulation by the investigator in the laboratory. It does not, however, imply that such a neoplasm has arisen without a cause. Viral agents, carcinogenic chemicals, and so on, and various other influences are undoubtedly involved, so that the category of spontaneous neoplasms should be considered to be neoplasms that occur without intentional manipulation, but not as neoplasms whose cause is of an entirely different order. Now, specifically, the concept that such spontaneous tumors are nonantigenic or very poorly antigenic is no longer tenable. During the last number of years, it has been shown very clearly by a number of investigators that such tumors are antigenic. There will be further discussion at this meeting on this point, and I believe that their antigenicity can be subsumed by the dialectic presented by Dr. Bennette as well as the antigenicity of the so-called artificially induced ones.

DR. GREENE: May I just mention, Dr. Bennette, that I was reminded during your talk of a remark by Dr. L. C. Johnson, a very physiological pathologist at the Armed Forces Institute of Pathology, who indicated that everyone will develop cancer if he lives long enough. Would you like to comment on this discussion?

DR. BENNETTE: Regarding the question of spontaneous tumors, I am thinking particularly of the biographical episode of cancer in man, in which it is very often extremely difficult to assert that specific carcinogenic hazards have been directly involved. I agree with Dr. Weiss that one should not make distinctions between spontaneous tumors and induced tumors, as if they were two entirely different things. I did try to convey the concept that anonymity and the failure of the malignant cell to be recognized at all may be only one possibility. There is, of course, a much greater possibility that the malignant cell is a foreign entity, but that its foreignness is tolerated. May I leave your question, Dr. Greene, for discussion later.

IMMUNOLOGICAL PARADOXES: THEORETICAL CONSIDERATIONS IN THE REJECTION OR RETENTION OF GRAFTS, TUMORS, AND NORMAL TISSUE

Jonas Salk

The Salk Institute for Biological Studies
San Diego, Calif.

I am very pleased to have been exposed to such a wide variety of viewpoints here. It seems to me that the conference has been extremely successful in bringing together individuals who, although from such diverse points of view, have a common interest. The remarks that I have to make are of two kinds: First, to comment upon what I heard this morning, regretfully, without time for sufficient quiet thought such as one would like to have in pondering the information presented this morning, and, second, to present a few thoughts of my own that have developed over a number of years and that I think will fit into the context of this morning's discussion.

Dr. Bennette's remarks were rather poetic, and I believe describe a process that in fact does go on in nature. The problem with which the experimental scientist is confronted is to try to relate structure and function in biological systems, to try to define the actual mechanism that is involved, and especially in ways that can be manipulated. When Dr. Weiss pointed out that there really is no fundamental distinction between a spontaneous neoplasm and one that is induced experimentally, he could very well have been clarifying the use of the term "spontaneous" as applied to mammary tumors of mice, as if they were different from the tumors induced by the milk factor or by the mammary tumor virus.

The very brilliant analysis by Dr. Eva Klein should have revealed to you what can be done with a very heterogenous system, all lumped together under the same term "cancer" or "neoplasia," when carefully analyzed. And, therefore, it does illustrate what–not to use the word disparagingly–a reductionist approach can do in an attempt to isolate and identify the particular factors that are crucial even in systems in which a multiplicity of factors are involved. I hope to illustrate this a bit further myself.

What she was able to demonstrate is that certain laws do govern the relationships between structure and function. She showed very nicely how differently tumors induced by viruses behave from those that are chemically induced. She showed experimentally and quantitatively that 100% effects do not always occur. This tempts us further to try to look more precisely into the events that are involved. It says that we do not as yet have all the answers, and it is this that challenges the experimentalist who tries to find out much more precisely what variables are involved and tries thereby to reveal a means for controlling this natural phenomenon. Fundamentally, this is what we are all attempting to understand, and to be able to do, whether it be through the use of the tools of the immunologist, the virologist, or the psychiatrist. The problem with which this conference seems to be confronted is that of developing an understanding of the relative roles played by each of the multiplicity of factors that we presume, or that we know, are operative in neoplasia.

Dr. Bahnson's interests are broad, his bias is clear. At the same time, he does demonstrate an open mind in regard to the many factors that undoubtedly play a role in a disease process, the exact or precise nature of which is not yet clear either with respect to single or multiple predisposing and precipitating factors.

I was interested in the enormous compilation by Dr. Solomon of data and of evidence to which he himself has contributed by asking the question about the relationship between psychological factors, stress, and the behavior of the immunologic system.

One thought went through my mind as I listened to some of the discussion this morning, and that concerns the method of approach. I had occasion, when presenting a talk in which I made the remark to which Dr. Solomon referred in his discussion, to say that answers preexist, and that it is the question that needs to be discovered. It is the question, and especially the form of the question, that is so vitally important. We are all interested in the problem of cancer; each of us chooses a different question to ask. And, through pursuit of these questions, an answer will eventually be revealed.

If this conference keeps questions and questioning in mind, rather than preconceived answers, I believe that the value and contribution of the conference will be greatest.

As I thought about the problem with which this conference is confronted and about my own contribution to it, I realized how large and complex is the question that is being posed and how necessary it is to reduce it to manageable proportions.

The question may be expressed in the following forms: (1) Is there a cause-and-effect relationship between psychological states and neoplastic diseases? (2) If such a relationship exists, what is the mechanism whereby it is mediated?

In considering the first question, regarding cause and effect in the psychopathogenesis of cancer, there seem to be two schools of thought. One school is of the opinion that there is a direct connection between the psyche and the target tissues; another school is of the opinion that psychic effects are mediated through such systems as the endocrinologic and/or the immunologic.

Since the exact cause of each of the various forms of cancer in man is not yet established, and since seemingly identical circumstances do not always produce the same effect, both schools of thought accept the idea of direct and of contributing factors. So long as the causative factors of a particular disease of man remain unknown, the field is open to all kinds of conjectures. And, until the pathogenesis of cancer is more precisely established, this field will remain one in which hypotheses will be rampant. The need, of course, is for rigorous observations, rigorous experimentation, and rigorous proof. The purpose of this conference, in part, it seems to me, is to reveal where such exist, and to distinguish between hard facts and soft facts or between facts and impressions.

I will not address myself to the evidence, hard or soft, relative to psychogenic contributions to cancer, because I really have not taken the time to study the subject sufficiently. I would accept the plausibility of the view that systemic factors play a role in the initiation of the clinical process and in the clinical course. Moreover, some of these systemic factors are nervous and psychologic in origin. But the systemic factors that I have thought most about are the immunologic and the endocrinologic.

In order to establish hard facts in this area of inquiry, model systems are necessary; and we have heard comments about this earlier. These model systems are either experimental or clinical, and we heard of both kinds today. For this, each investigator chooses a set of conditions that he subjects to test. The result is a message, or an answer, of some kind; a take-home lesson that is either clearly affirmative, clearly negative, or may even be clearly unsettled!

We can look at the immunologic side of the problem of cancer, since this may be useful to those who think about or investigate psychophysiological factors in cancerous conditions. I will do so by illustrating experiments done some time ago with monkeys, because this illustrates the relationship between the immunologic system and the neoplastic process. My purpose is to discuss certain immunologic paradoxes that should be taken into consideration by those who think about psychophysiologic factors in the pathogenesis of cancer.

I was particularly pleased to hear the attention given to the idea of paradoxes, because they are quite clearly applicable here, and, also, to the very thorough discussion of what appears to be a paradox–the evidence for the existence of the enhancement phenomenon to which Dr. Klein referred when she pointed out that sometimes it produces an enhancing effect. It was precisely this that arrested our attention some time ago and resulted in the development of some ideas that I should now like to talk about.

At the conference, slides were shown in order to present the observations upon which these ideas were developed. Since the transcription of the discussion of the slide material could not contain the visual part of the message and would not be very coherent without a fuller elaboration and without inclusion of all of the graphic material, an alternative and simpler way of conveying the sense of the discussion was proposed; i.e., to insert here the full text of an unpublished lecture.* This is followed by the concluding remarks that followed the slide presentation at the present conference. The text is as follows and includes selected figures to illustrate some of the points made in the text.

The immunologic mechanism was first discovered performing the function of protecting the organism against invasion by parasitic agents. It was soon noted that other foreign substances induced "immunologic" reactions and that the host's response, at times, was exaggerated and harmful to self, and even fatal. Thus, the immunologic system was not an unmixed blessing–it could be useful or harmful, and at times it could be both.

The term "allergy" to denote "abnormal reactions" was proposed by Clement Von Pirquet, in 1906.[1] He noted that individuals who recovered from infections reacted to the causative organism, or its products, in an abnormal fashion: the tuberculous patient developed a delayed reaction to an injection of tuberculin into the skin. The patient treated with an immunizing serum from an animal often developed a "serum disease" that began about ten days later. After that, a skin test with the same serum caused an immediate local reaction, whereas a similar test before treatment was negative. In each case the normal reaction was altered, and Von Pirquet called it *allergie*.

Thus began a long era, which had been introduced still earlier by others, in which the problems and questions in immunity and allergy began to be defined. Experimentation soon advanced to the point where important practical tools became available for manipulating the immunologic system.

There continues to be a need for developing further understanding of the complex structure of the immunologic system and the many functions it performs, so that the armamentarium of the practicing physician may be enlarged still further for dealing with problems of hypoactivity as well as hyperactivity, and for dealing with problems caused by antigens of internal origin as well as antigens of external origin.

* Immunological Paradoxes: Theoretical Considerations in the Rejection or Retention of Grafts, Tumors, and Normal Tissue, presented as the Von Pirquet Lecture at the Eastern Seminar on Allergy on May 24, 1965, at Grossinger, N. Y.

The general statement may be made that the immunologic system, comprised of many parts in "proper balance," provides the natural means for developing and maintaining identity and integrity of self, in the immunologic sense. Either too much reactivity or too little reactivity–too much "intolerance" or too much "tolerance"–may lead to disease or death. The immunologic system must, therefore, be thought of as contributing to the maintenance of homeostasis in relation to factors that arise from within as well as from without.

In this sense, the immunologic system needs to be comprehended as a whole in relation to the problems of disease and of health with which it is involved. There are a number of paradoxes, the existence of which imply that the orthodox way of looking at the immunologic system leaves something to be desired.

It is the purpose of this paper, in part, to support a point of view that tends to reduce the number of paradoxes and, therefore, the number of otherwise unexplainable or unpredictable observations. The usefulness of this point of view remains to be judged and will be measured (1) by the degree to which it explains facts otherwise difficult to explain; (2) by the degree to which it can unify as yet unclassified facts and observations; and (3) by the degree to which it provides direction for observation and experimentation of theoretical and practical importance.

The basis for the hypotheses to be proposed, and the theme that connects them, began to be developed as a result of certain apparently paradoxical observations made several years ago.

Delayed Allergy in Tuberculous Monkeys: Observations on "Tumor-Cell Tolerance"

The accidental occurrence of tuberculosis in a colony of monkeys under study for "other reasons" provided the opportunity to make the paradoxical observations to which reference has just been made. The ideas that developed subsequently emerged in the course of a search for an explanation for the observed phenomena.

The studies for "other reasons" had been undertaken to determine the neoplastic potential for the monkey of a continuously propagating cell derived from a culture of normal monkey heart tissue. This cell line[2] was first established, late in 1955, by Miss Elsie Ward. It was considered as a possible substitute for kidney tissue from intact monkeys,[3] as a medium in which to culture polio and other viruses for conversion into vaccines for human use. Before using a continuously propagating cell in this way, it was thought desirable to determine whether or not the intact cell, or extracts of such cells, possessed the capacity for inducing neoplasms–at least in monkeys. This was the motivation behind the first manipulations that led well beyond this first intention.

Although, usually, a small cell mass developed in the inoculation site and regressed in two to three weeks, it was occasionally found (FIGURE 1) that a large tumor mass developed that reached a peak in about six weeks and regressed by three months. Reinoculation of cultured cells in such animals resulted in normal or accelerated rejection. Large tumors were observed in about one out of 20 monkeys, and for no apparent reason; at no time were tumors caused by extracts of such cells injected either subcutaneously or intravenously; nor were tumor masses ever observed after intact, living cells were given intravenously–tumors were observed only when given subcutaneously (the dosage range studied was 1×10^6 to 50×10^6/ml inoculum).

In the course of such observations, one of the monkeys that developed a

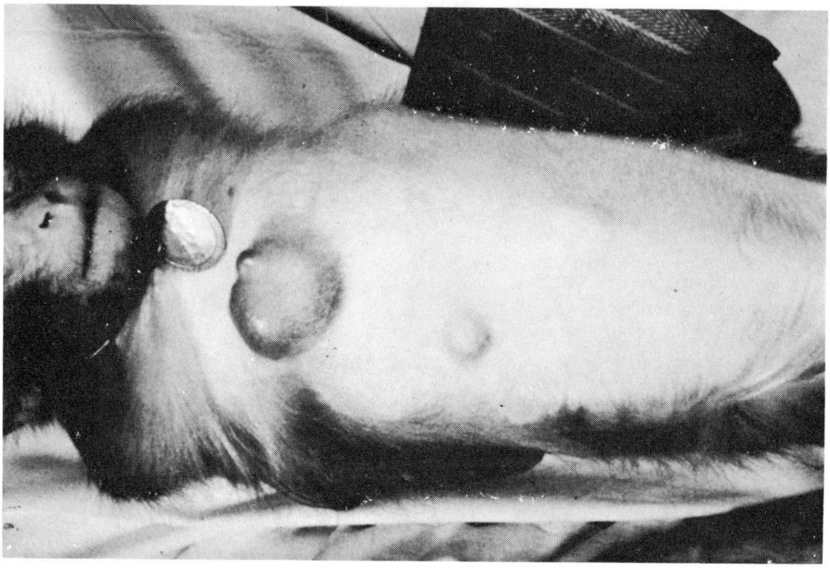

FIGURE 1. Large tumor mass in a monkey inoculated with a continuously propagating cell from a culture of normal monkey heart tissue.

subcutaneous tumor (FIGURE 2) became ill and emaciated. At autopsy this animal was found to have extensive tuberculosis (FIGURE 3). As a result of this finding, and the recognition of unsuspected tuberculosis in the colony (which had heretofore been clean in this respect), the Von Pirquet test for tuberculin allergy was performed. Groups of skin-test-positive and skin-test-negative monkeys were then inoculated subcutaneously with cultured cells and were observed for the occurrence of tumor formation. The *a priori* assumption was made that tumors would be found in the group that exhibited a positive tuberculin skin test and not in those with negative skin tests. The surprising fact was that the reverse was observed.

Animals in the tuberculin-negative group, in which tumors appeared, were then observed over a period of time until a substantial mass developed; at autopsy these animals, even though tuberculin-negative, were found to have extensive tuberculosis. This observation suggested the possibility that the first monkey observed to have a tumor mass and in which tuberculosis was found at autopsy, may also have had a tuberculous infection with a negative skin test.

The failure of "tumors" to develop in monkeys with a positive tuberculin skin test and the development of "tumors" in tuberculous monkeys with a negative skin test suggested that, if it were possible to observe the stage of conversion of the tuberculin skin test from positive to negative, conversion to "tolerance" to the cultured cell would also be observed.

To test this hypothesis, monkeys with a tuberculin-positive skin test were repeatedly skin tested and were repeatedly inoculated with living cultured cells. In three instances in which conversion from a positive to a negative skin test was actually observed, the animals concomitantly developed "tolerance" to the cultured cell that had been repeatedly rejected previously but that now multiplied rapidly at the site of subcutaneous inoculation.

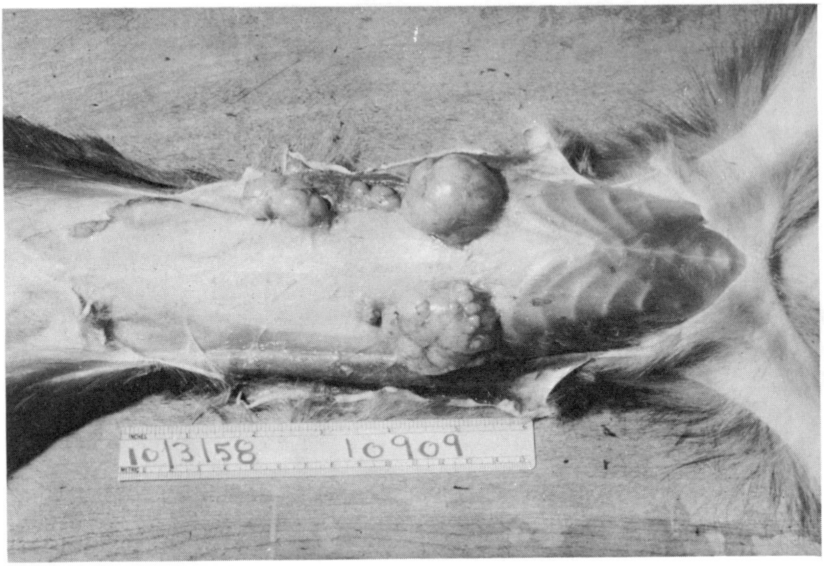

FIGURE 2. Subcutaneous tumor in a monkey inoculated with intact, living cells from a culture of normal monkey heart tissue.

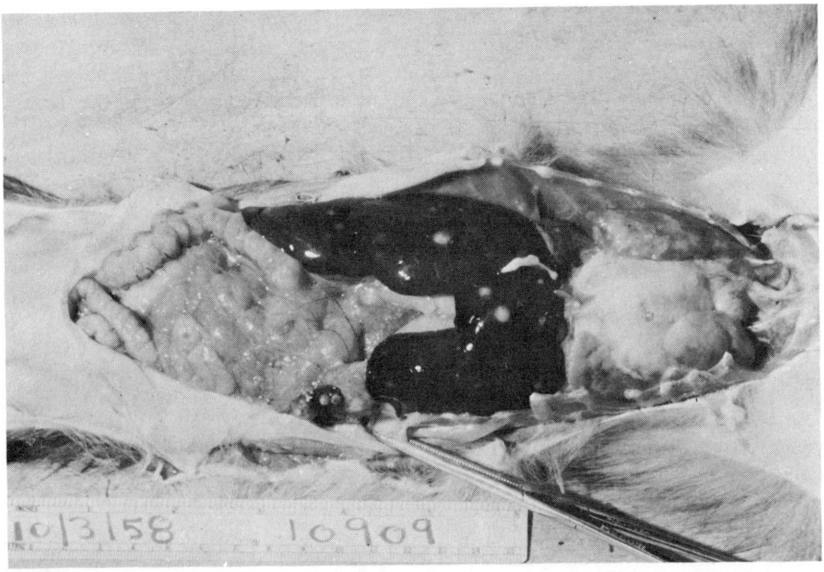

FIGURE 3. Extensive tuberculosis found at autopsy in the monkey shown in FIGURE 2.

Thus, it seemed that depression of the previously positive delayed hypersensitivity reaction to the tubercle bacillus, in these instances, was accompanied by a depression of the normal "homograft reaction" to a continuously propagating cultured cell that now formed a "tumor mass."

The first surmise was that the tuberculous infection had depressed the immunologic system totally to the point of loss of reactivity not only to the tubercle bacillus, but to other antigens as well. However, when serum samples were tested for antibody to the cultured cell, it was clear that the humoral antibody mechanism was active even though the tumor-rejecting mechanism was "inactive." Serum samples tested for tbc antibody, using the tanned cell method of Boyden[4] were also positive, even though the skin-test reaction was negative. Thus, one part of the immunologic system (delayed allergy) was depressed for both antigens, while the humoral antibody system remained active (TABLE 1).

TABLE 1
CORRELATION BETWEEN SEQUENTIAL TBC SKIN TESTS, REJECTIONS OF CULTURED CELLS, AND HUMORAL ANTIBODY LEVELS IN MONKEYS

TBC Skin Test	Cultured Cell Rejection	Humoral Antibody
++++	++++	+
++++	++++	+
++++	++++	+
0	0	+++
0	0	++++

It was obvious from these findings that the delayed hypersensitivity system and the humoral antibody system were operationally distinct; these observations strongly suggested that a controlling relationship might exist in which augmented humoral antibody levels depressed the "tumor"-rejection mechanism. The obvious possibility was considered that depression of the tuberculin-delayed hypersensitivity reaction may have been facilitated by the continued presence of the antigen as well as by an elevated humoral antibody level to tuberculin, and that the same mechanism was operative in depression of tuberculin skin reactivity and in "tumor" rejection, and may have had a reinforcing effect upon each other.

A number of unexpected effects were observed in these studies. The first was the development of a large tumor mass (FIGURES 4 & 5) in an animal in which similar injections given previously resulted in "rejection"; it was expected that the repeated treatments given earlier would have increased, rather than decreased, the reaction of rejection (FIGURE 6). Thus, the development of a tumor mass under circumstances such as here prevailed needed explanation.

A second unexpected effect was the multiplication of cultured cells with formation of a tumor mass in spite of the promptly developed and increasing titer of cytotoxic serum antibody (FIGURES 7 & 8). It was expected that cytotoxic serum antibody would, of itself, have brought about rejection. However, it appears from these observations that the cytotoxic effect of the serum, easily demonstrable *in vitro*, was relatively ineffective *in vivo*. This is reminiscent of the seemingly paradoxical effect of the phenomenon known as immunologic "enhancement" of tumors that occurs following treatments that are expected to have a contrary effect. Apart from the fact that there is a need to explain the

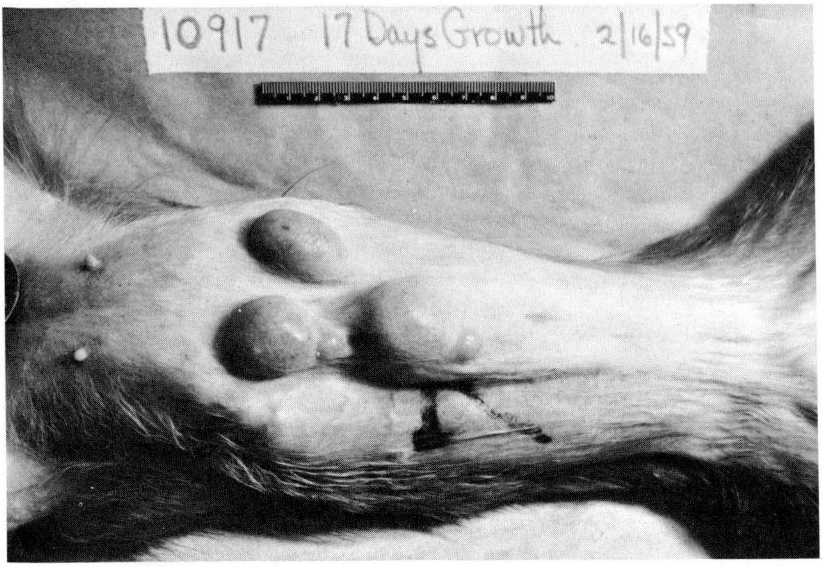

FIGURE 4. Subcutaneous tumors that appeared in a tuberculous monkey following inoculation of living cultured cells after conversion had occurred from a tuberculin skin test positive state to a tuberculin skin test negative state. (Rhesus monkey No. 10917)

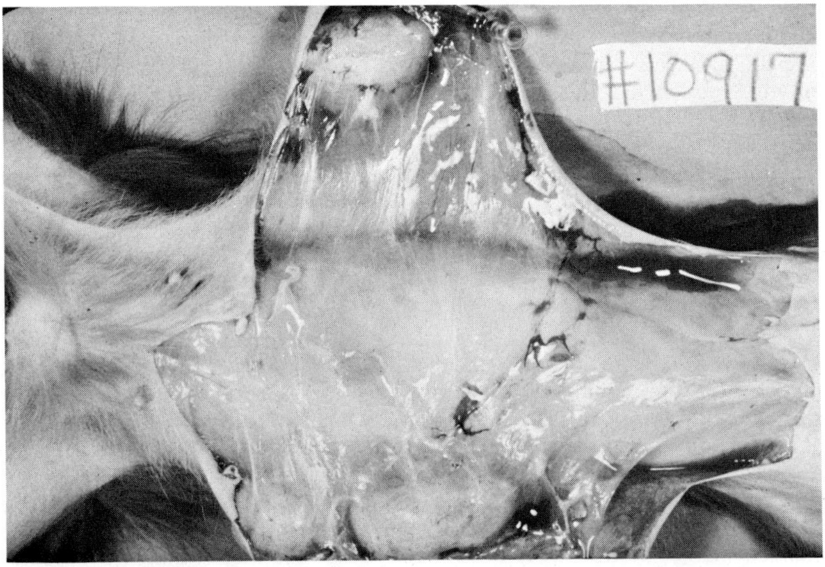

FIGURE 5. Exposure of subcutaneous tumors in monkey shown in FIGURE 4.

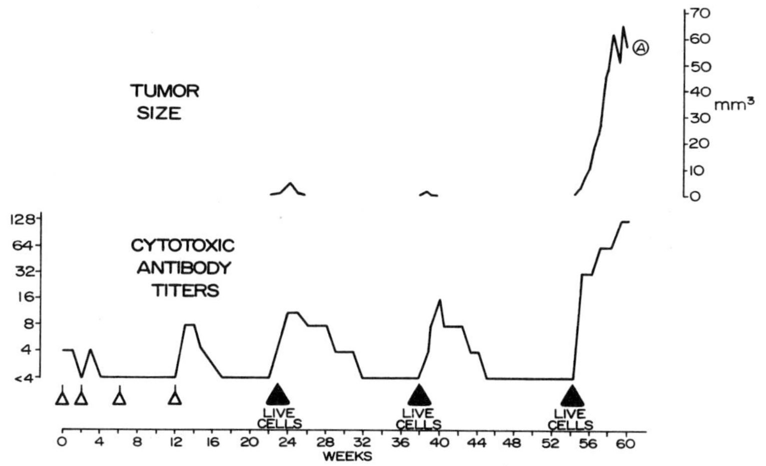

FIGURE 6. Comparison of cultured cell-tumor size and cytotoxic antibody levels in rhesus monkey no. 10917.

particular effects here observed, a fully satisfactory explanation for the phenomenon of immunologic enhancement has still not been provided.[5]

"Tolerance" in Delayed Allergy: A Two-Factor System

The distinction between the two parts of the immunologic system revealed in the observations made in 1958 in the tuberculous monkeys is similar to the distinctions that have since been shown to exist between that part of the immunologic system controlled developmentally by the thymus gland and that part controlled by the bursa of Fabricius, or its equivalent.[6] Not only are there two parts to the immunologic system distinguishable ontogenetically, but the two parts seem to be interrelated, as revealed by studies on delayed allergy in which it

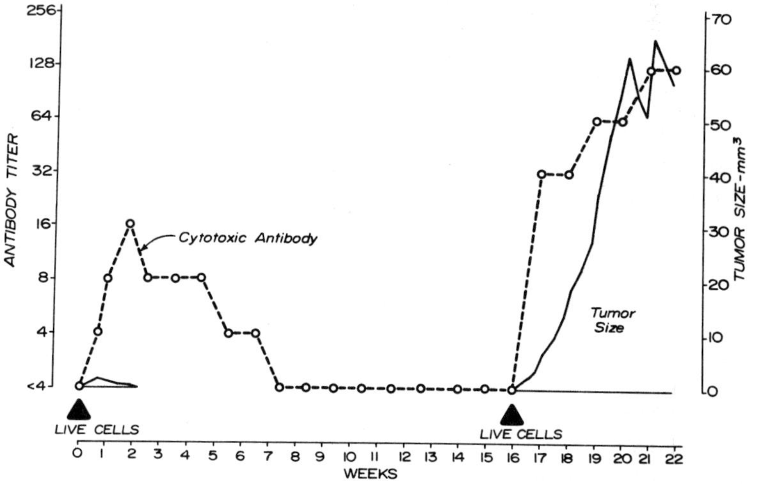

FIGURE 7. Cultured cell-tumor formation vs cytotoxic antibody development in rhesus monkey no. 10917.

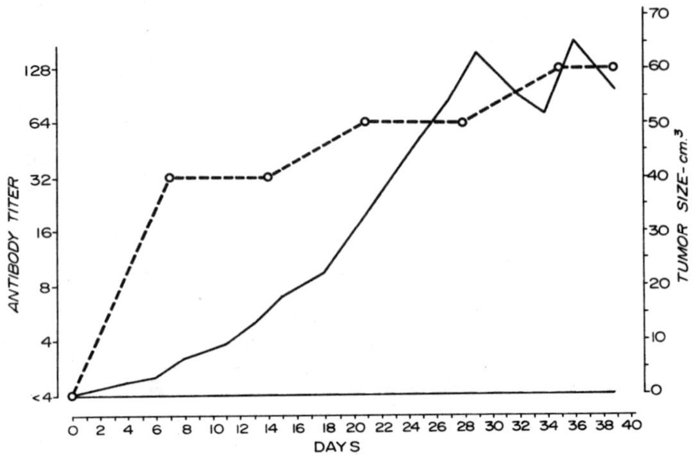

FIGURE 8. Cultured cell-tumor formation vs cytotoxic antibody development in rhesus monkey no. 10917.

appears that a specific humoral antibody factor has a depressing effect upon the corresponding delayed-allergy reaction.

To narrow our focus, and to extend the discussion, let us draw attention to the two kinds of skin reactions with which immunologists and allergists are concerned, and to which reference was made earlier. These are of the immediate type and of the delayed type.[7] The two are different not only in the time of their appearance, following the injection of an appropriate antigen into the skin, but they are distinctly different as revealed in passive-transfer experiments. Reactions of the immediate type are passively transferable to normal recipients by serum derived from a sensitive individual, whereas the delayed type is readily transferable by lymph-node cells or peripheral white blood cells derived from a sensitive individual, and not by serum[8] (TABLE 2).

The foregoing distinction between delayed- and immediate-type reactions has been known since Landsteiner and Chase first demonstrated the difference between serum and cells in the passive transfer of the delayed reaction to the tubercle bacillus.[9,10]

All delayed-allergy reactions have in common the fact that they are passively transferable by means of a suspension of sensitized lymph-node cells, whereas

TABLE 2

SENSITIVITY REACTIONS IN PASSIVE-TRANSFER EXPERIMENTS

Skin Sensitivity	Serum Transfer	Cell Transfer*
Immediate	+	0
Delayed	0	+

* White blood cells or lymph-node cells.

serum from a sensitized animal seems not to contain the substance readily capable of passively transferring delayed allergy. From the evidence to which reference has been made, and from a vast amount of additional information, it appears that serum, at an appropriate stage in immunization or sensitization, contains a substance that has a specific anti-delayed-allergy property, and is actively inducible and passively transferable.

The explanation for the seeming paradoxes to which reference has been made has been postulated to lie in the contrary effects induced on the one hand by sensitized lymph-node cells, and on the other, by antiserum. By way of further description, and in the remainder of this discussion, we will refer (a) to the lymph-node cell factor as the delayed-allergy factor, and (b) to the serum factor as an anti-delayed-allergy factor. Reactions included under the term delayed allergy are (1) the delayed hypersensitivity reaction of the tuberculin type; (2) contact dermatitis due to chemicals; (3) graft rejection; (4) tumor rejection; and (5) such autoallergic phenomena as, for example, experimental allergic encephalomyelitis.[8,11–14]

Included under the term "anti-delayed-allergy factor" are those that act (1) in the prevention of tumor rejection, i.e., the phenomenon of immunologic "enhancement" of tumors; (2) in the protection against the development of EAE; (3) in the prevention or the reversal of a positive tuberculin skin test; and (4) as one of the humoral factors that is here postulated to be associated with induced tolerance to homografts. The precise role of antigen persistence in the anti-delayed-allergy phenomenon is not yet clear; whether antigen has a direct effect, whether its effect is mediated through a humoral antibody factor, or whether both mechanisms operate synergistically, remains to be determined.[5,13,15,16]

Stated in another way, it would appear from the foregoing that induced "tolerance" in delayed-allergy systems is due, in part at least, to the presence of a serum factor that depresses the activity of the specific factor responsible for "intolerance." Such "tolerance" is regarded not as an expression of the "absence of intolerance," but rather as due to the active presence of an "anti-intolerance" factor. "Tolerance," or "retention," in instances involving delayed-allergy phenomena, from this point of view, is due not to immunologic "paralysis," "indifference," or "inactivity"; on the contrary, it appears to be due, in part, to the presence of a specific immunologically active serum factor. Acquired "tolerance" to soluble antigens, on the other hand, which is expressed as a depressed or absent humoral antibody response, is due to an operating mechanism different from that seen in the particular delayed-allergy phenomena to which reference is made here. It is important to recognize this distinction not only for theoretical reasons, but for practical reasons, if one is to employ an understanding of the mechanisms involved for any potential clinical benefit.

The hypotheses that have been proposed in the discussion thus far are (1) that the term "tolerance," used to describe immunologic "nonreactivity," implies a different operating mechanism in these delayed-allergy phenomena, as compared with humoral antibody-response phenomena; (2) that "tolerance," in these delayed-allergy phenomena, is due, in part, to the presence of a serum factor, which seems to be a specific antibody; (3) that delayed-allergy effects can be depressed in the presence of specific antigens without evident impairment of the humoral antibody response mechanisms, and therefore, (4) that a serum antibody seems to have a depressing effect upon the corresponding specific delayed-allergy reaction, by an as yet unrevealed mechanism.

The inference to be drawn is that "tolerance" in the delayed-allergy systems here referred to is an "active process" operating by inhibiting reactions of "intolerance," and that the inhibiting effect is mediated, in part, by a humoral antibody. The cellular system responsible for humoral antibody response is different from the cellular system responsible for the delayed-allergy phenomena; each has a different ontogenic development and each is controlled by a different set of genes.

Two Factors in Other Delayed-Allergy Systems

It has been shown (by Paterson and his associates)[15,17] in EAE, and (by others) in immunologically induced thyroiditis and aspermia that tissue damage is induced by passively transferable sensitized lymph-node cells (LNC) and that a humoral antibody factor appears to be associated with the prevention of these immunologically induced tissue changes.[18,19] The effect of humoral antibody may well be similar to that observed in the phenomenon of "tumor enhancement"—and all of these together might be looked upon as the effect of an anti-delayed-allergy factor in the serum that acts by preventing the development of the delayed-allergy effect. The practical usefulness of an anti-delayed-allergy phenomenon is clear for conditions in which "rejection" or "tissue damage" is the pathological state. However, in the case of tumors, if persistence of tumor is related to the phenomenon of "immunologic enhancement," the anti-delayed-allergy factor would aid and contribute to the pathological state. In such instances, from the practical point of view, depression of the humoral anti-delayed-allergy factor, and potentiation of the delayed-allergy factor, would be expected to produce the desired clinical effect.

To substantiate the foregoing hypotheses, in regard to therapy or prophylaxis, it would be necessary to know the nature of the response as expressed in the formation of humoral antibody (of the 7S and the 19S varieties) in relation to the induced response of sensitized cells responsible for the delayed-allergy reaction. If the humoral response and the net sensitized-cell response are in some way linked, and the relative time of appearance of an effective concentration of the first in relation to the second determines whether delayed allergy or anti-delayed allergy dominates, then we need to understand the quantitative parameters within which such qualitatively different effects are produced that are as different as "rejection" or "retention."

The following distinction is made between (1) the nature of "tolerance" such as is observed between identical twins and (2) the nature of "tolerance" that might be induced under nonisogenic conditions. In isogenic conditions, as in the case of identical twins or their equivalent (i.e., inbred mice), "tolerance" seems to be due to the absence of "intolerance." Under nonisogenic (i.e., allogenic) conditions, it is proposed that "tissue tolerance" may be controllably induced and maintained by attention to the quantitative details needed for a balance in favor of factors for "retention," or "tolerance," as opposed to factors for "rejection" or "intolerance," and that this can be accomplished by maintaining a just-sufficient dominance of the anti-delayed-allergy factors, one of which is postulated to be a serum antibody. Such dominance can be brought about either by a relative increase in an anti-delayed-allergy serum factor or by a relative decrease in one of the delayed-allergy factors or through such effects simultaneously in both systems.

Methods presently in use for immunosuppressive purposes do not deliberately make this distinction, and yet those that have been effective may well have been so for reasons that have just been suggested. The late reversal of apparently successful "transplants," with consequent rejection, may be due to a shift in balance in which "recovery" from an "immunological crisis" had not occurred soon enough; "recovery" from an "immunological crisis" might well be due to a successful shift in favor of dominance of an anti-delayed-allergy effect. Anti-delayed-allergy effects, due to serum antibody, may, at times, induce a direct immunotoxic-tissue effect. Thus, in some instances, there may be a fine line between an anti-delayed-allergy effect and a direct tissue or cytotoxic serum effect that might accompany the humoral factor that appears to be responsible for the anti-delayed-allergy effect that results in "retention" or "tolerance."

For inducing "tolerance" in the foregoing sense, the ideal method would be one in which suppression of the specific delayed-allergy system is effected without otherwise altering other specific reactivities—either delayed-allergy or humoral antibody. The extent to which this ideal may be possible will have to be determined for each particular antigen-host system in the same way that it is necessary to work out the particular details for immunization against a given infectious disease or the details for desensitization in a given allergy. What appears to be needed is a proper concentration of the appropriate antigen presented in a form and in a way that will induce the formation of the "anti-DA" (i.e., "retention" or "tolerance") factor without inducing "delayed allergy" (i.e., "rejection" or "intolerance.") At times it may be necessary to depress the delayed-allergy system—either specifically, if possible, or nonspecifically—just sufficiently to permit the humoral antibody response to dominate, at least early enough for the initial reaction of "acceptance" or "retention" to be sustained long enough, until "active tolerance" is established, and becomes self-sustaining by the mechanisms that have been suggested.

It may be necessary, from time to time, to reinforce the "tolerance-maintaining" effect by administration of the appropriate antigens if these are not introduced into the circulation sufficiently from within the graft, for example; and it may, from time to time, be necessary to reinforce the "tolerance-maintaining" factor, for the purpose of suppressing the relapse of an autoallergic disease. The need here is for biological preparations essentially free of undesirable side effects; i.e., preparations less capable of enhancing "delayed-allergy" than of enhancing "anti-delayed-allergy" effects.

For clinical usefulness, the need is for an understanding of the degree to which the desired effects of a "tolerance-inducing antigen" can be brought about with little or no aid from manipulations that cause suppression of immunological activity generally. In the case of the tuberculous monkeys, it would appear that the reversal of the tuberculin skin test from positive to negative was associated with a reduction in the population of cells that are carriers of specific delayed hypersensitivity reactivity and that this resulted in general depression in the population of cells involved in delayed allergy, and that this may have facilitated the expression of the "immunological enhancement" effect made possible, in part, by the prior sensitization of the monkeys with the cultured cell. The relative advantage thus provided to the humoral antibody system, previously sensitized by the cultured cell, set in motion a sequence of events that led to the dominance of the anti-delayed-allergy factor and thereby resulted in "tolerance" to the cultured cell that previously, and consistently, evoked a reaction of "rejection" or of "intolerance." Thus, it would seem that, at least in the adult animal, and in the presence of a mixture of antigens capable of inducing delayed allergy on the one hand, and humoral antibody response (i.e., anti-delayed allergy) on the other, that (1) antigen form and concentration and (2) competence of the host to react, in both systems, would determine whether the net effect was one of "retention" or "rejection"– these terms being used in the broad sense to include the various categories of delayed-allergy reactions.

The problem, therefore, seems to be one of establishing conditions for use of the appropriate antigens, relative to host reactivity, in relation to the time of application of an organ transplant, for example, or in anticipation of a relapse of an autoallergic disorder.

In regard to neoplastic tissue, which is, in general, sufficiently similar to host tissue to account for the absence of strong delayed-allergy reactions, the reasoning here presented suggests the possibility that "tumor tolerance" may, in part, be maintained by anti-delayed-allergy factors such as have been suggested above. Drugs that are effective in treatment of cancer, even for a time, could, in some instances, conceivably operate through a relatively greater suppression of the anti-delayed-allergy factors, if an effective delayed-allergy response can occur, because there does exist a sufficient antigenic difference between tumor tissue and host.

The question of recognition of antigenic differences as a factor in the expression of delayed allergy is distinct from the question of the capacity of the host to respond dominantly with a delayed-allergy or with an anti-delayed-allergy reaction, either because of disease affecting the immunologic system or for genetic reasons.

Genetic Factors in Delayed Allergy And Anti-Delayed Allergy

It is simply accepted as a fact that wide degrees of individual differences exist in immunologic reactivity; that different species tend to react characteristically; and that within species, inbred lines may be characterized by one kind of immunologic reactivity or another. For example, guinea pigs are, in general, good delayed-hypersensitivity responders; in some inbred strains a strong delayed-allergy reaction can be induced, and in others, such effects are only weakly demonstrable. Similarly, some inbred strains of mice are susceptible to the induction of experimental allergic encephalomyelitis (EAE), while others are resistant. The familial tendencies in man, with respect to allergic disease, is generally acknowledged, and it may be assumed that this is also genetically determined. The question arises as to what it is that one would look for, and what is already known about differences in strains of mice or other animals known to be different from one another in delayed-allergy reactivity.

In this regard, attention is drawn to the studies that have been done by Schneider and by Lee, in two inbred lines of mice, one of which (BSVS) is highly susceptible to the induction of EAE and the other of which (BRVR) is resistant. Their observations on EAE parallel earlier observations on Salmonella resistance and susceptibility. If it were possible to develop a simple marker for the significant difference in immunologic reactivity between these two lines of mice, such a marker might serve to distinguish individuals in whom delayed-allergy syndromes can be expected to occur as distinct from those in whom this would be unlikely.

The genetics of the resistance and susceptibility to EAE have been worked out by Schneider[20] and reveal the existence of two genetic factors for resistance, both of which are dominant; resistance is conferred by the presence of either one alone. Thus, homozygosity for susceptibility is necessary for the manifestation of susceptibility to EAE; the heterozygote is resistant. The two factors to which reference has been made in the present paper may serve to explain the patterns of reactivity that are observed, and the possibility is suggested that the delayed-allergy component is under the control of one gene and the humoral antibody mechanism is under the control of another gene. The simultaneous occurrence of low-humoral antibody reactivity and high delayed-hypersensitivity reactivity would result in an animal susceptible to EAE.

Summary

The value of the hypothesis that a two-factor system is operative in delayed allergy phenomena can be further tested by a discussion of many other examples in which a delayed-allergy reaction is operative. Suffice it to say, in summary of this preliminary account, that the hypothesis that the delayed-allergy system is counterbalanced by an anti-delayed-allergy system, which is maintained through a humoral factor, accounts for facts that are paradoxical according to other hypotheses; it unifies a variety of seemingly different and unrelated phenomena, and it provides direction for observations and for experimentation of theoretical and practical importance. It is necessary to apply the acid test of experimentation to dissolve or to substantiate the broadly outlined view of a two-factor mechanism in rejection or retention of grafts, tumors, and normal (self) tissue.

My purpose in presenting the foregoing ideas was to try to view the problem through a wide-angle lens. It is necessary to look at the details while at the same time looking at the problem as a whole. Rather than look for a single hypothesis that would explain everything in the very heterogeneous and diverse systems that are involved, I would rather try to look for a few unifying ideas.

The notion that cancer has a single cause, or that there is a single set of factors (i.e., psychological factors that when undisturbed keep cancer under control) seems rather unlikely. It seems much more likely that the problem of cancer must continue to be dissected, and we will have to continue to try to understand the relationships among the various systems involved. The most useful approaches and the most useful present attitude is to admit and accept the fact that a great deal still needs to be learned to help clarify our thoughts about the problem.

In my own view, at the moment, the contributions that have been made by Dr. George Klein, Dr. Eva Klein, and others, and by Dr. David Weiss and those who are working in the field of immunology, have shed an enormous amount of light on what just a few years ago was a problem of utter and complete confusion. I look forward with tremendous interest to the years ahead, to seeing to what extent separate but perhaps interrelated psychological factors can be discerned such as have been demonstrated immunologically and for the incitants of neoplasia.

References

1. Von Pirquet, C. V. 1906. Allergie Munchen. Med. Wochschr. **53**: 1457.
2. Salk, J. E. & E. N. Ward. 1957. Some characteristics of a continuously propagating cell derived from monkey heart tissue. Science **126** (3287): 1338.
3. Salk, J. E. 1958. Discussion—Studies on cultured mammalian cells. *In* Poliomyelitis: Papers and Discussions Presented at the Fourth Annual Poliomyelitis Conference : 289. Lippincott. Philadelphia, Pa.
4. Boyden, S. V. 1951. The adsorption of proteins on erythrocytes treated with tannic acid and subsequent hemagglutination by antiprotein sera. J. Exp. Med. **93**: 107.
5. Kaliss, N. 1958. Immunological enhancement of tumor homografts in mice. Canc. Res. **18**: 992.

6. Good, R. A., A. E. Gabrielsen & M. D. Cooper. 1964. The role of the thymus and bursa of Fabricius in the development of effector mechanisms. Ann. N. Y. Acad. Sci. **129:** 130.
7. Crowle, A. J. 1962. *In* Delayed Hypersensitivity in Health and Disease. N. Kugelmass, Ed. : 5. Chas. C Thomas. Springfield, Ill.
8. Waksman, B. H. 1959. *In* Cellular and Humoral Aspects of the Hypersensitive States. H. S. Lawrence, Ed. : 123. Paul B. Hoeba, Inc. New York, N. Y.
9. Landsteiner, K. & M. W. Chase. 1942. Experimental transfer of cutaneous hypersensitivity to simple compounds. Proc. Soc. Exp. Biol. Med. **49:** 688.
10. Chase, M. W. 1945. The cellular transfer of cutaneous hypersensitivity to tuberculin. Proc. Soc. Exp. Biol. Med. **59:** 134.
11. Kligman, A. M. & W. L. Epstein. 1959. *In* Mechanisms of Hypersensitivity. J. H. Shaffer, G. A. LoGrippo, and M. W. Chase, Eds. : 713. Little, Brown & Co. Boston, Mass.
12. Lawrence, H. S. 1959. Homograft sensitivity: An expression of the immunologic origins and consequences of individuality. Physiol. Rev. **39:** 811.
13. Alvord, E. C. Jr. 1965. Pathogenesis of experimental allergic encephalomyelitis: Introductory remarks. Ann. N. Y. Acad. Sci. **122:** 245.
14. Kies, M. W. & E. C. Alvord. 1959. *In* "Allergic" Encephalomyelitis. M. W. Kies and E. C. Alvord, Eds. : 293. Chas. C Thomas. Springfield, Ill.
15. Paterson, P. Y. & S. M. Harwin. 1963. Suppression of allergic encephalomyelitis in rats by means of antibrain serum. J. Exp. Med. **117:** 755.
16. Uhr, J. W. & A. M. Pappenheimer. 1958. Delayed hypersensitivity. III. Specific desensitization of guina pigs sensitized to protein antigens. J. Exp. Med. **108:** 891.
17. Paterson, P. Y. 1960. Transfer of allergic encephalomyelitis in rats by means of lymph node cells. J. Exp. Med. **111:** 119.
18. Rose, N. R., J. H. Kite, *et al.* 1965. Studies on experimental thyroiditis. Ann. N. Y. Acad. Sci. **124:** 201.
19. Brown, P. C., L. E. Glynn & E. J. Holbrow. 1963. The pathogenesis of experimental orchitis in guinea pigs. J. Path. Bact. **86:** 505.
20. Schneider, H. A. 1959. Genetic and nutritional aspects of experimental "allergic" encephalomyelitis. *In* "Allergic" Encephalomyelitis. M. W. Kies and E. C. Alvord, Eds. : **130**. Chas. C Thomas. Springfield, Ill.

Part II. Early Experience, Psychopathology, and Cancer

PSYCHOSOCIAL FACTORS MODIFYING HOST RESISTANCE TO EXPERIMENTAL INFECTIONS*

Stanford B. Friedman, Lowell A. Glasgow, and Robert Ader

Departments of Pediatrics, Microbiology, and Psychiatry
University of Rochester School of Medicine and Dentistry
Rochester, N. Y.

We have attempted over the past six years to develop an animal "model" that would help elucidate the physiologic mechanisms by which psychologic and social factors influence host resistance to disease processes. In our work, numerous diseases and pathogens have been studied, though this report will include only those of an infectious or neoplastic nature.

Our orientation from the onset has been that it cannot be predicted whether a specified experimental stimulation will increase, decrease, or not influence host resistance on any a priori grounds. Rather, it has been our view[1] that whether or not a given form of stimulation is detrimental to the host depends upon the particular infectious agent (or disease process) to which the animal is subsequently subjected. Therefore, it seems best to avoid, whenever possible, the very use of the word "stress," since it connotes, to many, a deleterious effect on the organism. It may be helpful to recall, as an analogy, that the stress of nutritional deficiency leads to decreased resistance to some microorganisms and increased resistance to others[2] and that change in resistance is further complicated by the finding that the chronicity of the infection must be considered.[3]

The studies to be reported utilize one of three methods of modifying the animals' environment: combinations of programmed light and electric shock stimulation, various forms of stimulation early in life, and differential housing. Under each of these conditions, the ability to change host resistance to a number of infectious agents will be discussed, and we also have included data from experiments using a transplantable rat tumor, Walker-256 sarcoma.

Programmed Light-Shock Schedules

Electric shock, with or without a preceding warning signal, has frequently been used as a noxious stimulus in the field of experimental psychology. We were interested in whether such stimulation might modify host resistance, particularly the effect of pairing a warning signal to the shock stimulation and the relative influence of periodic versus aperiodic presentation of these stimuli. A preliminary parametic study[4] showed that the periodic presentation of light-shock stimulation resulted in a greater loss of body weight in young BALB/c mice than shock or light stimulation alone, or than the aperiodic presentation of the light-shock stimulus. Figure 1 is a schematic representation of this stimulation, which occurred for 15 hr on seven consecutive days. The results of this study were used as a guide in examining the influence of light and shock stimulation upon resistance to Cox-

* The studies described in this report were supported by USPHS grants MH-06163, MH-06352, MH-03655, K3-MH-18,542, F1-MH-35,517, and K3-MH-6318 from the National Institute of Mental Health and AI-06388 from the National Institute of Allergy and Infectious Diseases.

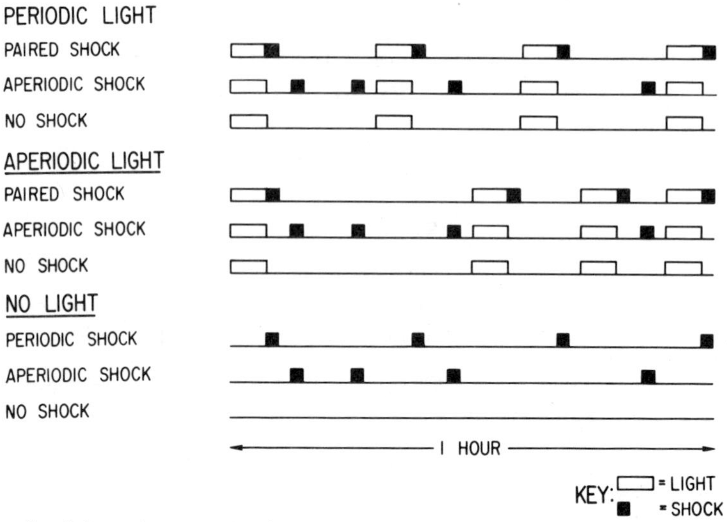

FIGURE 1. Schematic representation of experimental conditions. The light stimulus was 15 sec in duration; the electric shock of 0.6 ma was presented for 2 sec. By permission of the authors and Psychosom. Med. 1965. **27:** 28.)

sackie B-2 virus. Although adult mice are relatively resistant to this strain of Coxsackie virus, preliminary work demonstrated that it was possible to use loss of body weight as an index of the severity of infection.

To reduce the weight loss due to change in housing condition per se, an adaptation period was introduced that consisted of a seven-day period when the mice lived in the experimental cages, but received no light or shock stimulation. Different groups received three days of periodic light-shock, shock, or light stimulation alone. All mice then were inoculated intraperitoneally with Coxsackie B-2 virus and subjected to four additional days under these experimental conditions. FIGURE 2 includes data from a typical experiment, showing that the periodic presentation of light-shock stimulation resulted in increased disease susceptibility as compared to shock or light stimulation alone or to animals continuously housed in standard laboratory cages.[5] All animals that died were from the light-shock group, and though statistically significant, the mortality rate was low. This high recovery rate was not surprising, since adult mice are relatively resistant to this virus, but it was disappointing in terms of our interest in uncovering possible physiologic mechanisms that might account for the observed difference in susceptibility. This model with Coxsackie B-2 virus was not further developed, as it appeared advantageous to alter mortality to a greater extent if differences in physiological mechanisms were to be detected.

The desire to produce greater mortality differences led to additional experiments using other infectious agents. The first approach was to utilize a strain of Coxsackie B-1 (Conn. -5) virus that had been found to be virulent for adult mice.[6] Three experimental conditions again were investigated (light-shock, shock, and light stimulation) and a fourth group of mice remained in standard laboratory

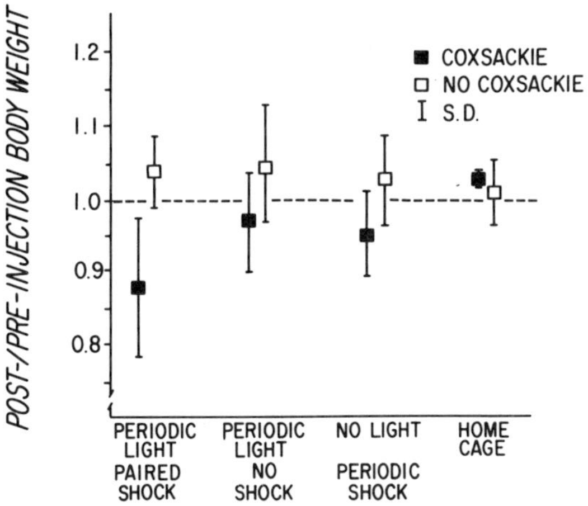

FIGURE 2. Weight loss in mice inoculated with Coxsackie B-2 virus while subjected to varying forms of stimulation or allowed to remain in standard laboratory cages (home cage). (By permission of the authors and Psychosom. Med. 1965. **27:** 365.)

cages. In brief, it was noted that at high dosages of the virus all, or nearly all, the mice succumbed, while at a lower dosage approximately equal numbers of animals died from the three experimental groups but none from those living under standard housing conditions. Thus, all experimental conditions investigated resulted in enhanced susceptibiltiy to Coxsackie B-1 virus, and no further modification of resistance was noted by pairing the light and shock stimulation.[5]

It then was decided to use the identical forms of stimulation as a way of modifying susceptibility to encephalomyocarditis (EMC) virus in CD-1 mice (Charles River). EMC virus was selected because other studies[7,8] in our laboratory had shown that resistance to this virus could be readily modified and that these alterations in resistance were associated with changes in the pathophysiology of the infection. However, no differences in mortality were ever noted in numerous experiments, which included changing the schedule of stimulation, time of inoculation, and virus dosage. Thus, it was again impossible to generalize our findings with Coxsackie B-2 virus to other viral agents.

Most recent work, done with Mr. Michael Plaut, who is a graduate student in our laboratory, has been with *Plasmodium berghei,* a parasite that produces malaria in rodents. In these experiments, identical forms of stimulation were used, but they were presented in sessions of 6 hr alternating with 6 hr of "rest." Following one week of no stimulation in the experimental cages, the mice were inoculated i.p. with blood containing approximately 1×10^6 parasitized red cells from a donor animal. The mice then were subjected to the experimental conditions or left in standard cages until death occurred. The mean survival time was 20.2 days for the mice in the light-shock group, 20.7 days for the shock group, 19.1 days for the light group, and 16.8 days for the animals in the experimental cages receiving no stimulation. The mice living in standard laboratory cages died with a mean survival time of 16.7 days. Statistical analysis disclosed that all stimulated groups differed from the unstimulated animals in both the experimental and laboratory cages. The mortality rates are shown in FIGURE 3. Thus,

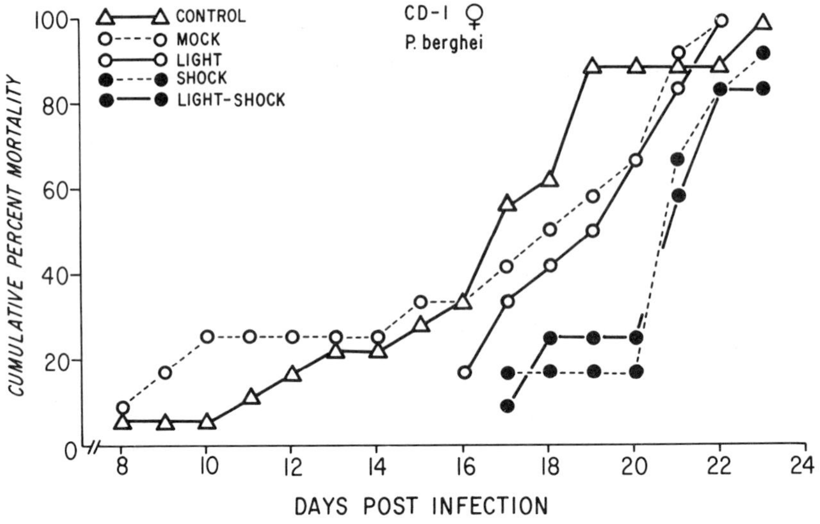

FIGURE 3. Cumulative mortality due to *P. berghei* in mice subjected to varying forms of stimulation or allowed to remain in standard laboratory cages (control).

stimulation had the effect of *prolonging* the mean survival time of mice injected with *P. berghei.* This effect was eliminated if the time of inoculation was postponed until the animals were subjected to two days or more of stimulation adaptation, the schedule that is more analagous to the Coxsackie studies.

In summary, a schedule of light-electric-shock stimulation was found to increase susceptibility of mice to Coxsackie B-2 virus, as compared to animals subjected to either the light or shock stimulation alone or to no stimulation. When a more virulent strain of Coxsackie B-1 virus was used, the light-shock schedule had no unique effect, in that all stimulated animals differed from those living in standard laboratory cages, and this was true only if the dosage was carefully adjusted. All attempts to modify resistance to encephalomyocarditis virus by use of these programmed light-shock schedules have thus far been unsuccesful. The resistance of mice inoculated with *P. berghei* and subjected to similar stimulation was modified regardless of whether the stimulus was light or shock, alone or paired, but in this case stimulation resulted in decreased susceptibility.

Stimulation Early in Life

Numerous studies have shown that relatively simple and brief stimulation early in life has long-term effects on the behavior and physiology of the animal. Commonly, the stimulation consists of several minutes of electric shock per day or merely placing the animal in a different environment. The latter procedure is usually referred to as "handling," which in our laboratory consists of holding the animal gently in the experimenter's hand. Our original work in this area involving a neoplastic or infectious process was with Walker-256 sarcoma, a rat neoplasm in which subcutaneous tumors characteristically develop at the site inoculated with a suspension of viable tumor cells.

Rats were either handled or subjected to electric shock (3 min per day) during the first, second, or third week of life or throughout the three-week preweaning period.[9] When 45 days old, all animals, including an unmanipulated control group, were inoculated with a suspension of tumor cells. Growth rate of the tumor and mortality attributable to the neoplasm were recorded. In terms of tumor development, only those rats handled throughout the preweaning period differed from the control group, with the handled animals showing a retarded rate at which the tumors reached 2 cm in diameter. However, further differentiation emerged when one examined mortality (FIGURE 4). Among the handled

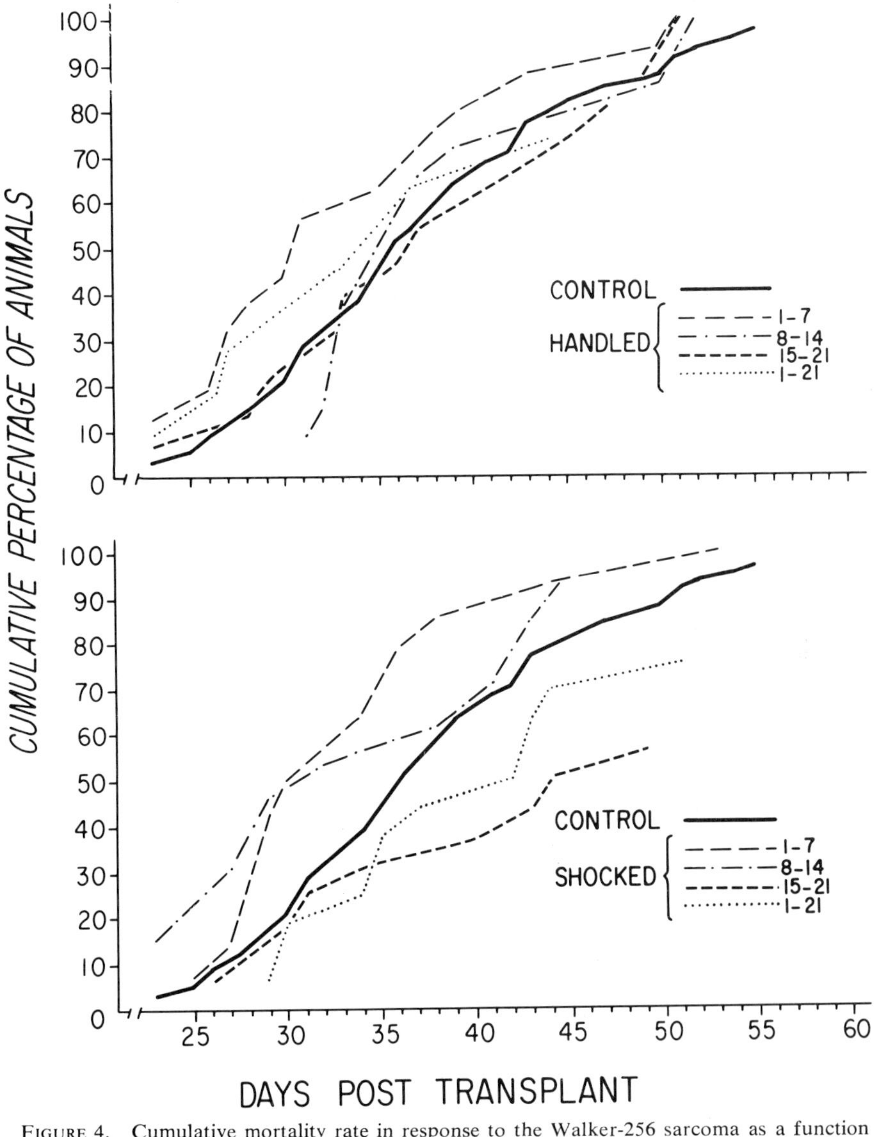

FIGURE 4. Cumulative mortality rate in response to the Walker-256 sarcoma as a function of early experience and the period of life during which the experience occurred. (By permission of the authors and J. Comp. Physiol. Psychol. 1965. **59**: 361.)

animals, those manipulated during the first week of life died at a faster rate than the controls, but none of the other subgroups of handled animals differed from unmanipulated animals. Electric shock during the first week of life, like handling, resulted in an increased mortality rate. Unlike handling, shock administered during the third week of life, or throughout the preweaning period, decreased the death rate relative to control animals. The effects of early stimulation upon resistance to Walker sarcoma depends, therefore, upon the nature of the stimulus and when in the preweaning period this stimulation occurs. Further, the interpretation of whether the course of the disease has been altered is greatly influenced by what measurement is used, namely, the rate in which tumors reach 2 cm in size or the rate of death due to the tumor.

The effects of handling and shock stimulation upon the development of murine leukemia were studied in AKR/J mice, a strain in which the majority of animals spontaneously develop a characteristic leukemia. Mice obtained from Jackson Laboratory were mated, and the offspring either handled, subjected to electric shock (0.2 increased to 1.0 ma over 21 days) for 3 min twice daily, or unmanipulated. These manipulations were performed from day 1 through day 21 (weaning) *or* from day 56 through day 76. At 90 days of age, all animals were tested for "emotionality" by the standard open-field method, and latency, the number of squares traversed, and defecations were recorded. No differences in "emotionality" could be attributed to prior experience with handling or electric shock at day 90. All mice were housed three to seven per cage until death, at which time an autopsy was performed whenever possible. Though virtually all animals appeared to have leukemia at the time of death, neither handling or shock stimulation altered the mortality rate. In contrast to the previous work with Walker sarcoma, these forms of stimulation, irrespective of when they occurred, did not modify the animal's response to this neoplastic disease.

Similar experiments also have been done in the preweaning period with polyoma virus, an agent that typically produces tumors at multiple sites in the mouse. Unfortunately, our studies with this virus have always been complicated by serious technical difficulties. In one study, mice were either handled, shocked, or unmanipulated for the first 2, 7, 14, or 21 days of life and then, immediately following stimulation, inoculated s.c. with polyoma virus. Of those animals manipulated during the first two days of life, tumors developed in 28% (6/21) of those handled and 17% (5/30) of those shocked. The rate of tumor development in all other groups was less than 7%, including the control groups. It is the low rate of tumor development in this study that makes it necessary to view the results with caution, though it appears that further invesigation of the effects of stimulation during the first few days of life upon resistance to polyoma virus would be promising.

Resistance to encephalomyocarditis virus also has been investigated in young mice subjected to handling or electric shock. Animals were handled or subjected to electric shock (0.2 to 1.0 ma) for 3 min twice a day, or they were unmanipulated, from day 1 to day 21 (weaning) or day 42 to day 62. Immediately following the last manipulation, all groups were inoculated intraperitoneally with EMC virus (2×10^3 PFU). The animals were then housed four to six per cage and checked at least once per day for deaths. The sex of the animal was carefully recorded, as previous work revealed a marked difference in mortality between males and females.[7] It may be seen in FIGURE 5 that there were no differences in the frequency of deaths in those animals stimulated from day 1 to day 21 and the unmanipulated controls. For purposes of later discussion, however, it should be

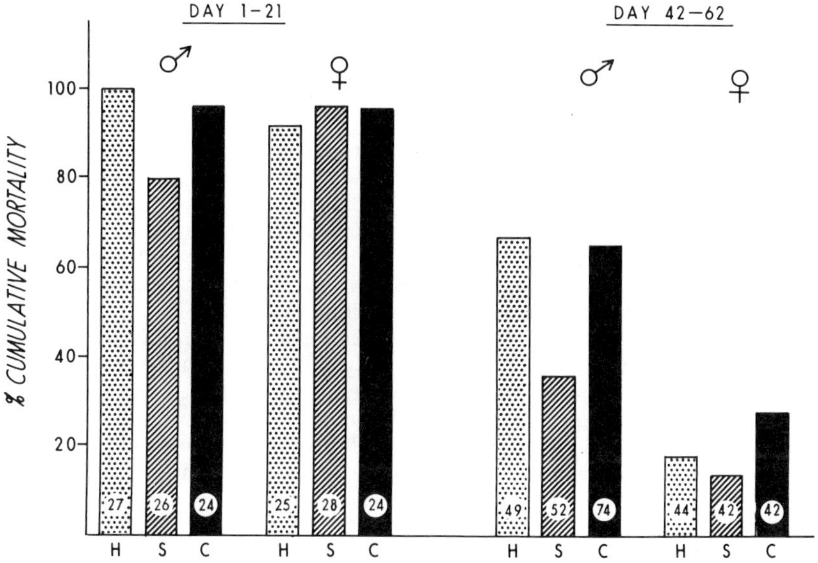

FIGURE 5. Frequency of deaths due to encephalomyocarditis virus in handled, shocked, and unmanipulated male and female mice. Manipulations occurred from day 1 to day 21 or from day 42 to day 62. Animals were inoculated with 2×10^3 PFU of EMC virus.

noted that the shocked animals had a lower mortality that was not significant. The right-hand portion of FIGURE 5 represents data collected from four replications of the same experiment. In each of the four replications, the male mice subjected to shock from day 42 to day 62 had a lower mortality rate than either the handled or manipulated animals; this difference was significant when the data from all four studies were combined. This increase in resistance in animals subjected to shock was not observed in females.

The effects of early (days 1–21) handling and electric shock stimulation were further examined, as it was thought that potential differences in resistance might have been masked by the high mortality in all groups. A lower inoculum of EMC virus (2×10^2 PFU) was therefore inoculated into cotnrol mice and animals subject to electric shock from day 1 to day 21. In each of three replications, the male mice in the shock group tended to have a lower mortality rate, but the differences never reached statistical significance. Two studies using a further tenfold dilution (2×10^1 PFU) gave conflicting results; in one, the shocked animals had an unexpected higher mortality, and in the second experiment, the mice subjected to shock again appeared to be more resistant. We have no explanation for this single reversal and cautiously conclude that early shock stimulation does tend to increase resistance to EMC virus, but that this change in host resistance is not nearly as consistant as that observed in animals subjected to shock from day 42 to day 62. From a theoretical point of view, it is of interest that a noxious stimulus, such as electric shock, can exert a protective effect on animals later challenged with a potential pathogen. This is direct evidence of the danger of equating noxious stimulation, or stress, with deleterious influences upon the organism.

Handling and electric shock stimulation, therefore, have varying effects upon disease susceptibility. In the studies involving Walker sarcoma, modification of disease was dependent upon both the form of stimulation and the time period in the animal's life when stimulation occurred. Neither handling nor electric shock appeared to modify the natural course of the leukemia that spontaneously develops in AKR mice, and the results in animals inoculated with polyoma virus are inconclusive. In male mice subjected to electric shock in the postweaning period (days 42–62), there is a significant decrease in susceptibility to EMC virus, a change in resistance that as yet has been impossible to clearly demonstrate in animals manipulated in the preweaning period or in female mice. Also, no change in resistance to EMC virus, relative to controls, was noted in mice that were handled.

Animals may be manipulated prenatally as well as during postnatal life. One way in which this has been done is by handling the pregnant animal and then observing the offspring during postnatal life. Our only work in this area involving neoplastic diseases consisted of handling pregnant AKR/J mice twice daily for 10 min. Appropriate fostering was done to control for possible postnatal maternal effects. Litters were weaned at 21 days of age, and at approximately 60 days of age they were inoculated with a suspension of homogenized spleens from leukemic donor mice. The inoculation procedure was used to accelerate the development of leukemia, and it results in virtually a 100% mortality. The survival time of the offspring of the handled mothers tended to be longer than that of the offspring of unmanipulated mothers, though this difference did not reach significance ($p < .1$).

Another manner of manipulating the early life experience of an animal is to introduce weaning at varying ages. Premature weaning in animals has been shown to influence subsequent behavior and physiology.[1,10,11] In our work with Walker sarcoma,[12] one group of rat pups were weaned at 15 days of age and maintained in the nesting cage with shallow trays containing food and water. A second group of pups were weaned at the usual age of 21 days. At 45 days of age, all rats were injected with a suspension of tumor cells. The number of animals that developed tumors did not differentiate between early-separated and control animals, and in both groups the tumors reached 2 cm in diameter at the same time. There was, however, a significant difference in the rate at which the animals died; early-separated animals died a median of 21 days following inoculation, as compared to 25 days for the controls. FIGURE 6 shows the cumulative mortality rate in this experiment. Similar studies with EMC virus in mice have, as yet, failed to demonstrate any differences in early-separated and normally weaned offspring that are later injected with virus.

Differential Housing

Housing animals in groups of varying size has a profound influence upon a number of physiologic and disease processes.[13,14] Such studies are often referred to as "isolation" or "crowding" experiments, though in many cases this appears to reflect certain value judgments on the part of the investigator as to the meaning of the experience to the animal. Our early work again used Walker sarcoma as the challenging agent.[15] Rats were housed from weaning either individually or in groups of five to seven animals per cage. Prior to inoculation with tumor cells at 120 days of age, all animals were subjected to tests of "emotionality." Though the differential housing situation resulted in behavioral differences, there was no influence of housing upon the frequency or rate at which tumors developed. A similar study was performed with AKR/J mice with animals housed either individually

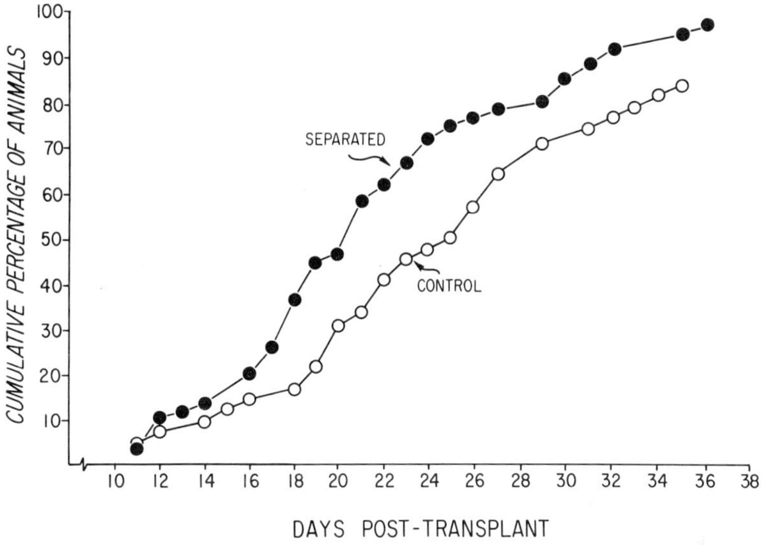

FIGURE 6. Cumulative mortality rate in response to Walker-256 sarcoma in rats separated at 15 days of age (separated) and in animals weaned at usual time of 21 days (control). (By permission of the authors and Psychosom. Med. 1965. **27:** 121.)

or in groups of five from the time of weaning. Again, although group-housed animals were less "emotional" at 90 days of age, the animals died of spontaneous leukemia at identical rates. Thus, in at least these two neoplastic diseases, differential housing did not have any detectable influence upon disease susceptibility or mortality rate.

Significant modification of host resistance was observed in our housing studies involving EMC virus. In one typical experiment, female CD-1 mice (Charles River) were obtained at 21 days of age and housed either individually or in groups of five in standard 6 × 10-inch clear plastic cages; cardboard was placed between the cages of those mice housed alone. At 110 days of age, all mice were inoculated with EMC virus. As shown in FIGURE 7, the death rate of those animals housed individually is greater than that of those housed in groups. Additional studies have shown that similar results are obtained with male CD-1 mice and with BALB/c mice housed in this fashion. Increasing the size of the grouping to as high as 20 mice per cage does not further alter susceptibility to this viral agent. There does not appear to be any significant differences between individually and group-housed mice in basal corticosterone levels nor in their ability to produce interferon or antibody, so that at this time we have no insight into the possible underlying physiologic mechanism(s) responsible for the observed modification of host resistance.

Opposite results, from the point of view of disease susceptibility, have been noted in differential housing experiments using *P. berghei.* In FIGURE 8 are the results of a typical study with this pathogen, showing that, in contrast to the EMC experiments, mice housed individually for three months are less susceptible than animals housed five per cage. Also differing from the EMC virus studies is the finding that as the number of mice per cage is increased, the rate of death increases

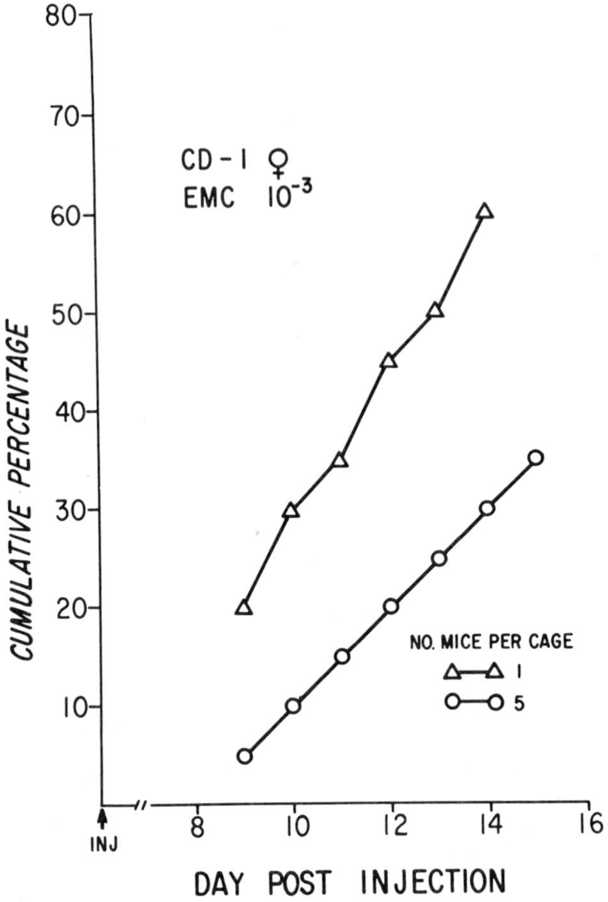

FIGURE 7. Cumulative mortality due to encephalomyocarditis virus in mice housed individually and in groups. Animals were inoculated with 2×10^4 PFU (0.2 ml of 10^{-3} dilution) of EMC virus.

in progressive fashion. Currently, studies are underway to determine whether these findings are related to differences in temperature in the cages, population density, or the availability of social interactions.

Differential housing experiments, therefore, clearly demonstrate that a given condition may be judged as being detrimental or helpful to the organism only if one specifies the pathogenic agent or disease under investigation. In the studies briefly cited in this review, differential housing had no effect upon two disease processes, and in two others, host resistance was modified in opposite directions.

Conclusion

In this paper, we have reviewed our attempts to develop a model suitable for studying the effects of psychosocial factors upon host resistance to infectious disease. Foremost in our efforts has been the search for a host-parasite relation-

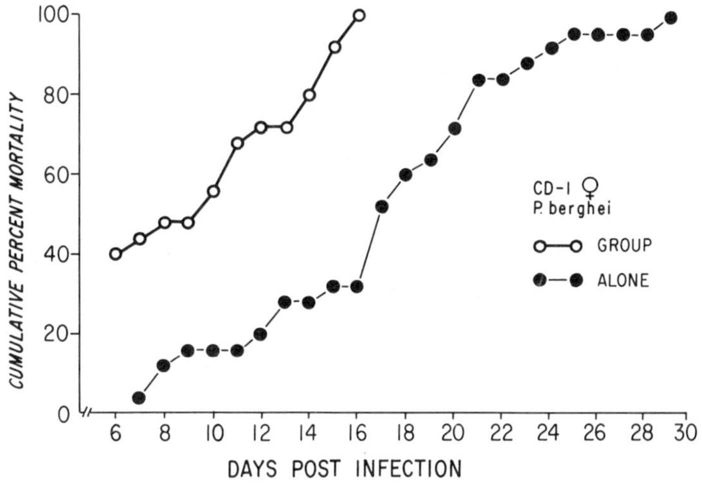

FIGURE 8. Cumulative mortality due to ***P. berghei*** in mice housed individually and in groups of five.

ship that not only may be modified by a number of environmental manipulations that appear to be mediated by the central nervous system of the organism, but also will offer the potentiality of defining the associated physiologic mechanisms. From the experience included in this report and the many studies of other investigators reviewed elsewhere,[16] it now appears certain that environmental factors of a psychosocial nature can modify resistance to a number of infectious and neoplastic diseases. Further studies that merely demonstrate this fact cannot, therefore, significantly advance our state of knowledge. With this in mind, we have discontinued earlier work with certain diseases, such as Walker sarcoma in the rat, as they did not appear to further our understanding of the physiologic changes that must accompany the modification of resistance.

The data clearly indicate that whether a given environmental manipulation will influence disease is a function of the type of manipulation and when it occurs in the life of the animal, the dosage or intensity of the pathogenic insult, how one chooses to measure the course of the disease, and what disease entity is under study. It also appears that no available single theory of stress can predict the effects that a particular form of stimulation will have upon host resistance and that even the direction of change in susceptibility is dependent upon the disease that the organism is experiencing. We believe that such findings also have implications for those investigating similar problems at the clinical level, in that life situations judged stressful, such as the loss of a loved one, might be expected to predispose to some disease states and have a protective effect in others.

References

1. ADER, R. & S. B. FRIEDMAN. 1964. Psychological factors and susceptibility to disease in animals. *In* Medical Aspects of Stress in the Military Climate. : 457–470. April 22–24. Walter Reed Army Institute of Research.
2. SPRUNT, D. H. & C. FLANIGAN, JR. 1960. The effect of nutrition on the production of disease by bacteria, rickettsiae, and viruses. Advances Vet. Sci. **6:** 79–110.

3. SPRUNT, D. H. & C. C. FLANIGAN, 1956. The effect of malnutrition on the susceptibility of the host to viral infection. J. Exp. Med. **104:** 687–706.
4. FRIEDMAN, S. B. & R. ADER. 1965. Parameters relevant to the experimental production of "stress" in the mouse. Psychosom. Med. **27:** 27–30.
5. FRIEDMAN, S. B., R. ADER & L. A. GLASGOW. 1965. Effects of psychological stress in adult mice inoculated with Coxsackie B viruses. Psychosom. Med. **27:** 361–368.
6. GRUNBERG, E. & H. N. PRINCE. 1963. Lethal infection of adult mice with Coxsackie B-1 virus. Proc. Soc. Exp. Biol. Med. **114:** 494–496.
7. GLASGOW, L. A. & S. B. FRIEDMAN. 1967. A model for the investigation of host resistance to virus infection. Presented at the 37th Annual Meeting of The Society For Pediatric Research. Atlantic City. April 28–29.
8. MURPHY, B. R. & L. A. GLASGOW. 1968. Factors modifying host resistance to viral infection. III. Effect of whole body x-irradiation on experimental encephalomyocarditis virus infection in mice. J. Exp. Med. **127:** 1035–1052.
9. ADER, R. & S. B. FRIEDMAN. 1965. Differential early experiences and susceptibility to transplanted tumor in the rat. J. Comp. Physiol. Psychol. **59:** 361–364.
10. KRAUS, M., J. ANDEL, H. DLOUHA, V. FLANDERA, J. KRECEK, J. KRECKOVA & J. ROKOS. 1960. The development and length of life of rats weaned normally and prematurely and living on a free choice of electrolyte solutions. *In* The Development of Homeostasis. E. F. Adolph, Ed. Academic Press, Inc. New York, N. Y.
11. SEITZ, P. R. D. 1959. Infantile experience and adult behavior in animal subjects. II. Age of separation from the mother and adult behavior in the cat. Psychosom. Med. **21:** 353.
12. ADER, R. & S. B. FRIEDMAN. 1965. Social factors affecting emotionality and resistance to disease in animals. V. Early separation from the mother and response to a transplanted tumor in the rat. Psychosom. Med. **27:** 119–122.
13. ADER, R. 1967. The influence of psychological factors on disease susceptibility in animals. *In* The Husbandry of Laboratory Animals. M. L. Conalty, Ed. Academic Press, Inc. (London), Ltd. London, England.
14. CHRISTIAN, J. J. & D. E. DAVIS. 1964. Endocrines, behavior, and population. Science **146:** 1550–1560.
15. ADER, R. & S. B. FRIEDMAN. 1964. Social factors affecting emotionality and resistance to disease in animals. IV. Differential housing, emotionality, and Walker-256 carcinosarcoma in the rat. Psychol. Rep. **15:** 535–541.
16. FRIEDMAN, S. B. & L. A. GLASGOW. 1966. Psychologic factors and resistance to infectious disease. Pediat. Clin. N. Amer. **13:** 315–335.

DISCUSSION OF THE PAPER

DR. WEISS: I will address myself to the use of the Walker sarcoma as a tumor challenge. The comment I should like to make is the following. Whenever one uses a population of neoplastic cells that is either not isogenic to the strain of animals in which it is employed (that is, is not of the same genotype as the animals in which it is tested), or if one employs a population of neoplastic cells that has arisen originally many, many transplant generations earlier, once it has been dealing with a system in which the dissimilarity between tumor-cell population and host is sufficiently marked, then it becomes quite likely that any subtle but still significant difficulty such as the one that may be tested in terms of psychophysiological effects could well be obscured. I throw this out because I think that in some of these experiments the use of the recently arisen isogenic tumor might perhaps give more clear-cut results than work done with the old warhorse tumor that cannot be considered to be isogenic, and where one can question whether this does represent a bona fide population of neoplastic cells or some kind of cell population that has been selected over and over again for its ability to grow at a predictable rate in a given state of the animal.

In other words, I wonder what your reaction would be to attempts at similar experiments, but with the use of a neoplastic challenge that would more closely approach the natural circumstances of neoplasia.

DR. FRIEDMAN: I must admit that to a large degree this is what led us to give up work with this neoplasm. It was highly artificial, and, furthermore, did not lend itself to an understanding of the underlying physiologic mechanisms.

DR. ALFRED AMKRAUT (*Stanford University, Palo Alto, Calif.*): I wonder if you have looked at all into the effect of your stresses on phagocytosis? The reason I am asking this is that there are obviously diseases that are combatted by cellular immunity versus those combatted by humoral immunity. Now, if you are dealing with cellular immunity, decrease in phagocytosis may be very important in permitting the disease to establish itself, whereas when you are dealing with humoral immunity, decrease in phagocytosis, which may, in fact, permit the antigen to stick around for somewhat longer and get into the proper kinds of cells, may be instrumental in increasing antibody production.

We have done some experiments in stressed rats in which we find that removal of tagged red cells from the peritoneal cavity is very significantly increased under stress. I was wondering, first of all, how you inject your material, and second, whether you have looked at this particular parameter (phagocytosis).

DR. FRIEDMAN: We usually use the intraperitoneal for the virus work. We have not done any such studies on phagocytosis, but hope to get into the very area you mention.

One problem, and I am sure you're aware of it, is the manipulations that are needed to get good yields of white cells from the peritoneal cavity. Such manipulation may itself interact with the environmental conditions to modify resistance to disease further. This is always a problem in work of this type.

DR. SOLOMON: I should first of all like to compliment Dr. Friedman on his exposition of the enormous complexities of this area, which is very easy to oversimplify. In terms of early experience, Seymour Levine pointed out that various dosages of red cells will alter the occurrence of differential antibody responses as a result of differential early experience. Nonmanipulated rats showed greater production of hemolysin after injection with two percent sleep red cells but less antibody response when 0.5% sleep cells were used. Similarly, our own experiments on early experience and antibody response showed that primary response was modified considerably more than secondary response by handling in early life in the rat; whereas, the stress experiments, if anything, showed a greater effect on secondary response, so that all of these observations are just complexities added to complexities, if you will.

PSYCHOLOGICAL AND SOMATIC VARIABLES ASSOCIATED WITH THE DEVELOPMENT AND COURSE OF MONOZYGOTIC TWINS DISCORDANT FOR LEUKEMIA*

William A. Greene and Scott N. Swisher†

Departments of Medicine and Psychiatry
University of Rochester Medical Center
Rochester, N. Y.

Introduction

Other than that in the novelty of the occurrence, interest in leukemia developing in one of identical twins has focused on the relevance of a genic determinant,[1,2] the feasibility of therapeutic bone marrow transplantation from the well to the sick twin,[3-5] and more recently on the finding of abnormal chromosomes in chronic myelocytic disease, the significance of which may be clarified by chromosomal studies of the leukemic and the nonleukemic identical twin.[6-10] There have been no studies, to our knowledge, of psychosocial variables that may account for psychological differences in monozygotic twins discordant for leukemia and that may contribute, along with congenital experience,[2] somatic illness,[11] and environmental circumstances, to the development of the disease in only one of the twin pair. This is a report of studies over the past 10 years of three sets of monozygotic twins discordant for leukemia. All were males and were 19, 17, and 15 years of age at the time of development of chronic myelocytic, acute myeloblastic, and chronic myelocytic leukemia, respectively.

Method

Data on the diagnosis and disease course were obtained by the usual hematological diagnostic procedures, including bone marrow examinations. Chromosome study of the bone marrow and peripheral blood in both sets with chronic myelocytic leukemia showed the Ph^1 chromosome in the sick twin only. Data on the gestational circumstances, the past illness experience, personality development, social characteristics, including family interrelationships and determination of dominance, activity, and intelligence of each twin pair were obtained by extended interviews with each twin, the mother in all three sets, and the father in the 17-year-old pair. This information was confirmed by information from the hematologist's histories, the local physician, the high school guidance counselor, and reference to hospital birth records.

Investigation of these twins was not carried out *de novo*. Rather, we had certain focuses of interest and hypotheses based on our previous studies of psychological variables in persons who developed leukemia: first, that the circumstances prodromal to the manifest development of the disease would include states of despair, hopelessness, or discontinuity on the part of the patient incident to separation from significant objects or goals,[12,13] including frustration of reproductive goals in men[14] as well as women; secondly, that the past psychological experience and the past reticuloendothelial functioning of the individual separ-

* Supported in part by USPHS Program Project Grant MH-11668 from the National Institute of Mental Health.

† Dr. Swisher's present address: Department of Medicine, Michigan State University, East Lansing, Mich.

ately and together might differentiate the uniqueness of the individual developing the leukemia;[15] thirdly, that in regard to the child or adolescent (and all of these twin pairs were adolescents), the mother's pregnancy might be associated with a significant loss and emotional reaction on her part, influencing, perhaps independently, the gestational morphogenesis of the fetus and also the quality of the mother-child relationship.[16,17] Therefore, in keeping with the title of this section of the monograph, we will be focusing on these twin pairs' recent experience, early experience, and earliest experience. We will not, in this presentation, go into the details of the close relationships and the striking similarity of interests in school subjects, athletics, hobbies, work, and recreation of the members of each twin pair throughout their childhood and adolescence.

To make the presentation easier, and we hope clearer for the reader, we will present three or four tables for each twin pair, showing chronologically the social and illness experience of each twin along with the course of the mother. In these tables, time will run from top to bottom. Focus is on the gestational circumstances, then the possibly differentiating illnesses during childhood and early adolescence, and later the prodromal circumstances. In keeping with the custom of giving twins assonant names, each twin pair will be referred to as Luke, the sick twin, and Aluke the nonleukemic or well twin. The twin pairs will be differentiated by a number (19, 17, or 15), which is the age at which the manifest disease developed and happens to be the order in which they came under observation.‡

TABLE 1A shows the 19 family – 19 being the age at which the affected twin developed his leukemia. On the right is Luke, in the middle is Aluke, and on the

TABLE 1A
GESTATIONAL, BIRTH, AND INFANCY CIRCUMSTANCES FOR ALUKE AND LUKE 19
(CHRONIC MYELOCYTIC LEUKEMIA)

AGE	MOTHER-19	AGE	ALUKE-19	LUKE-19
25	MARRIED		CAESARIAN	CAESARIAN
28	STILLBIRTH GIRL		1ST BORN	2ND BORN
29	STILLBIRTH BOY			
36	BUSINESS DEPRESSION		6 lbs. 6 oz.	5 lbs. 15 oz
39			CIRCUMCISED	CIRCUMCISED
40	DAUGHTER, BORN CAESARIAN		FATHER'S NAME	MATERNAL G.F. NAME
42	HUSBAND NEPHRITIS BP↑			
44	TWINS; TUBES TIED			
45	HUSBAND "STROKE" + 3 MONTHS HUSBAND DIED + 6 MONTHS	1	TO MATERNAL GRANDPARENTS	TO MATERNAL GRANDPARENTS
46		2		
47		3		

‡ Two of these three sets of twins have been previously reported – Luke and Aluke 19[7] and Luke and Aluke 15[10] – in reference to Ph^1 chromosome studies. The twins Luke and Aluke 17 have not been previously reported.

left is the mother. A year after marriage the mother had a stillbirth girl and then a stillbirth boy. After 10 years she ventured another pregnancy at age 39 and had a daughter by caesarian section. Two years later her husband developed nephritis and high blood pressure. At age 43 she again became pregnant and had the twins by caesarian section, and her tubes were tied. Needless to say, in each of these pairs of twins, one was born first, one was born second, and one weighed more than the other. Perhaps of more importance in emphasizing the fact that twins, even monozygotic twins, may be quite different at birth, as evidenced by the usual weight difference, is the fact that Aluke was named after the father, Aluke 19 the ninth, and Luke was named after the maternal grandfather. Three months after birth of the twins, the mother's husband, the father of the twins, had a stroke, and he died six months after their birth. This mother, who never remarried, still cried 19 years later in talking about the death of her husband, and she referred to the "miracle" of having twins who replaced the two stillbirths and also the loss of her husband.

After the death of the father, the twins were sent to live with the maternal grandparents – a move that was said to be logical and gratifying for everyone, because the grandparents had never had any sons of their own. During the growing up of these twins there was a family attitude that Luke, named after the maternal grandfather, was more the son of the grandparents, whereas Aluke was the son of his mother and his father. Throughout their childhood, the twins lived with the maternal grandparents as mother and father, although they frequently visited their mother and the older sister, who stayed with the mother. So much for the gestational circumstance.

TABLE 1B shows the course of the twins during the intervening years, in particular their differentiating illnesses and social circumstance. They both had a tonsillectomy and adenoidectomy at age five, measles and then mumps at age six, and chickenpox at age seven. However, at age five Luke had had scarlet fever and Aluke did not have it – a fact that was commented on and known as family folklore by the twins and the mother and had been commented on by the doctor. Whether this was a reflection of some difference in the immunologic makeup of the twins at age five or served as a subsequent differentiating immunologic characteristic of the twins is open to conjecture.[11] When the twins were 11, the maternal grandmother died, and two years later the grandfather died. The twins then returned to live with their mother and sister.

As shown in TABLE 1C, shortly thereafter the older sister graduated from high school and was married. The mother and both twins commented on the fact that Luke had had considerably more frequent streptococcal throat infections than Aluke had had. By age 17, both twins graduated from high school. In the meantime, their older married sister had had two sons.

We will not go into the problem of how twins adjust to separation from one another except to point out that one of the ways is for each to get a girl friend. Aluke had planned to go to an arts college and Luke had planned to go to a technical college, which separation would have been the first for the twins. A month after graduation from high school, Luke married. At the end of the summer, Aluke went off to college in the city, and Luke followed him with his wife and took a menial job. Shortly thereafter, Luke's first child, a daughter, was born. In the city, Luke found that, particularly in view of his job, he was traveling in circles that were entirely different from those of his twin brother. Feeling left out, he moved back to the home town, following which he had a severe and prolonged streptococcal infection and penicillin therapy. In the meantime, Aluke lost his girl friend.

TABLE 1B
COURSE OF CHILDHOOD AND EARLY ADOLESCENCE FOR ALUKE AND LUKE 19 (CHRONIC MYELOCYTIC LEUKEMIA)

MOTHER-19		ALUKE-19		LUKE-19
48*		4*		
49		5	NO SCARLET FEVER T & A	SCARLET FEVER T & A
50		6	MEASLES MUMPS	MEASLES MUMPS
51		7	CHICKEN POX	CHICKEN POX
52		8		
53		9		
54		10		
55	MOTHER DIED	11	GRANDMOTHER DIED CORONARY	GRANDMOTHER DIED CORONARY
56		12		
57	FATHER DIED	13	GRANDFATHER DIED LUNG CANCER TO MOTHER'S	GRANDFATHER DIED LUNG CANCER TO MOTHER'S

* The numbers in this column specify years of age.

TABLE 1C
COURSE OF ADOLESCENCE FOR ALUKE AND LUKE 19 (CHRONIC MYELOCYTIC LEUKEMIA)

MOTHER-19		ALUKE-19		LUKE-19
58*	DAUGHTER GRADUATED HIGH SCHOOL DAUGHTER MARRIED	14*	TO HIGH SCHOOL	TO HIGH SCHOOL
59		15		
				STREP THROAT - PEN.
60	DAUGHTER'S SON	16		
61	DAUGHTER'S SON	17	TETANUS TOXOID GRADUATED HIGH SCHOOL	NO TETANUS TOXOID GRADUATED HIGH SCHOOL MARRIED
			TO COLLEGE IN CITY	TO CITY
62		18		DAUGHTER BORN BACK TO TOWN STREP INF.-PEN.
			LOST GIRL FRIEND	

* The numbers in this column specify years of age.

He became neurotically depressed and consulted a psychiatrist, and three months later he married another girl, as shown in TABLE 1D.

Luke felt that his brother's marriage was the final evidence of their going their separate ways. Shortly after this, his wife had their second child, another daughter. (Luke, Aluke, and the mother all emphasized his disappointment that this child was not a boy.) He then became very anxious to conceive another child. During this time he developed what was probably a transient two-hour episode of priapism.

In the meantime, Aluke's first child, a son, was born. He was named Aluke 19, the tenth. Shortly thereafter, Luke had a second episode of priapism, lasting some 24 hours. He had a prolonged, irreversible episode of priapism two months later and was admitted to the hospital, where the diagnosis of chronic myelocytic leukemia was made. He continued to try to conceive a son, and his wife actually became pregnant, but she aborted spontaneously during the course of his illness. His illness, with exacerbations and remissions with appropriate treatment, lasted approximately three years. Late in his disease, both of the twins were studied for Ph^1 chromosome in the leukocytes in their peripheral blood and bone marrow. It was present in Luke, but not in Aluke. Shortly thereafter, preparation was made for bone marrow transplantation, but Luke died before this could be attempted.

TABLE 1D

PRODROMAL CIRCUMSTANCES AND DEVELOPMENT AND DURATION OF CHRONIC MYELOCYTIC LEUKEMIA DISCORDANT FOR ALUKE AND LUKE 19

MOTHER-19		ALUKE-19		LUKE-19	
63*	DAUGHTER'S DAUGHTER	19*	TO PSYCHIATRIST		
			MARRIED		
					DAUGHTER BORN
				SEPT	PRIAPISM
64		20	SON BORN	NOV	PRIAPISM
				JAN	
				MAR	PRIAPISM HOSP Dx LEUKEMIA
				MAY	
			HE & WIFE WORKED - 1 YR	JULY	
				SEPT	
65	PNEUMONIA	21		NOV	
				JAN	WIFE 2 MONTHS PREGNANT
	CEREBRAL HEMORRHAGE		DAUGHTER BORN	MAR	WIFE MISCARRIED
				MAY	
			HE & WIFE TO COLLEGE	JULY	
				SEPT	
66		22		NOV	
				JAN	
				MAR	
				MAY	
			HE & WIFE GRADUATED	JULY	
				SEPT	
67		23		NOV	
				JAN	ACUTE BLASTIC CRISIS
				MAR	PNEUMONIA
			NO (Ph') CHROMOSOME	MAY	(Ph') CHROMOSOME
				JULY	
				SEPT	TRANSPLANT ?- DIED

* The numbers in this column specify years of age.

Aluke has been followed now for 10 years without evidence of disease. He had one subsequent examination for Ph^1 chromosome, but no evidence of it was found.

In TABLE 2A we present Luke and Aluke 17. Here the mother had had two full-term pregnancies previously, with spontaneous deliveries of a daughter and a son. Her father died when she was 27 years old. She then bore the twins, who she said had been born "nine months to the day" after the death of her father. Following the birth of the twins, she had what was called a "nervous breakdown," which sounded like a moderately severe postpartum depression, for which she was treated by her local physician and from which she recovered after about six months. The twins were born by spontaneous delivery. Again, one was born first, and Aluke weighed more than Luke. These twins had no special names.

This was a typical northern New York farm family of a number of generations. The father of the twins first worked on his father's farm and then moved in order to become the overseer of somebody else's farm. Eventually he acquired his own farm. During their childhood the twins had the same contagious diseases, the first being measles. At age four Aluke suffered a mangled right hand when his brother turned on the mangler unexpectedly, and he still had a significant scar when he was seen years later.

As shown in TABLE 2B, they went to kindergarten at the same time, and they both repeated the third grade when the family moved to their own farm. Luke apparently had difficulty seeing the blackboard and was treated with glasses, which he wore for five years, and then it was decided that he did not need them after all. At age 13, Aluke fell and broke his arm. Diagnostic x-ray for this was the only instance of x-ray exposure, prenatal or postnatal, for any of these three sets of twins.

At age 15, both of the twins began high school, as indicated in TABLE 2C. Shortly thereafter, the father was first approached about an expressway coming

TABLE 2A

GESTATIONAL, BIRTH, AND EARLY CHILDHOOD CIRCUMSTANCES FOR ALUKE AND LUKE 17 (ACUTE MYELOBLASTIC LEUKEMIA)

AGE	MOTHER-17	AGE	ALUKE-17	LUKE-17
22	MARRIED		SPONTANEOUS	SPONTANEOUS
23			2nd BORN	1st BORN
24	1st DAUGHTER BORN		6 lbs. 5 oz.	5 lbs. 14 oz.
25	1st SON BORN		CIRCUMCISED	CIRCUMCISED
26			NO SPECIAL NAME	NO SPECIAL NAME
27	FATHER DIED			
28	TWINS			
29	"NERVOUS BREAKDOWN"	1		
30	MOVED TO OTHER FARM	2		
31		3	MEASLES	MEASLES
32		4	MANGLED RIGHT HAND	

TABLE 2B
COURSE OF CHILDHOOD AND EARLY ADOLESCENCE FOR ALUKE AND LUKE 17
(ACUTE MYELOBLASTIC LEUKEMIA)

MOTHER-17		ALUKE-17		LUKE-17
33*		5*	CHICKEN POX KINDERGARTEN	CHICKEN POX KINDERGARTEN
34	2nd SON BORN	6	MUMPS	MUMPS
35		7	RUBELLA	RUBELLA
36		8	3rd GRADE	3rd GRADE GLASSES (5 YEARS)
37	MOVE TO OWN FARM	9	REPEAT 3rd GRADE	REPEAT 3rd GRADE
38		10		
39		11		
	HUSB. HERNIATED DISC			
40		12		
			BROKE ARM	
41		13		
42	2nd DAUGHTER BORN	14		

* The numbers in this column specify years of age.

through the middle of his farm. The entire family was apprehensive and angry, and they did all they could to fight this development. But approximately a year later the expressway was started several miles away, coming toward their farm. A few months later the father developed a bleeding peptic ulcer, the first symptom of an ulcer that he had ever shown. By the time the twins were 17, the family's land was actually taken over, with the road crews moving in equipment and occupying the farm land.

In this family, as is customary in many northern New York State farm families, the twins over the years had been given a calf to raise and sell. They had also been given a plot of land that they could work and harvest and from which they could keep any profit. It happened that the land that was taken by the expressway included that of Luke, but did not include that of Aluke. The twins were distressed by this, and Aluke tried to halve his plot with Luke. Luke refused, saying that his father had dealt with the loss of much of his land and he could deal with the loss of his. Early in his 17th year, Luke developed nosebleeds, without any other particular symptoms except some degree of fatigue and enlargement of his lymph nodes. He came into the hospital three weeks later, and a diagnosis of acute leukemia was made. He died in two weeks. Since then, the family has carried on

TABLE 2C
PRODROMAL CIRCUMSTANCES AND DEVELOPMENT AND DURATION OF ACUTE MYELOBLASTIC LEUKEMIA DISCORDANT FOR ALUKE AND LUKE 17

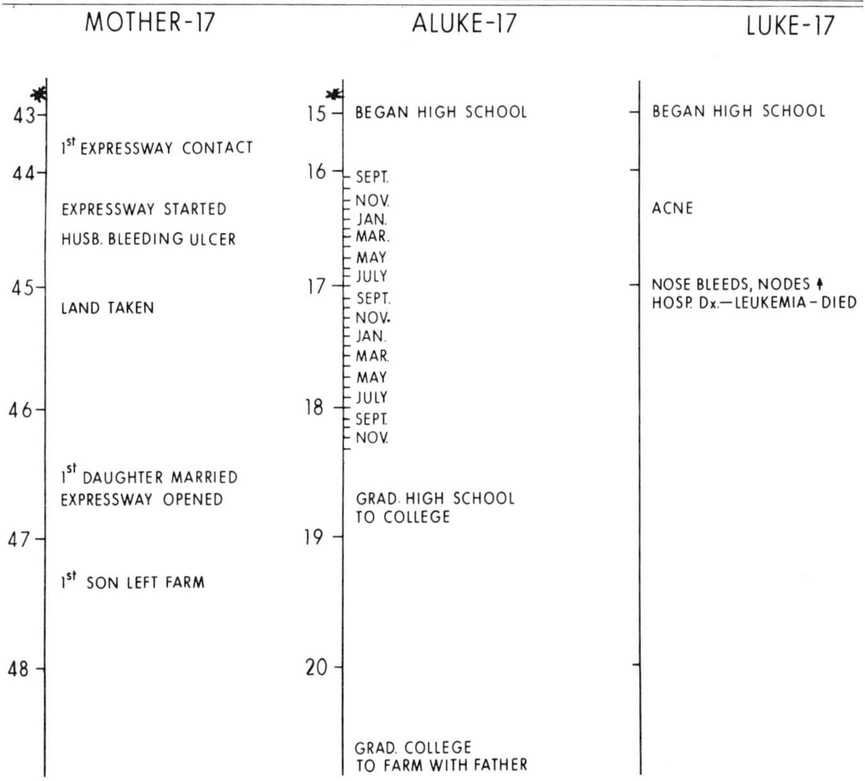

* The numbers in this column specify years of age.

with the expressway through the middle of their farm. Aluke has gone to a two-year college, majoring in agriculture, and has returned to work with his father on the farm.

Next we come to the third set of twins – the 15-year-olds – Luke and Aluke 15, shown in TABLE 3A. In this family, the mother had married at age 19, and approximately a year later she had her first child, a daughter, who was very severely brain-damaged. She cared for this daughter at home and could not part with the child for nearly eight years. She was married to a ne'er-do-well alcoholic, who was usually at home and cared for the children while the mother worked. This woman was a very aggressive, effective, hysterical personality who generally held two jobs – one in a factory and the other doing domestic work. Two years after the birth of her daughter, she had a son born by spontaneous delivery. She again became pregnant two years after that and, much to her surprise, had the twins. She was anxiety-ridden during the pregnancy, worrying about how she was going to take care of another child – much less two. Luke was a spontaneous delivery and Aluke was born by breaching extraction. Luke was born first, and

TABLE 3A

GESTATIONAL, BIRTH, AND EARLY CHILDHOOD CIRCUMSTANCES FOR ALUKE AND LUKE 15 (CHRONIC MYELOCYTIC LEUKEMIA)

AGE	MOTHER-15	AGE	ALUKE-15	LUKE-15
			BREECH EXTRACTION	SPONTANEOUS
			2ND BORN	1ST BORN
19	MARRIED			
20	1ST DAUGHTER BRAIN DAMAGED		5 lbs 6 oz.	6 lbs 11 oz
21	SON, SPONTANEOUS		NOT CIRCUMCISED	CIRCUMCISED
22			FATHER'S MIDDLE NAME	FATHER'S FIRST NAME
23				
24	TWINS			
25	2ND DAUGHTER BORN	1		HOT WATER BURN, CAST
26		2	MEASLES MUMPS	MEASLES MUMPS
27	STILL BIRTH-BOY TUBES TIED	3		
28	1ST DAUGHTER TO INSTITUTION	4		

he was a pound heavier than Aluke. Luke was given the father's first name and Aluke had the father's middle name. In spite of the marked similarity between the twins, Luke was more identified and associated with the father than Aluke was, partly because he was the first born and partly because he had the father's first name.

A second daughter was born a year after the twins. During the week the mother was waiting to go to the hospital for the delivery, while she was feeding the twins one morning, Luke sustained severe burns on his chest and abdomen when a kettle of hot water was tipped over. He was taken to the hospital, where he was confined in a shell body cast for immobilization. He was hospitalized for a month and apparently healed reasonably well in spite of some secondary infection. He was then immobilized at home for another month, under the care of the mother and various friends. In the meantime, the mother had gone to the hospital for the delivery of the new baby and was at home with the new baby when Luke returned from the hospital.

Subsequently, the twins both had measles and mumps at the same time. Next the mother had another pregnancy and delivered a still-birth boy, following which her tubes were tied because, as her physicians told her, she should certainly not have any more children. They also warned her that she would die of overwork if she did not institutionalize her brain-damaged daughter. Therefore, after considerable conflict, she institutionalized her daughter, but she continued to go to see the girl several times a year over the subsequent years.

She repeatedly expressed her feeling that having the twins somehow made up for the misfortune of her brain-damaged daughter and the still-birth son.

After beginning kindergarten the twins had chickenpox, as shown in TABLE 3B. When they were eight years old, the mother, keeping all the children with her, separated from the father. This was a difficult time for the twins as well as for the

TABLE 3B

COURSE OF CHILDHOOD AND EARLY ADOLESCENCE FOR ALUKE AND LUKE 15
(CHRONIC MYELOCYTIC LEUKEMIA)

MOTHER-15		ALUKE-15		LUKE-15	
29*		5*	KINDERGARTEN CHICKENPOX		KINDERGARTEN CHICKENPOX
30		6			
31		7			
32	SEPARATED	8			
33	MOVED TO TOWN	9	T & A		T & A
34		10			
35		11			
36		12			
37	1ST SON TO HIGH SCHOOL	13			
38		14		JAN	
	1ST SON TO FATHER			MAR	
			THRU GRADE SCHOOL	MAY	THRU GRADE SCHOOL
				JULY	
			BEGAN HIGH SCHOOL	SEPT	BEGAN HIGH SCHOOL
				NOV	

* The numbers in this column specify years of age.

other children, since the father had had considerable contact with them in the home. A little over a year later, the mother and the children moved to another town. This she described as having been an even more difficult time, during which the children would cry for their home town as well as for their father. But after a year they settled down. Later her first and older son began high school. In his sophomore year in high school, he returned to the father, to whom he had been more attached than had anyone else in the family. The twins both finished grade school and began high school.

During these years, the mother became aware that her older son was moving away and that the twins, beginning high school, would eventually be moving out. For these reasons, she said, she decided that she would divorce her husband, the twin's father, so that she could marry again if she wished. At that time she had no particular person in mind. In the early summer she started divorce proceedings, as indicated in TABLE 3C. During the same summer, Aluke was the first of the twins to begin to "go steady" with a girl, and Luke began to experience what was later described as fatigue and lethargy. He lay around the house much of the time then, according to the mother, not knowing what to do with himself. She

TABLE 3C

PRODROMAL CIRCUMSTANCES AND DEVELOPMENT AND DURATION OF CHRONIC MYELOCYTIC LEUKEMIA DISCORDANT FOR ALUKE AND LUKE 15

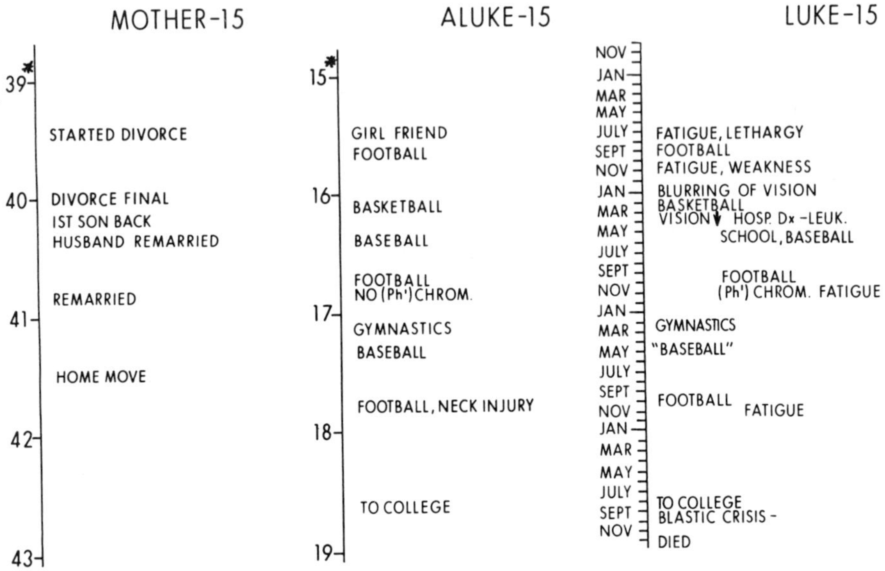

* The numbers in this column specify years of age.

attributed this to Aluke's having a girl friend, which left Luke at loose ends since the twins had always done everything together. During the fall of this year, in the football season, Luke noticed that he was not able to run as fast as his brother and he tired more easily. He had some questions about his qualifications to fulfill the role of quarterback on the team. Also during the football season he probably had some transient blurring of vision. This, however, did not interfere with his going out for basketball later, along with his twin. In January, near the end of the twins' 15th year, the mother's divorce became final. She felt that the twins accepted this but that Luke was more troubled about it than Aluke. A week after the mother's divorce became final, Luke developed acute blurring of vision, which he mentioned to no one. Two months later his vision was suddenly further impaired, and he was hospitalized. The diagnosis of chronic myelocytic leukemia was first made then.

The father remarried approximately six months later, and the mother remarried about a year after that. We will not go into the details of Luke's course with leukemia here except to point out that he had an initial complete remission with splenic irradiation and several other excellent responses to radiation when he relapsed. Approximately a year after the development of his leukemia, studies for the Ph^1 chromosome in the peripheral blood leukocytes and bone marrow were made on the twins, showing the Ph^1 chromosome in Luke's blood but not in that of Aluke. Luke continued to participate actively and effectively along with Aluke in each season in the various athletic endeavors in which they excelled. At age 18 they both left home for the first time to go to a two-year college. Luke

TABLE 4

COMPOSITE OF SEVERAL BIRTH, ZYGOSITY, IDENTITY, ILLNESS, AND SURVIVAL CHARACTERISTICS FOR THE THREE SETS OF TWINS

	CHRONIC MYELOCYTIC LEUKEMIA		ACUTE MYELOBLASTIC LEUKEMIA		CHRONIC MYELOCYTIC LEUKEMIA	
	LUKE-19	ALUKE-19	LUKE-17	ALUKE-17	LUKE-15	ALUKE-15
BIRTH ORDER	SECOND	FIRST	FIRST	SECOND	FIRST	SECOND
BIRTH WEIGHT	5 LBS. 15 OZ.	6 LBS. 6 OZ.	5 LBS. 14 OZ.	6 LBS. 5 OZ.	6 LBS. 11 OZ.	5 LBS. 6 OZ.
DELIVERY	CAESARIAN	CAESARIAN	SPONTANEOUS	SPONTANEOUS	SPONTANEOUS	BREECH EXTRACT.
CIRCUMCISION	YES	YES	YES	YES	YES	NO
BLOOD GROUPS	ANTIGENS/SYSTEMS 11/4		16/7		27/11	
PLACENTA	MONOZYGOTIC BY HISTORY		NO DATA		MONOZYGOTIC BY RECORD	
APPEARANCE	SAME		SAME		SAME	
HANDED	RIGHT	RIGHT	RIGHT	LEFT	RIGHT	RIGHT
IDENTITY SCAR	FOREHEAD CUT			MANGLED HAND		BROKEN NOSE
DOMINANT	–	+	+	–	+	–
ACTIVITY-10+ SCALE	6+	4+	6+	5+	8+	9+
INTELLIGENCE-10+	7+	9+	6+	8+	3+	2+
X-RAYS	0	0	0	Dx. BROKEN ARM	0	0
DIFFERENT ILLNESS	SCARLET FEVER STREP INFECTIONS			MANGLED HAND BROKEN ARM	HOT WATER BURN	BROKEN NOSE
Ph^1 CHROMOSOME	+	0	NO DATA		+	0
TWIN SICK	†3 1/2 YEARS		†5 WEEKS		†3 YEARS	
TWIN WELL		10 YEARS		4 YEARS		3 1/2 YEARS

developed a blastic crisis and died two months later, three years after diagnosis of his illness.

Composite of Findings

TABLE 4 shows a number of types of information on the three sets of twins, consolidated into several categories. The characteristics of the twins in regard to birth order, birth weight, and type of delivery are presented first. There seems to be nothing of striking significance. Next is a group of factors related to zygosity. The twins were the same on all blood groups studied. These were obtained in progressively increasing numbers for each set we have seen: 11 antigens in four systems for twin set 19, 16 antigens in seven systems for twin set 17, and 27 antigens in 11 systems for twin set 15. In the third category, nothing significantly differentiating was found with respect to dominance, activity, or intelligence in comparison of the sick to the well twin. Fourth, a group of possibly differentiating biological factors in terms of development of the leukemia are listed. It is emphasized that throughout their lives none of these twins were exposed to x-rays except Aluke 17, who had diagnostic x-ray at the time of his broken arm. None of the mothers had had prenatal x-ray for diagnosis of twins. In both patients with chronic myelocytic leukemia, there was a previous differentiating inflammatory illness – streptococcal infections in Luke 19 and the hot-water burn in Luke 15. Both the twins with chronic myelocytic leukemia showed the Ph^1 chromosome, and the well twin did not. As indicated in the last section of this table, both of the twins with myelocytic leukemia survived approximately three years, and the twin with acute myeloblastic leukemia survived only five weeks. The three well twins have now been followed 10 years, four years, and three and a half years respectively without evidence of any disease.

Discussion and Summary

Before concluding, we would like to say something about the twin method of investigation. In a recent report by Miller[18] on the epidemiology of those with a high risk of leukemia he states, "Recognition of the extraordinary risk of leukemia in the young child whose identical twin has developed the disease provides investigators with the opportunity to study the as yet unaffected twin in regard to cell kinetics, immunity, virus status, and chromosomes with the expectation that on the average in one out of five instances the child will develop the disease within a short time. Retrospective investigation may reveal why eighty per cent of co-twins escape the disease although both members of a pair are genetically identical and share the same environment." This statement is based on the recent survey of a large population by MacMahon[1] showing 22 cases of identical twins with leukemia, only five of whom were concordant. In all instances, the second twin became ill with the disease within a year. Concordance for leukemia has generally occurred only in twins below the age of seven years.

In research using the twin method, there is a tendency to overemphasize the similarity of twins and to deny the fact that their congenital experiences are probably different, as evidenced by the simple fact that nearly all twins are different weights at birth, and there is particularly a tendency to deny that their postnatal environments are dissimilar, even though they have very different social assignments, and therefore interpersonal experiences, and therefore personality developments. We suggest the possibility that if the psychological reaction of the individual in adjusting to disruption of a significant object relationship is of significance in time of manifest development of leukemia, or any other disease, the frequency of development of the same disease in both members of a pair of monozygotic twins may be in part a function of the reaction of twins to separation from one another, which is probably unique in interpersonal experience. The loss or threat of loss for the well individual whose twin has developed some disease may be as important in disease concordance as similarity in genic endowment. This factor may be less significant after age seven in development, when psychological and interpersonal differentiation of the twins is relatively more complete.

In summary, it should be emphasized that these three sets of discordant twins did not all have the same type of leukemia; acute myeloblastic leukemia, we assume, is a different type of disease than chronic myelocytic leukemia. The finding of the Ph^1 chromosome in each twin with chronic myelocytic leukemia, and not in the well twin, suggests that this is a postzygotic, acquired chromosomal abnormality, congenital or postnatal, but it does not completely exclude the possibility of a predisposing factor or factors for the induction of the Ph^1 chromosome.

In each twin pair, the symptoms of leukemia developed in a setting of major psychological stress – one that was stressful for the entire family, but particularly so for the affected twin: In set 19 the sick twin, after feeling left out when his brother went off to college and then married, became profoundly depressed when his second child was a girl rather than a boy; in set 17 an expressway was run through the middle of the family farm, taking land assigned to the sick twin but not that assigned to the well twin; and in set 15 the mother divorced the father.

The several types of information that have been gathered on these three sets of twins can be used in a number of ways and with varying degrees of emphasis in a consideration of the manifestation of leukemia in only one of the identical twins. It is our interpretation that the gestational circumstances, along with the ensuing role assignment, contributed to the magnitude and quality of the reaction to the acute, prodromal, stressful circumstances as a precipitating factor in the time of the manifest development of the leukemia. This interpretation in no way precludes the significance of undefined genic determinants, the likely contribution of previous differentiating physical illnesses, or the possibility of one or more undetermined mutagenic or viral agents. The course of each twin pair suggests that it may be fruitful to look at the psychological and social aspects of the prodromal circumstances along with psychological similarities and differences in each member developmentally, as well as the psychological aspects of the gestational circumstances. We strongly urge that this be done whenever there is an opportunity to study monozygotic twins who are either discordant or concordant for leukemia.

References

1. MacMahon, B. & M. A. Levy. 1964. Prenatal origin of childhood leukemia. Evidence from twins. New Eng. J. Med. **270:** 1082.
2. Hewitt, D., J. C. Lashof & A. M. Stewart. 1966. Childhood cancer in twins. Cancer **19:** 157.
3. Thomas, E. D., H. L. Lochte, Jr., J. H. Cannon, O. D. Sahler & J. W. Ferrebee. 1959. Supralethal whole body irradiation and isologous marrow transplantation in man. J. Clin. Invest. **38:** 1709.
4. Atkinson, J. B., F. J. Mahoney, I. R. Schwartz & J. A. Hesch. 1959. Therapy of acute leukemia by whole body irradiation and bone marrow transplantation from an identical normal twin. Blood **14:** 228.
5. Miller, D. G. & H. D. Diamond. 1961. The biological basis of bone marrow transplantation. Med. Clin. N. Amer. **45:** 711.
6. Nowell, P. C. & D. A. Hungerford. 1960. Minute chromosome in human chronic granulocytic leukemia. Science **132:** 1497.

7. Goh, K. & S. N. Swisher.. 1965. Identical twins and chronic myelocytic leukemia. Chromosomal studies of a patient with chronic myelocytic leukemia and his normal identical twin. Arch. Intern. Med. **115:** 475.
8. Sandberg, A. A., J. Cortner, N. Takagi, M. A. Moghadam & L. H. Crosswhite. 1966. Differences in chromosome constitution of twins with acute leukemia. N. Eng. J. Med. **275:** 809.
9. Jacobs, E. M., J. K. Luce & R. Cailleau. 1966. Chromosome abnormalities in human cancer. Report of a patient with chronic myelocytic leukemia and his nonleukemic monozygotic twin. Cancer **19:** 869.
10. Goh, K., S. N. Swisher & E. C. Herman. 1967. Chronic myelocytic leukemia and identical twins. Additional evidence of the Philadelphia Chromosome as postzygotic abnormality. Arch. Intern. Med. **120:** 214.
11. Osborne, R. H. & F. V. DeGeorge. 1967. Cancer and contagious disease in twins. Interrelation of host defense mechanisms. Cancer **20:** 263.
12. Greene, W. A. 1954. Psychological factors and reticuloendothelial disease. I. Preliminary observations on a group of males with lymphomas and leukemias. Psychosom. Med. **16:** 220.
13. Greene, W. A., L. E. Young & S. N. Swisher. 1956. Psychological factors and reticuloendothelial disease. II. Observations on a group of women with lymphomas and leukemias. Psychosom. Med. **18:** 284.
14. Greene, W. A. 1966. The psychosocial setting of the development of leukemia and lymphoma. Ann. N. Y. Acad. Sci. **125:** 794.
15. Greene, W. A. 1966. Discussion of the papers. Psychophysiological Aspects of Cancer. Ann. N. Y. Acad. Sci. **125:** 919.
16. Greene, W. A. & G. Miller. 1958. Psychological factors and reticuloendothelial disease. IV. Observations on a group of children and adolescents with leukemia: an interpretation of disease development in terms of the mother-child unit. Psychosom. Med. **20:** 124.
17. Greene, W. A. 1959. Role of a vicarious object in the adaptation to object loss. II. Vicissitudes in the role of the vicarious object. Psychosom. Med. **21:** 438.
18. Miller, R. W. 1967. Persons with exceptionally high risk of leukemia. Cancer Res. **27:** 2420.

DISCUSSION OF THE PAPER

Miss Denah Harris (*New York, N. Y.*): In relation to Luke, whose grandfather died of cancer and who had only girls, would his reaction, when he had a daughter, and also his reaction to the death of his grandfather, be related to the tendency to identify the expectation of experience with that of the person for whom he is named, and might his reaction also be related to the tendency that is very marked in the human race, to be constantly unsure of our identities?

Dr. Greene: I think this is possible. I think that there were certain very early differentiating assignments, particularly in the 19th pair, which you can think of in terms of multiple generations. One of the striking things in this pair was Aluke 19, having a son, Aluke 19 the 10th. Luke was very despairing, very angry about his brother's name and his brother's name compared to his own, which may have had something to do with the grandfather, the mother's father, compared to his own father, I'm not sure what.

Miss Harris: The mother, as I remember it, always cried about the death of the father, evidently giving Aluke the feeling that the man he was named for was very highly prized by her. Do you have any data on her attitude toward her father, by comparison? Because that too, might bear on the incident, the activation, the psychosomatic malfunction.

Dr. Greene: Perhaps.

Dr. Day: This interesting travelogue of some interesting twin pairs is a subject that I'm sure we will want to discuss as a model for learning during our discussion later.

A SPECULATIVE MATHEMATICAL MODEL OF THE PSYCHOPHYSIOLOGIC SYSTEM

Robert H. Riffenburgh

Department of Statistics
The University of Connecticut
Storrs, Conn.

General Remarks on Multidisciplinary Models

In the more mature, inductive stages of a developing science, the scientist usually makes use of his data only to accept or reject specific hypotheses. He is seldom willing to follow where the data lead, as was true of the earlier, descriptive stages in the science's development; he wishes to lead the data. The debility was well pointed out, if slightly bitterly, by Magoun (1963), about the reception given c. 1950 to the early RNA, DNA theorizing: "The Zeitgeist of that period was not a favorable one, however, for such enlightened views." The answer to this problem is that when a science reaches its inductive, or explanatory, phases, the scientist should continue to follow and speculate upon the path indicated by the data as well as to formulate his specific hypotheses. This is, of course, more easily said than done. The logical process of this scientific philosophy has been outlined elsewhere by the author (1966).

In order to pursue such a process, the evolving mathematical model (for what is such a model but the abstraction and conceptual repackaging of some subset of characteristics of the phenomenon in question?) must not spring from or even be tied to a "method," i.e., a restricted set of conceptual tools, but must be methodologically eclectic.

If we think of a model in the way just introduced, and let us do so for the remainder of this paper, the essence of science is the process of architecting a *set of evolving models*. If these evolutionary models are to have eclectic properties, they may most efficiently be formed by modeling multidisciplinary theory, not by "multidisciplinizing," or coordinating, extant narrowly defined specific models.

In addition, it should be clearly recognized that the logic and planning and the subsequent analysis and inference may well, and rightfully, exceed the data-gathering process in time spent. The opposite is too often the case; vast amounts of talent and funds are expended to gather data for purposes not clearly thought out in advance, and often much of the information that remains is cast down the drain by cursory or, worse, erroneous analytic techniques and sloppy inferential logic.

Let us consider several reasons for comprehensive modeling. These reasons will be listed but not discussed, since their meaning is obvious either immediately or upon a moment's reflection:

1. The most basic reason, implicit above in the "architecture of science" concept, has been said succinctly by Harmon and Lewis (1966): A model represents a "coherent, parsimonious description of nature."

2. A formal modeling effort forces clarity of thought and advance planning on the experimenter.

3. Through system modeling, the experimenter will find it difficult to divorce his work from its position in the organizational structure of major theories; he is

likely to find and retain the "big picture." Thus, studies on details may be coordinated and their quality assessed.

4. Vying for first-rank importance in reasons for system modeling is what might be called "cybernetic" or "white-box" experimentation. In many sciences – medicine and oceanography, to name two – the subject matter restricts the scientist from comprehensive experimentation. With the relevant characteristics of the system abstracted to a model, the scientist may experiment at will, utilizing the data that fate makes available to verify the efficacy of the model and its results.

5. "Cybernetic experimentation" may be conducted with new patterns of subsystems abstracted from their constraining physical orientations. Specifically in medicine, the model elements may be organized according to whatever functions are needed and not restricted to anatomic location or structure. (For example, in this paper the set of all sensor cells in the body compose a single functional location, or "white box," unrelated to their true anatomic distribution.)

6. When the system is organized into a comprehensive model, the most important elements relevant to some function of interest may be identified.

7. Following number 6 is the prediction of and/or control of system functions through measurement of and/or control of relevant elements.

8. A representative functional model may act as an estimating transducer in the sense that sometimes unknown values of elements must take on only certain ascertainable values in order for the model to function representatively. (In this paper, "transducer" is used in a general sense, not being restricted to strict electrical transducing, although electrical transducing remains one possible meaning.)

The Nature of a Psychophysiologic Model

When invited to give this paper, I took as a starting point the published papers of the last conference on psychophysiological aspects of cancer (Ann. N. Y. Acad. Sci. **125**, Art. 3, 1966.) Most of the studies involved one or two variables and little speculation as to the broad implications of the results. The plethora of this type of study throughout medicine was observed by Jonas (1966): "Present day medical thinking has tended to concentrate on the analysis of details, while at the same time the synthesizing propensity has fallen more and more into the background. This fragmentation has become the hallmark of both practical medicine and research." On the other hand, those who took the more "macro," or system-level, approach, and were thus able to make more sweeping generalizations, were unable to verify any part of their models except by reference to these very crucial "micro" studies. What impressed me particularly was that system coordination is almost impossible, because every study has its own set of underlying assumptions and unique frame of reference. What seems to be needed is a comprehensive system-level model into which the "micro" studies could fit as elements and the "macro" studies as subsets. I have not been able to find such a model in the literature.

What would be the characteristics of such a model? To satisfy the eight uses listed above, a system-level model must be (a) explicit, (b) measurable, (c) comprehensive, (d) communicable, and (e) repeatable (in both derivation and use) by others. One may find "conceptual models," as evinced in Grinker's (1953) chapter 3 heading: "Current Conceptual Models," but they fail requirements (a) and (b) and often (d) and (e). One may find "schematic models" in which a set of relationships are explicitly defined via some "scheme" or diagram, but (b) is lacking, since there is no measurement of system input/output or of the system components' effects on one another; Alexander (1950) is a good example of this. Perhaps closest to satisfying the requirements is a model of Bahnson and Bahnson (1964), in which they propose and discuss measurement, but explicitly derive none. Additionally, no model found involves an explicitly derived relationship of the system functions to the measurable physics of physiologic phenomena, which relationship would permit the "micro" studies of physiology – usually the most reliable scientifically – to enter as system elements.

With trepidation, I have attempted to form a speculative model, only pieces of which will be permitted by the space allowed here, designed to illustrate satisfaction of the criteria specified above. I wish to stress that this is *not* claimed to be the comprehensive model needed. My purpose here is to attempt the framework of a model capable of encompassing the psychophysiologic system relating even the "macro" and "micro" extremes of behavior and cell theory and perhaps to demonstrate the possibility and feasibility of such a model. It is stressed that this model is not claimed to represent the "is" of the system, but rather the "could be" of the system, in that it does not conflict with knowledge to date. In this sense, it is strictly a *speculative* mathematical model, no more.

If one takes the view that a psychologic stimulus is information fed into the system, which functions as a processing unit and outputs as physiologic activity, one is almost inevitably led to the cybernetic image of the psychosomatic complex as an information network replete with instructions, feedback, crossfeed, transducers, and noise. It is in this framework that I have considered the current model.

While such an approach may seem obvious in terms of today's sophistication, the early leap to such thinking two to three decades ago, primarily by McCulloch and his cohorts (e.g., McCulloch & Pitts, 1943, and Pitts & McCulloch, 1947), remains phenomenal. My thinking here appears to me not to have advanced significantly since McCulloch (1949) said of the "psyche" and "soma": "The real bridge we have is the science of signals, newly developed out of the art of communication. For a signal has a double nature; it is a physical event, which happens only once in a singular world, yet it is essentially capable of being true or else false." The primary difference today seems to be in the Zeitgeist, to recall Magoun's remark quoted earlier (Magoun, 1963).

The system model considered here will not be "physioanatomical," but rather "physiofunctional." As mentioned, the entire set of endocrine glands, for example, may be represented as a single function in a single model location, despite the fact that they are anatomically diverse and distributed.

A Sketch of the Model

A gross block diagram of the information network underlying the model as related to physiologic functional areas is presented as FIGURE 1. If the reader will follow the passage of information through the system originating at Source (top left), he will see that most of the paths are well recognized and long accepted. A few steps, however, should probably be documented.

The function of the sensors is rather well known. The signal is thought to go to the reticular system by collateral impulses (e.g. Magoun, 1963), which grades (in the electrical sense) the activity of the rest of the brain, operating as filter, integrator, and distributor. Noise, in the form of a variable membrane potential and random nerve firings, coexists with the signal (e.g., Vierstein & Grossman, 1961) and must be filtered out by a variable response to the signal-to-noise ratio. In addition, the most reasonable explanation for the phenomenon of habituation of neural cells is the gradual "classification" by the reticular system of the signal

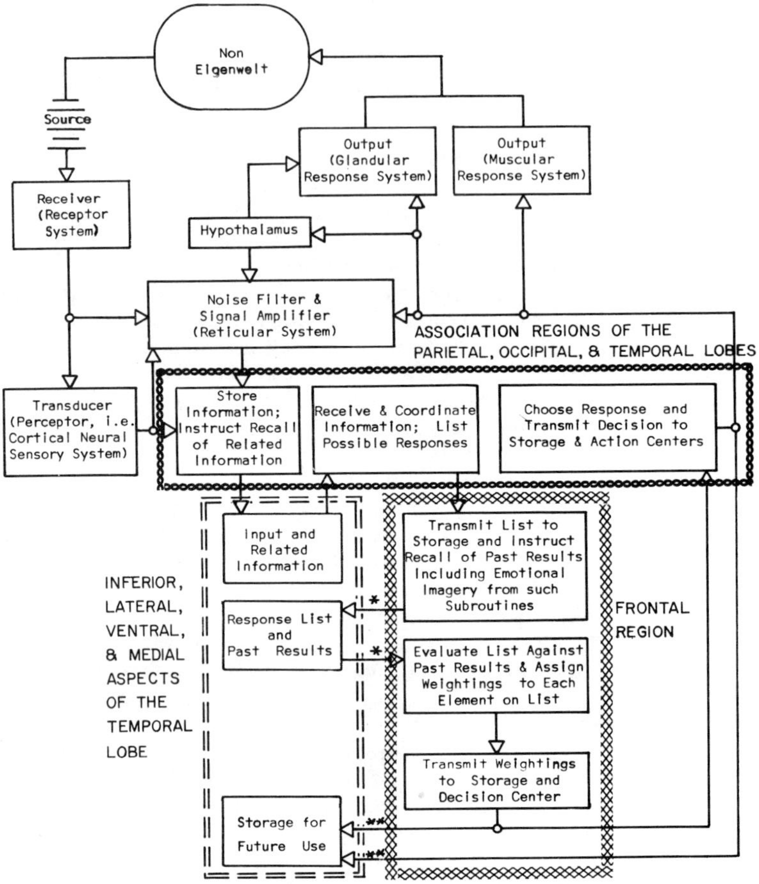

* Represents the recall of emotional imagery from storage. See text.
** This "store" instruction alters the memory of the "importance" of past events. See text.

FIGURE 1. Gross diagram of information network underlying model as related to physiologic functional areas with most cross-feeds and feedbacks not depicted.

as not worthy of transmission, i.e., as noise. The reticular system, then, amplifies or damps the signal and transmits the amplification or damping instructions to the association regions of the cortex as ancillary to the signal relayed from the perceptor. The perceptor, as the occipital region in the case of the visual stimuli, serves as a psychologic "transducer" putting the data into processable form, i.e., differentiating the type of stimulus, and transmitting it to the association regions of the cortex, which have logical processing as a function. In order to process the data in a logical fashion, this functional region must recall relevant information from storage – and of course, store the current information against possible future use. The recalled information enters the logic processing, and the set of possible actions is listed. Evaluation of possible action apparently occurs in the frontal region. The frontal region calls from memory the outcome of past decisions, including emotional imagery, similar to each element in the list.

One colleague feels that the frontal region is overstressed. This is probably correct, and if so, any overstress would be due to oversimplification. While some of the activity attributed to the frontal region occurs following ablation of this region, such activity is markedly reduced, which becomes crucial when it is noted that other activities that would be reduced if the reduction were just due to a general loss of large numbers of neural cells are little hindered. In particular, dealing with the visual circuit, Young (1964) says: "The circuit as a whole . . . can act as an amplifying device, in the sense of increasing the effectiveness of visual impulses in producing . . . [a correct response]. In particular, the lateral superior frontal itself seems to be necessary." More general is an earlier comment by von Bonin (1950): "One region of the brain, however, appears to be particularly adapted to forecasting. This is the frontal sector . . . the frontal lobe appears to be at least an important part of the forecasting mechanism, peculiarly unencumbered by other functions." Thus, probably much or most but not all of the activities here ascribed to the frontal region lie there. However, even if they do not, their functions are present and a simple renaming of the region performing these functions will retain the accuracy of FIGURE 1 with no change required of the model or its interpretation at the level here considered.

The asterisk footnote in the path will be referred to later, in the section entitled "Some Results of the 1965 Conference as Related to the Model." It represents the recall of emotional imagery from storage. The storage is apparently largely in the temporal lobe. There is evidence that the recall of emotional imagery redintegrates some of the original experience, perhaps in the closely related amygdala. Lesse (1960) found ". . . patterns of high voltage, rhythmic activity have been recorded from the region of the amygdala in human subjects during the recall of emotionally significant past experiences." Thus, the "call" instruction itself serves to redintegrate associated emotions, apparently, including general approach-withdrawal feelings in the system.

With its list of possible results from possible responses plus related memory, the frontal region proceeds to associate the "cost" of each possible result times the probability that it will occur associated with each element on the list. These "values" (perhaps subjective values – not necessarily directly relatable to a metric space) may be thought of as "weightings" for each list item, or the coefficients of Bayesian decision theory. Again, this speculation is not pure fancy. A common computer memory core (with random connection deletions but inhibitory as well as excitatory abilities to counteract the deletions) could be "twisted" and "shaped" (mathematically: mapped into a dual space) to match the dendritic patterns of neural connections. The addition of the ideas of facilitating neural junctions (by graded potentials) (Josephson, 1964) and of amplification-damping processes in resonant neural networks (Reiss, 1964) provides analog signals of a nature that would permit the derivation of a network mathematical submodel performing the capacities here speculated. Such a network model would have some properties similar to that of McCulloch and Pitts (1943), but would be stochastic, i.e., would involve probable paths rather than certain paths.

The weightings for the list elements are sent both to storage and to the decision center. The decision is made, and the result is sent both to storage and to the reticular system for relay into action.

The double-asterisk footnote on these last two "store" instructions will be referred to later, in the section entitled "Some Results of the 1965 Conference as Related to the Model." This store instruction alters the memory of the "importance" of past events, apparently by altering the potential and capacitance of the agglomeration of memory cells involved, and it is thus crucial in altering the accumulated resistivities of functional regions. The effect of a graded potential induced in varying numbers of cells and maintained by continued re-store instructions arising from continued awareness of the phenomenon remembered on the cellular RNA and eventually the nuclear DNA accounts for the long-term memory of some weightings and action outcomes and not others.

The hypothalamus is seen to intercept the response instructions from the decision center and crossfeed to the reticular system and glandular system. This is depicted to permit a crossfeed spiral (or "vicious" circle, ineptly named in that it may involve nothing that could be called vicious) between abstract/emotion areas of the brain and response without requiring a return through the stimulus-receptor-perceptor route. This relationship is documented by Ruch and colleagues (1961): "The posterior hypothalamus is . . . a way station in the *descending* system producing emotional display and in the *ascending* reticular system producing alertness and wakefulness."

The remainder of FIGURE 1 should be self-explanatory with the caution that most of the crossfeeds and feedbacks are not depicted, since such depicting would induce more confusion than the accuracy would add.

As if the "receiver-processor-transmitter" configuration were not enough to lead one to the electrical terms of physics, comments pervaded the first conference that stimulate one in this direction, although the speakers may not have intended electrical connotations. For example, Bahnson and Bahnson (1966) said "The matter of discharge routing becomes crucial." Feder (1966), in a panel discussion, observed a "gradual shift over a period of years from the idea of specific etiological factors to a consideration of the phenomenon of *altered host resistance* as the key in setting any disease off," and it seemed to him that "the concept of *host resistance* is a point where the physiologists, anatomists, chemists, psychiatrists, and psychologists can meet" (italics mine). He might even have included the physicists, engineers, and mathematicians.

Regarding FIGURE 2, if we think of a set or agglomeration of cells, each of

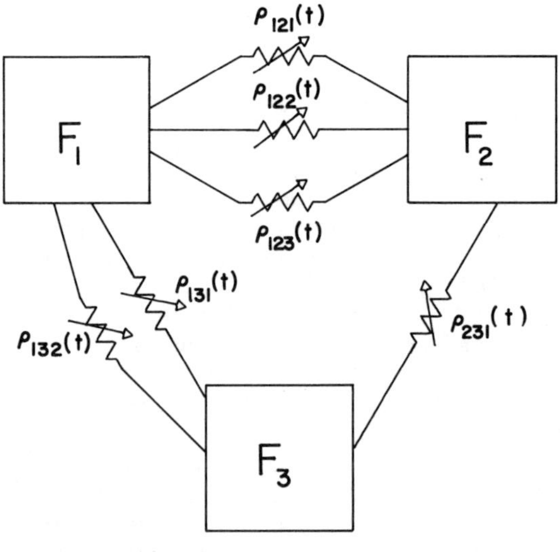

FIGURE 2. A diagram to illustrate function cell-sets and their related resistivities.

which has electrochemical properties, it must be obvious that the set will have electrochemical properties as a unit. Let F_i designate a set of cells combined conceptually by being involved in a common function. The i is an index. F_1 is the 1st such F named, F_2 the 2nd, etc. It can be seen that a certain cell could lie in two F's simultaneously if it is involved in two functions. Let $\rho_{ijk}(t)$ designate the resistivity (1/conductance) over the kth path between F_i and F_j at time t. For example, $\rho_{231}(t)$ is the resistivity over the first path between F_2 and F_3 at time t.

The following is a list of definitions for some symbols used:

Symbol	Definition
F_i	Set of cells combined conceptually by being commonly involved in the i:th function
$\rho_{ijk}(t)$	Resistivity over the k:th path between F_i and F_j at time t, $i \neq j$
$V_{ij}(t)$	Subsystem potential between F_i, F_j at t
$Q_i(t)$	Measure of subsystem charge in F_i at t
$C_i(t) = \sum_{j'} \frac{Q_i(t)}{V_{ij}(t)}$ $\begin{cases} j'=j \text{ if } i,j \text{ connected}, i \neq j, \\ j' \text{ not counted otherwise} \end{cases}$	Measure of capacitance in F_i at t
$p_{ijk}(t)$	Endoreticular: random generator for probability of path k between F_i, F_j at time t; Exoreticular: unity (1)
$R_{ij}(t) = \sum_k p_{ijk}(t)\,\rho_{ijk}(t)$	Resistance between F_i, F_j, $i \neq j$, at time t over all paths
$I_{ij}(t) = V_{ij}(t)/R_{ij}(t)$	Current between F_i, F_j, $i \neq j$, at t, all paths
$P_{ij}(t) = I_{ij}(t)\, V_{ij}(t)$	Power in ij:th functional pair, $i \neq j$, at time t over all paths

The first two have already been defined, and all but one of the remainder (viz. potential, charge, capacitance, resistance, current, and power) will be recognized as standard electrical relations, if one accepts the cell-set concept. This one exception is a probability, or randomly generated path choice.

All neural cells exhibit random phenomena (e.g., Harigawa, 1954). When only a relatively few cells are involved, the phenomenon is not significant enough to include in a system-level model; thus, the probability is taken as "one" in these neural regions. However, in the higher neural centers (or "endoreticular," as depicted in FIGURE 1), there are enough cells to require a probability factor in the model. Von Bonin (1950) concurs: "'Punctate' cortical regions will, in such a theory, be replaced by 'probability regions.'" The introduction of random neural processing in "man – that most improbable of all structures!" (Boulding, 1964) appears more an imposition of evolution than a coincidence. In the immediate view, random pathway selection seems to be requisite to maintain neural system tonicity; in the longer view, it is requisite for the survival of the species. If there were no random experimentation with new or not commonly used mental pathways, the organism would soon achieve too high a state of mental homeostasis, lose adaptability, and become easy prey for predators or destructive chance events.

Now what we should like to do is to tie the system properties of the information network of FIGURE 1, via our electrical symbolism, to psychophysiologic phenomena to obtain system criteria capable of explaining some of the results of the previous conference on psychophysiological aspects of cancer. In keeping with the principle of parsimony, we wish the fewest criteria possible in order to explain the phenomena. Probably general psychophysiologic behavior is many-variabled, but it appears we can manage reasonable explanations of the phenomena with four variables I have developed for this purpose. Let us derive S, V, E, and C. This is done in the following continuation of the definitions list:

Symbol	Definition
$P(t)$	$\sum_i \sum_j P_{ij}(t)$
$\dot{P}(t)$	$\sum_{\substack{i \\ i \neq j}} \sum_j I_{ij}(t) \sum_k p_{ijk}(t)\ \rho_{ijk}(t)$ for all i,j such that $\frac{d}{dt}\rho_{ijk}(t) \geq 0$
$\ddot{P}(t)$	$P(t) - \dot{P}(t)$
$S(t)$	$b^{\dot{P}(t) - \ddot{P}(t)}$
$V(t)$	$\sum_i \sum_j V_{ij}(t)$
$\Pi_{ij}[k \mid R_{ij}(t)]$	Probability that an impulse travelling from F_i to F_j uses path k, given $R_{ij}(t)$
$E(t)$	$-\sum_{\substack{i \\ i \neq j}} \sum_j \sum_k \Pi_{ij}[k \mid R_{ij}(t)] \ln \Pi_{ij}[k \mid R_{ij}(t)]$
$C(t)$	$\sum_i C_i(t)$
S_{OI}, V_{OI}, E_{OI}, C_{OI}	$\frac{1}{t_1 - t_0} \int_{t_0}^{t_1} \left\{ \begin{matrix} S(t) \\ V(t) \\ E(t) \\ C(t) \end{matrix} \text{ respectively} \right\} dt$

If the simple summing of component electrical measurements into system measurements seems heretical, heed Grinker (1956): "From the single living cell to the cerebral cortex mantle, energy systems are in a constant state of flux, and apparent differences in directional flow are only indications of an algebraic sum at a given time since all directions are always concurrently present."

P(t) is summed to yield a power-in-the-system at time t. Then P(t) is partitioned into $\dot{P}(t)$ for power associated with homeostatic and decreasing resistivities and $\ddot{P}(t)$ for increasing resistivities. The difference, $\dot{P}(t)-\ddot{P}(t)$, represents homeostatic and relaxing power less tension power; the exponentiation to get S(t) is just for mapping convenience, and the constant base, b, will adjust the scale to the individual in question. The system potential, or voltage, at time t, V(t), is given by summing over component potentials. Summing over the conditional probabilities, π's, times their logarithms yields a momentary conditional entropy, E(t), for the system. At last, summing over component capacitances gives a system capacitance, C(t). S(t), V(t), E(t), and C(t) are all variables measured at a point in time. While sometimes the form of the function conditional upon time is of interest, more relevant to our current problem are the mean functions over an arbitrary period of time, which may be named t_0 to t_1. The mean function is given by the integral over the time period of the function divided by the time period. These four integrals define S_{01}, V_{01}, E_{01}, and C_{01}. We may speak of simply S, V, E, and C if we understand that each refers to itself properly subscripted, but shall specify subscripts or functional dependence otherwise.

Now let us consider what S, V, E, and C mean conceptually. All may vary from 0 to ∞, so only the first hexadecimant of the four-dimensional Euclidean space need be considered in mapping point-sets. We shall refer hereafter to such a space simply as the SVEC space. S might be thought of as a system resistance dimension, or a tension scale. The log of S is the power in the system devoted to activities involving homeostatic or increasing resistivities. If the totality of conductances is increasing, the system may process more information, i.e., engage in more neural activity and hence interaction with the non-Eigenwelt, for the same power. If the total resistance is increasing, the system requires greater power just to handle the same information processing. Thus, when the system resistance as a total pattern is increasing, the system uses more and more available power on the same level of accomplishment; the person is becoming tenser and less efficient per unit power and S is small. S approaches 0 asymptotically as the system resistance increases without bound. If the resistance increase just balances the conductance increase, $\dot{P}-\ddot{P}=0$ and $S=b$, the base for the individual. This can happen by $\dot{P}$ being small or by P being large but evenly partitioned between $\dot{P}$ and $\ddot{P}$; the latter is unlikely to be seen often and will probably show up in E or V, so we can get along without including P as another dimension for the moment. If the system conductance as a total pattern is increasing, the system has greater power to cope with its information input and recalled emotions; the person is becoming less overwhelmed and more serene and S is large. The idea of achieving great system power, including having extensive interaction with the environment and vivid emotions, and yet retaining serenity is delightful to contemplate both philosophically and psychologically. Thus, the S stands for a Serenity measure, although the "powerfully serene" position on S occurs only at a very large value, perhaps psychologically unattainable; the more usual positionings on S are in the lower values, where S may be more effectively considered a measure of tension or stress.

V is a totality of electrical potential in the system, resulting directly from a system-accumulated electrical driving force. It may be most simply conceived intuitively as a psychic kinetic drive force dimension. With low V, there cannot be much power in the system. With high V, there is force, but the power is inversely proportional to the resistance; there can be great force but little power if the resistance is high. A person with high V is psychologically very active; the person with low V is passive, although not necessarily relaxed.

E is an entropy measure. It deals with the variety of choice in responses open to the individual under normal circumstances. If the probability of any one pathway between F_i and F_j is the same as any other, for every pair i,j, then E is maximum, i.e., very large. In this state, the system is as likely to make one response to a stimulus as another, whatever the stimulus. If, at the other extreme, the probability of one path for each pair i,j is unity (and therefore 0 for all other paths for that pair), the value of E is 0. Thus, the greater the order and predictability of the system, the less is E. From this interpretation plus the similarity of the defining formula, we may name this variable Entropy – hence, E. However, there is a difference from engineering theory: While 0 entropy is ideal in electronic packages and servomechanisms, 0 entropy in our theory would imply exactly predictable behavior. In the neuromuscular subsystem, for example, 0 entropy would occur only in a state of catatonia if not coma. Moderate but not large entropy is a prerequisite of evolutionary survival and an interesting intellectual condition. "To define order as good," say von Bonin (1950), "does not imply to define randomness as bad. Bad is the destruction of order, not its absence. For there must be randomness if there is to be any novelty." Consider a case in which V is high and S is low. The current is branched to infrequently (under "normal" V and S) chosen pathways, resulting in aberrant behavior. If E is low, the aberrant behavior is repetitive; if E is high, the aberrant behavior is varied.

C might be thought of as a system frustration-capacitance dimension. (Note the difference between "capacity" and "capacitance." C is a measure of the amount of charge-to-potential accumulated, not a measure of the ability to accumulate it.) If C is low, the individual responds immediately to stimulus; he tends to be more aggressive and turns his responses outward. If C is high, the charge from external stimuli may build up considerably before capacitive discharge forces response. Consider again the case in which V is high and S is low; the individual is driven, but meets internal resistance at every turn. If C is low, the individual responds projectively, frustratedly. He may throw things and shout in anger, or in more severe cases, he may become paranoid. If C is high, the charge evoked by the stimuli may be accumulated and tolerated for some time. The person responds more quietly, becoming anxious; in more severe cases, he may become depressed.

It should be understood that these paragraphs on interpretation of S, V, E, and C do not constitute their definitions; their definitions were given as specific, exactly communicable formulas. These interpretations are intended to serve only the function of providing preliminary connotations, or "gut feelings," for those not at home with symbolic manipulation.

Any psychologic or psychophysiologic system of inferential theory may be based upon identifying a set of variables from a space such that the normal and various pathologic states are identifiable by positions and/or motions in the space. Only recently have there been overt attempts to organize such inferential theory in a precisely communicable fashion, and often associated measurements are made only on related variables, not the particular variables of the postulated system. Most such efforts begin at the gross-behavior level and attempt to refine, i.e., most do not arise as, a systematization of known, physiologic components basic at the atomic level. The system-level model here considered is composed of variables that are precisely communicable, and it has arisen from the most basic components. Its variables are theoretically precisely and repeatedly measurable, although some very sophisticated tools would have to be engineered for this purpose. Working with the model, I feel intuitively that it adumbrates a nonpareil psychophysiologic coordination. However, such foreshadowing can here be nothing more than intuitive; this model is based on a chain of logic having "could be" rather than "is" in many of its links and thus may be taken seriously for nothing more than its current purpose: to demonstrate the possibility and, one hopes, even the feasibility of a system model capable of relating psychologic and physiologic processes in an exact, communicable, measurable, and verifiable fashion.

Consider the SVEC space. A psychophysiologic state may be thought of as a region in the space (a probability density with centroid and dispersion about the centroid). On the other hand, a S(t), V(t), E(t), C(t) space may be considered with psychophysiologic processes taken as a function in hyperspherical coordinates (r, θ, ϕ, ξ, say), which would be similar to the region concept except that the centroid of the probability density is subject to motion and the dispersion matrix is a function of the centroid's transient location. Further, if it is desired to map discrete psychophysiologic states over discrete time periods, mappings of the vector $(S_{01}V_{01}E_{01}C_{01})$ into $(S_{12}V_{12}E_{12}C_{12})$ or $(S_{23}V_{23}E_{23}C_{23})$ for general times t_0, t_1, t_2, and t_3 may provide insights. In the continuous case, the use of the vector analysis methods of gradient and divergence appear amenable in analyzing the flows of probability densities.

It is difficult to depict points or point sets in four-dimensional space. Let us consider a subspace for a moment. FIGURE 3 illustrates the location and/or motion in the SVE space of some representative psychophysiologic states. The reader may relate these locations and motions to the definitions of S, V, and E. Since several aberrant states plus one end of the normal density lie in about the same value of V, let us remap them into the SEC space, to make use of C, remembering that V holds fixed. This remapping composes FIGURE 4.

The mapping of the whole system in SVEC space may seem too simple and gross to represent man's psychologic complexities. It is, of course. It was stated that only four of many possible variables were chosen for parsimony. However, an additional oversimplification must be admitted: There should probably be a multivariable space for each of several subsystems. Such subsystems may not even be time-unique; the list of component neurons in a neural network composing a subsystem might vary with time. This has long been recognized. McCulloch and Pitts (1943) say: "The crux of this ignorance is that inference from any sample of overt behavior to nervous nets is not unique." For example, in FIGURE 3, catatonia was characterized by having very low entropy. It is true that the muscular behavior of a catatonic is quite predictable; it is also true that the emotional behavior of a catatonic is quite unpredictable. This suggests that we should consider spaces for two or more subsystems. If we consider an m-dimensional variable space for each of n subsystems, we must then think of a psychophysiologic state as mapped in an $m \times n$ space. However, in view of the current state of the art, the purposes expounded here, and space-time limitations, it seems reasonable to tolerate the simplicity of the four-dimensional SVEC space for this first pass at the problem. To ascribe too much detail at this stage would tempt immanent errors, as predicted by Sholl (1956): "Such speculation is valuable insofar as it stimulates the production of new hypotheses that are experimentally testable,

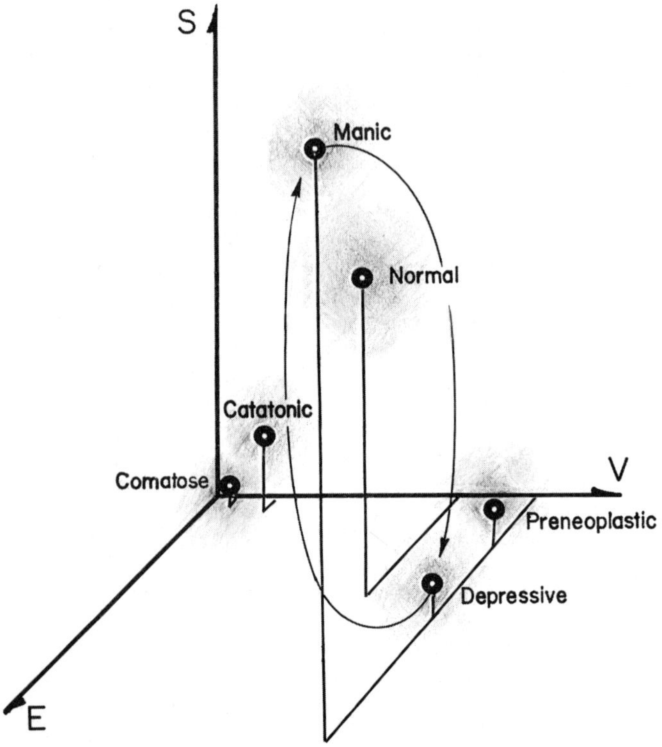

FIGURE 3. The SVE space with the location and/or motion of some representative psychophysiologic states illustrated.

but it is dangerous to devote time to the development of high-level hypotheses remote from experimental observation."

The question of the relation of this model to oncology has yet to be considered. In FIGURE 3, a "preneoplastic" personality was positioned as having a higher-than-normal V. In FIGURE 4, he may be seen in the SEC space as low S, low E, and high C. The high V indicates considerable drive and energy at work in response to inputs. The low E indicates very few channels for output. The low S indicates tension and high resistance for output in the few acceptable channels remaining. The high C permits the force to accumulate until it reaches a level at which the capacitive discharges will be intolerably high. Now let us invoke the Law of Conservation of Energy. The energy is conserved; the energy may not be released through overt behavior; the energy is large in amount; the energy must be released. The only solution admissible to physics is a somatic release at a continuingly high rate, with resulting somatic dysfunction. That such dynamics occur was suggested by Dunbar (1943) in a claim – perceptive for his time – that "psychic energy" (not in the form of electric energy) obeys the First Law of Thermodynamics. How and why neoplastic disease should be chosen from among the somatic dysfunctions is unknown (although often hypothesized). The following section offers some speculation on the subject.

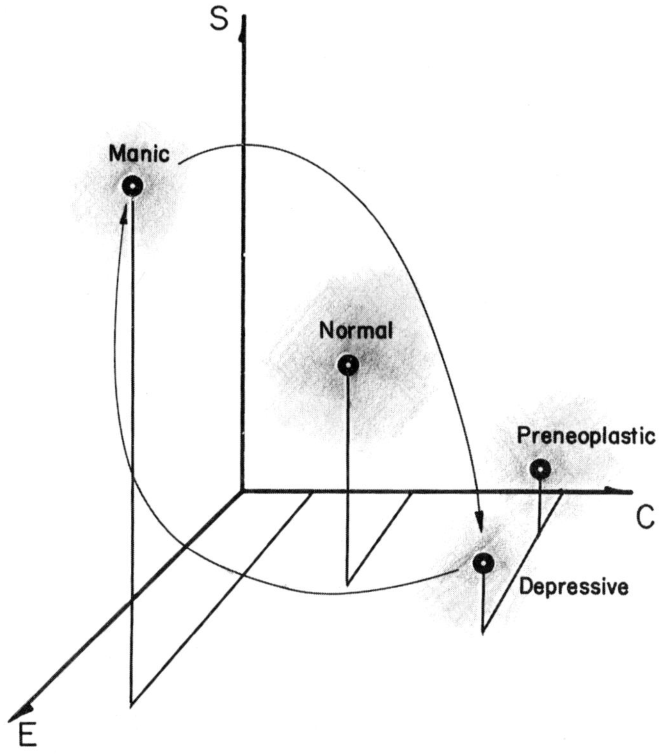

FIGURE 4. The SEC space with the location and/or motion of some representative psychophysiologic states illustrated.

Some Results of the 1965 Conference as Related to the Model

In this section, the major purpose is to show that a model can be comprehensive, coordinating various studies and permitting more extensive interpretation of detailed results.

Consider the ideas of LeShan (1966). When a young child experiences the loss of a loved one, a large class of previously rewarding interactions with the non-Eigenwelt is blocked. Pleasant emotional recall at the point indicated by the asterisk in FIGURE 1 becomes mixed with unpleasant, giving rise to high-cost, low-prior-probability Bayesian coefficients at the point indicated by the double asterisk in FIGURE 1. Rapidly increasing resistivities over large regions immediately follow. S plunges. The child is forced toward low entropy by denial rather than maturation. Eventually, he "adjusts," i.e., the current finds lower resistance pathways for dissipation and V increases to provide the additional power necessary for "acceptable" P levels. S increases again. The process of entropy decrease by maturation continues from its newly lowered base at a more rapid than normal rate due to the increased resistivities. The mature person appears to be normal, but has a higher V and lower E than normal. Given a second great personal loss, and tracing the same circuit effects, the S and E become very small, the V large. The person is now high-pressured, but low-powered. His entropy is very low, as is his S. Note the position of the preneoplastic individual in FIGURE 3.

Now let us compare our patient to Kissen's (1966) observations. Kissen found a poor outlet for emotional discharge in cancer patients. Such people tend to have a high C. The high resistance constrains the patient from perceiving (internally) many of the actions his system would like to take (i.e., from perceiving what would increase S), and the Bayesian coefficients constrain him from choosing to act on the remainder (i.e., from attempting to reduce E). The patient goes through the motions of life, feeling empty and unfulfilled. He is climbing a mountain that has no top. He can "top" the mountain only by increasing S, C, and E, which would also serve to reduce V, since a lower V would then permit the same power in the system.

Now let us take our patient to Bahnson and Bahnson (1966). The system cannot tolerate the high voltage. If C were low, so that the capacitance of the system were exceeded, the current would "surge," "blowing" resistors, and the "short circuits" would be manifested in psychopathic behavior, which would be interesting to consider when more space is available. However, this patient already has a high C and low E, so this mode of discharge is unlikely. Where is the current to go? Remember our random path generator $p_{ijk}(t)$. With the more mature levels of behavior blocked, $p_{ijk}(t)$ will sooner or later instruct the current to attempt pathways on a level below that resisted on the cortical and parietal levels, i.e., instruct it to try "regressed" pathways, bypassing upper-brain judgment on appropriateness and feasibility of response. The current passes directly from the reticular to the temporal storage region and returns. Bizarre, uncoordinated instructions reach the hypothalamus, passing on in turn as uncalled glandular discharge. Occasionally a "grow" instruction is issued from the pituitary to some randomly selected site. The site may respond if the signal is strong and frequent enough, especially if it has been irritated by external sources and desires an instruction as to how to respond, as for example with smoke-irritated lungs. Thus cell proliferation and dedifferentiation, the most regressed manifestation of somatic discharge, results and the patient develops a neoplasm.

Grinker (1966) concurs: ". . . growth and development leading to pride, productivity, and creativity are significant antidotes to disease." That is, if the patient were able to increase S and E, the neoplasm might be avoided. In addition, Grinker states: "On the contrary, failures in growth and development associated with shame-anxiety are facilitative toward illness." Anxiety is certainly associated with low S. He points out that age and maturity predispose the multivariable etiology of disease. Note the V, E pattern in relation to the maturity of our patient.

Shands (1966) points out that the system seeks to process new information in old programs – a low-entropy characteristic. The bypassed upper brain, i.e., the misdirected message, may provide feedback that the low entropy processes into a pattern of response, favoring whatever paths result in a reduced voltage; a random result may be thus self-reinforcing, a cross-feed spiral.

Paloucek and Graham (1966) would say that a model must be able to vary with the individual's genetic and cultural background. Does ours here? The basic building blocks of all four variables are cell potentials and resistivities that vary from cell to cell and individual to individual for any reason desired. The answer is yes.

Hagnell (1966) postulated the basis of a model, giving four dimensions of personality. Do they mesh with the proposed model here, or do they conflict? Hagnell first proposes a Capacity Factor: intellectual ability of the individual. This factor relates to b, the base in S for the individual, and probable domain, i.e., a stochastic interval, in P or S. He does not consider a measure of the use one makes of this capacity, either in the total (P or S) or in partitions relating to the improvement or homeostasis ($\dot{P}$) and the degradation of ($\ddot{P}$) of the system. He next postulates a Stability Factor: tracking capability of the CNS (abstraction, emotional control, coolness). This factor is clearly closely related to our entropy, E, or more precisely, to its inverse. His third factor is a Solidity Factor: inertia of the nervous system functioning; degree of lability and suggestibility in intellectual and emotional life. This factor is closest to C, but is clearly not independent of E or of V. It appears to be a linear function of C, E, and V, most heavily weighted on C, or at least such a linear function would give much the same information. Hagnell's fourth factor is a Validity Factor: the amount of energy supply for nervous system functioning; the amount of energy investment available. This factor appears to be almost identical with V. It is satisfying and somewhat relieving to find that my proposed model, quite naive with respect to psychiatric practice, agrees rather well with the modeling efforts of a man guided by experience and practice.

Acknowledgment

The author acknowledges with gratitude the invaluable assistance received from Drs. Claus Bahnson (Jefferson Medical College), Gilbert Glaser (Yale Medical School), and Charles Loeser (University of Connecticut Medical School) in the preparation of this paper.

References

ALEXANDER, F. 1950. Psychosomatic Medicine. W. W. Norton & Company, Inc. New York, N. Y.

BAHNSON, C. B. & M. B. BAHNSON. 1964. Cancer as an alternative to psychosis: A theoretical model of somatic and psychologic regression. *In* Psychosomatic Aspects of Neoplastic Disease. D. M. Kissen & L. L. LeShan, Eds. Sir Isaac Pitman & Sons, Ltd. London, England.

BAHNSON, C. B. & M. B. BAHNSON. 1966. Role of the ego defenses: Denial and repression in the etiology of malignant neoplasm. Ann. N. Y. Acad. Sci. **125** (Art. 3) : 827–845.

BOULDING, K. E. 1964. The Evolutionary Potential of Quakerism. Pendle Hill. Pendle Hill, Pa.

DUNBAR, H. B. 1943. Psychosomatic Diagnosis. Hoeber. New York, N. Y.

FEDER, S. L. 1966. Quoted from Panel Discussion: Retrospects and prospects. Ann. N. Y. Acad. Sci. **125**(Art. 3): 1032.

GRINKER, R. R. 1953. Psychosomatic Research. W. W. Norton & Company, Inc. New York, N. Y.

GRINKER, R. R. 1956. The intrapersonal organization. *In* Toward a Unified Theory of Human Behavior. R. R. Grinker, Ed. Basic Books, Inc., Publishers. New York, N. Y.

GRINKER, R. R. 1966. Discussion of the papers. Ann. N. Y. Acad. Sci. **125**(Art. 3): 874–875.

HAGNELL, O. 1966. The premorbid personality of persons who develop cancer in a total population investigated in 1947 and 1957. Ann. N. Y. Acad. Sci. **125**(Art. 3): 846–855.

HARIGAWA, S. 1954. Analysis of internal fluctuation of the sensory nerve impulse. Jap. J. Physiol. **4**: 234–240.

HARMON, L. D. & E. R. LEWIS. 1966. Neural modelling. Physiol. Rev. **46**(3): 513–591.

JONAS, A. D. 1966. Theoretical considerations concerning the influence of the central nervous system on cancerous growth. Ann. N. Y. Acad. Sci. **125**(Art. 3): 946–951.

JOSEPHSON, R. K. 1964. Coelenterate conducting systems. *In* Neural Theory and Modelling. R. F. Reiss, Ed. Stanford University. Stanford, Calif.

KISSEN, D. M. 1966. The value of a psychosomatic approach to cancer. Ann. N. Y. Acad. Sci. **125**(Art. 3): 777–779.

LESHAN, L. 1966. An emotional life-history pattern associated with neoplastic disease. Ann. N. Y. Acad. Sci. **125**(Art. 3): 780–793.

LESSE, H. 1960. Rhinencephalic electrophysiological activity during "emotional behavior" in cats. Psychiat. Res. Rep. Amer. Psychiat. Ass. **12**: 224–237.

MAGOUN, H. W. 1963. The Waking Brain. Charles C. Thomas, Publisher. Springfield, Ill.

McCULLOCH, W. S. 1949. Physiological processes underlying psychoneuroses. Proc. Roy. Soc. Med. **42**: 71–84.

McCULLOCH, W. S. & W. H. PITTS. 1943. A logical calculus of the ideas immanent in nervous activity. Bull. Math. Biophys. **5**: 115–133.

PALOUCEK, F. P. & J. B. GRAHAM. 1966. The influence of psycho-social factors on the prognosis in cancer of the cervix. Ann. N. Y. Acad. Sci. **125**(Art. 3): 814–816.

PITTS, W. H. & W. S. McCULLOCH. 1947. How we know universals: the perception of auditory and visual forms. Bull. Math. Biophys. **9**: 127–147.

REISS, R. F. 1964. A theory of resonant networks. *In* Neural Theory and Modelling. R. F. Reiss, Ed. Stanford University. Stanford, Calif.

RIFFENBURGH, R. H. 1966. On problems of sampling and decision in exotic environments. Cybernetica No. 2 : 109–117.

RUCH, T. C., H. D. PATTON, J. W. WOODBURY & A. L. TOWE. 1961. Neurophysiology. W. B. Saunders Company. Philadelphia, Pa.

SHANDS, H. C. 1966. The informational impact of cancer on the structure of the human personality. Ann. N. Y. Acad. Sci. **125**(Art. 3): 883–889.

SHOLL, D. A. 1956. The Organization of the Cerebral Cortex. Methuen. London, England.

VIERSTEIN, L. J. & R. G. GROSSMAN. 1961. Neural discharge patterns in the transmission of sensory information. *In* Information Theory (Fourth London Symposium). C. Cherry, Ed. Butterworths. London, England.

VON BONIN, G. 1950. Essay on the Cerebral Cortex. Charles C. Thomas, Publisher. Springfield, Ill.

YOUNG, J. Z. 1964. A Model of the Brain. Oxford University. Oxford, England.

DISCUSSION

Lawrence LeShan

Mills College of Education
New York, N. Y.

For a long time we have had increasing evidence of the relationship between genetic factors and stress. Earlies studies of lymphoma and leukemia show how well a synthetic approach, combining various approaches to study the same data, can work; longitudinal, genetic, constitutional, and psychological studies taken together can strengthen our understanding considerably.

For example, Greene points to a period of time largely ignored in most cancer studies and in studies in the psychosomatic area. He points to the importance of the time between the early infantile experiences and the "specific" predisposing event that seems to trigger off the cancer. The long life-history that goes between these two periods is of vital importance to the individual himself, yet, most studies have tended to ignore it.

Greene points up that we can ignore this long time-period only at the risk of severely distorting and limiting our data. To my knowledge, outside of the work of Booth, only one other study has referred specifically to this period and pointed up its importance. That is the study, very little known in this country, a cross-cultural study of leukemias, done by Hans Baltrusch a few years ago.

Friedman's paper shows, I think, how well the analytic and single-correlation approach can work, if used to study in detail one narrow area that would then increase the possibility of our making generalizations and synthesizing larger concepts. For example, a very valuable contribution is made when it is pointed out that noxious stimuli in childhood or afterward cannot be equated with the increased statistical likelihood of cancer. The important thing seems to be how the noxious stimuli play a part in determining the organism's perception or response to his environment. This is the crucial factor, rather than the noxious stimuli themselves.

Graham Bennette has pointed out that a strong stimulus can be either a challenge or a threat, depending upon the individual's ability to cope with it. I hope that this crucial point can be amplified further.

The same that is true of the noxious stimulus is true of the individual and group housing. I think all of us remember the early Andervont and other studies that would seem to point out that animal housing played a part in the development of cancer. We are gradually learning to appreciate, that the effect of the housing (and how this effects group host resistance) seems to be a factor concerned with the animal and the disease themselves rather than just the housing as a factor. We are reminded here of Vincent Ginsberg's work and the data Booth pointed to so strongly. Ginsberg raised three strains of mice. In one strain, if you gave them early gentling, later in life they were affectionate, warm and friendly. In the second strain, if you gave them early gentling, later in life they were aggressive and scrappy. In the third strain, it did not matter whether you gave them early gentling or not; whatever you did, they went right on in their own way and developed in their own manner.

Perhaps we should learn from all of this a new definition of the term "spontaneous." When we hear anybody use this term applying it to the appearance of the malignancy or to its regression, this should be a clear signal that whatever frame that individual is using is much too narrow for the problem. We should use it both in signaling to ourselves that the frames of reference are too narrow, and in referring to those of anyone else.

Riffenburgh's paper is a little difficult to sum up here. It is a bold and complex attempt at a theoretical model, and through using it we try to show the coherence and relatedness of various studies in the field. It is a type of tool that we need. I am afraid, however, that it is a type of tool that no one can respond to after hearing such a brief presentation. This is the kind of thing one must read, study, and experiment with, rather than just answer and discuss after hearing it for the first time. To respond too quickly to such a concept as this would be, I think, both superficial and arrogant.

Personally, I find a lack in it of the peculiarly human element. There does not seem to be much place for a human being in it. But this may well be because I understand so little of it at this time.

Perhaps one thing we can learn from this afternoon's session is that specific data are necessary, but only really useful when seen in a larger context, when used synthetically. The synthesis then presents new fields of data, new ideas, new places to look for hypotheses, and it goes on and on. We need two types of thinking.

Raymond Pearl, who was probably America's greatest biometrician, once pointed out the limitations of a scientific method as it is generally conceived. What he really meant was the analytic reductionist method of thinking, the 1-to-1 correlation method, what we used to call the method of concomitant variation. He said: "The scientific method in this sense is not a way of getting new ideas or new concepts. It is useless for this point. It is often a very useful way of testing ideas and testing hypotheses that we get through quite other methods of generating knowledge."

Max Wertheimer once caricatured the difference between the American and the German psychology laboratories. The American laboratory, he said, was full of mechanical and electrical equipment from plethysmographs to chemical testing devices. The equipment in the German's laboratory consisted of an easy chair and a pound of shag tobacco. We really need both types to go on.

I am going to end by stealing a leaf from Graham Bennette's notebook this morning, in quoting Abraham Meyerson. Meyerson said that the true scholar is like a pin. He has to have a sharp end and a round end. The sharp end, the point, drives and analyzes. The round end contemplates and synthesizes. If he has only a sharp end, he is a pedant. If he has only a round end, he is a dilettant. We need scholars in this field.

DISCUSSION

David W. Weiss

Department of Immunology, Hebrew University-Hadassah Medical School
Jerusalem, Israel

The central question before us is whether psychodynamic states can influence the genesis or development of neoplastic processes. Assuming that a causal relationship between certain psychic states and neoplasia can be demonstrated, attention has been focused today on a second core question: Are the means of such causality in the realm of immunological reactivity?

Do we, in fact, possess clear information pointing to a link between psychic phenomena–stress, repression, depression–and the abnormal patterns of cellular proliferation that are named, collectively, neoplasia? I have read the abstracts and some of the papers that reached me, and have examined some of the background literature made available to me in recent months by Dr. Bahnson and Dr. Solomon. While I am impressed by the fact that many reported observations point to some correlation between certain types of psychic conditions or events and neoplasia, I am not as yet satisfied that a true causal relationship has been demonstrated beyond doubt. It is still possible to play devil's advocate and to suggest that the correlation between psychic and cell-proliferative changes is not at all causal, and that some entirely extraneous, nonpsychodynamic factors concomitantly and independently affect alterations in psychological and cellular-growth equilibria. If you ask me whether I actually believe this to be the case, my answer would be "No!" The circumstantial and suggestive evidence for a causal link between pathology of the psyche and pathology of growth is quite persuasive--but there still remains the difference between strong suggestion and proof. Suggestion that the operative hypothesis of this conference is valid, we have; proof and certainty, I hold, still remain to be adduced.

With this consideration in mind, I view with particular interest this afternoon's communication dealing with the three sets of Luke and A-Luke twins–the system on which this study is based is of singular importance. If one deals with monozygotic twins, one equalizes to a very large extent both genetic and environmental circumstances of a nature other than what we would call frankly psychic. Hence, in a study of monozygotic siblings discordant for a neoplastic illness, one has a situation in which psychodynamic factors are lifted out from the huge background of all other factors that may play a role in neoplasia, and can thereby be given the significance that we believe, but do not yet know for certain, they merit. Further studies with monozygotic twins are thus of cardinal importance, and will, I think, bear a great deal of fruit.

I am very conscious of the strictures that must be imposed on the word "psyche" when we speak of emotional processes in man, and I doubt whether one can really employ the term, to speak of events involving "soul" or "feeling" or "higher consciousness," in designating processes and reactions in animals. I question, therefore, the validity of animal studies as truly pertinent models of psychological behavior in man. Nonetheless, I should strongly suggest the undertaking of experiments in animals standing in the same genetic relationship to each other as do human identical twins, as long as it is remembered that one deals with essentially unsatisfactory models, and that any extrapolation of results must be exceedingly conservative. With this serious reservation in mind, it may be possible to isolate sufficiently and pinpoint certain stress factors in experiments with isogenic mice, guinea pigs, and other species; that is to say, with animals of essentially identical genetic and experiential background, to supplement and perhaps extend the information as to the relevance of such factors to neoplasia that will come from further observations in human monozygotic twins.

If we now turn to the immune response as a possible matrix, or medium, for the translation of psychic and psychic-like circumstances to determinants of neoplastic events, what do we find? For one, there can be little doubt today that the immune response has a very direct bearing on neoplasia, and I say this not because I am an immunologist, but because the data before us are convincing. In several papers to be seen in this monograph, these data will be presented and analyzed in some detail, and if I am permitted to hazard a brief summary now, I would say that there is no reasonable doubt left by the middle 1960's that it is possible, at least in animals, to induce significant states of specifically acquired resistance against neoplastic cells. This means, in effect, that neoplastic cells are recognized by the organism as being in one way or another qualitatively different from analogous normal cells. An immediate corollary of this fact is the expectation that the individual should be able to handle autochthonous neoplastic cell variants immunologically; i.e., to attack and destroy them as foreign tissue. But progressive neoplasia is a sad and only too common reality, and therefore we are led to ask: Perhaps cancer is the manifestation of an underlying, preexisting immunological disability? And, indeed, there is before us an increasing amount of information pointing in this direction. A causal interaction between the immune response and the progressive development of neoplastic cells thus appears to be a strong likelihood—but I shall shortly introduce some necessary qualifications and reservations.

Before doing so, however, I must turn my attention to the other side of the hypothetical process: psychic state⟶immunological responsiveness⟶neoplasia, and must ask: Is the immune apparatus affected *directly* by psychogenic stimuli? Here, again, certainly is still not within our grasp. There is, indeed, some recorded information suggesting that animals subjected to certain stresses have an altered ability to recognize and to respond to antigens, but it remains essentially unknown whether the immunological end effect is reached by virtue of the psychic-like consequences of the stress experience, or whether such experience impinges directly on lymphoid tissue and without any reference to psychological mediation.

At this point, it is necessary to introduce an important word of caution, already alluded to by Dr. Klein, but of sufficient relevance to our discussion to justify repetition and elaboration: In speaking of the significance of the "immune response" in any biological context, one must take into consideration the extreme lability and multifaceted aspect of this response. It would be absurd for an immunologist to speak in 1968 of immunological responsiveness as if this were a single entity or event. In consequence of quite small changes in the total environmental background or in experimental parameters, immunological reactions that might have led to a state of resistance can lead to a state of enhancement, or to specific tolerance or paralysis in place of the specific creation of antibodies. Indeed, such opposite manifestations of immunological recognition can exist in the same animal at the same time against the same antigenic configurations—resistance against normal cells and enhancement vis-a-vis neoplastic variants of the same donor or even tissue, responsiveness toward antigen in one physiochemical state and tolerance toward the same antigen in another state. The parameters of immunization and challenge, the state of the target tissue, the relative cellular and humoral immunological ability of the host and his relative capacity to make different categories of immunoglobulins—all these and other parameters determine whether an experience with a foreign tissue will result in rejection or acceptance of that tissue subsequently, or after a second such experience. More than this, the circumstances under which an organism experiences an antigenic stimulus determine whether there will be any response at all—thus, for example, an otherwise quite strong antigen may not be reacted against if it is introduced in conjunction with a number of other antigens.

The immune response is always to be seen as a multicompartmental entity, not only divisible into cellular and humoral components, but, within each of these major subcategories, into molecular species of antibodies and families of immunocompetent cells with reactivities of different biological implication. It would be a large and dangerously misleading oversimplification, therefore, to speak of the immune response in relation to neoplasia without specifying the circumstances, the possible mechanisms, and the various expectations held of such a postulated relationship. In short, the immune response is not by any means necessarily on the side of the angels with regard to host resistance against cancer cells.

Precision must therefore be introduced at all levels of the postulated interconnections between psychic state, immunological reactivity, and neoplasia. Precisely what kind of psychodynamic imbalance will affect precisely which aspects of a total immune response toward a given antigenic entity, and to what precise biological manifestation will the altered immunological reactivity lead in a host-tumor context?

The major virtue of any scientific discussion is that it may lead to new and better experiments, and thereby to a closer approximation of reality. From this perspective, I consider our discussions today to have been highly useful. If nothing else, the papers and comments presented so far, and those still to come at this meeting, underline both the great intrinsic interest of this area of psychophysiological aspects of cancer, and the unusually great dangers and difficulties of remaining on an even scientific keel when attempting to provide new observational and experimental data in this field. The importance of elevating to the level of detectability psychodynamic factors from the background of genetic and environmental circumstances has been stressed, and this points, in turn, to the necessity of dealing with highly inbred animals in many types of experimentation. The necessity of considering the total ecological aspects of neoplasia and of psychic state is being emphasized, and this leads to a critical examination as to whether the "stress" experiences to which laboratory animals are commonly subjected are indeed even distant models of the stresses that a living creature experiences in the course of its natural history.

In summary, then, I can no longer question a significant role of immunology in neoplasia, but I am only beginning to see specific cause-and-effect relationships within this configuration. I am rather persuaded to believe that there exist direct psychodynamic facets in the etiology of cancer and in the progressive development of a neoplastic process, but I require additional information before I can be certain that my predilection is correct. And if it proves to be, I would view the inherent susceptibility of the immune response to modulation by a variety of factors, and the existing evidence suggesting relationships between certain psychic states and immunological responsiveness, as sufficient stimuli to warrant careful further study towards elucidation of immunological pathways between pathologies of the psyche and the pathologies of the cell collectively spoken of as neoplasia.

COMMENT

Claus Bahne Bahnson*

Department of Psychiatry, Jefferson Medical College
Philadelphia, Pa.

DR. DAY: Dr. Bahnson, would you care to make comments at this point in the conference?

DR. CLAUS BAHNSON: The meeting today has been very gratifying. I think that our plan to get workers together who talk quite different languages has proved its value. When we started to organize this conference, we thought, at first, that it might be helpful to segregate out participants as one usually does, in order to have each group of researchers present in its particular area, enabling researchers to communicate with their own kind but not to cross-communicate with each other from field to field.

I think that we all felt a certain strain, moving from existentialism on the one hand to exact and refined studies in immunology on the other, but I do hope that during the next days to come, this boldness in planning will pay off, in the sense that scientists have tried to listen to each other and may be able to put forward an effort to communicate on this basis, even in areas where they have not previously been on speaking terms.

Many theoretical formulations have been put forward here, but all of them have to do with a few crucial points. One has to do with affective depression, hopelessness, and withdrawal; a second centers on coping mechanisms, control, or organization; and a third, and slightly different, problem, which Dr. Bennette particularly has raised, is related to the concept of alienation that originated in sociology (Durkheim introduced it during the last century) and that now has spread to other disciplines. This concept is not identical with depression and not with repression either. It represents, in a way, the "third party." And, as so often is the case, maybe the "third party" will play a crucial role in the progress of our proceedings.

I also wish to thank all those who have come today for their patience in listening to people who talk in languages quite different from their own. There have been no hostile feelings at all, of which we all were afraid. I hope we can proceed in the same vein.

* Present address: Eastern Pennsylvania Psychiatric Institute, Institute of Pennsylvania Hospital, Philadelphia, Pa., and University of Connecticut, Storrs, Conn.

PART III. EMOTION, IMMUNOLOGY, AND CANCER

IMMUNOLOGICAL PARAMETERS OF THE HOST-PARASITE RELATIONSHIP IN NEOPLASIA*

David W. Weiss

Department of Immunology, Hebrew University-Hadassah Medical School
Jerusalem, Israel

The natural history of neoplastic diseases resembles in essential aspects the interactions of host and microbial parasite in chronic infectious diseases. In both instances, the outcome of the relationship between the host and a population of pathogenic living cells is determined by complex interactions governed by the genetic potentials of both partners and influenced by internal and extrinsic environmental factors. Indeed, neoplastic cells, growing beyond the architectural configurations and spatial patterns of normal tissues, unresponsive to the stimuli that govern normal rates of cellular growth, death, and differentiation, often distinguished by new physiological or morphological characteristics, and causing pathological changes in their host, must be considered as essentially independent parasitic organisms even though they represent variants that originated in one way or another from among the normal cellular constituents of the host.

There may be appreciable advantage to considering neoplasia as properly falling within the category of host-parasite relationships. In recent years, the focus of emphasis in the study of host-microbial-parasite relationships has turned sharply away from the parasite as the only really significant factor in such associations, determining largely by itself their duration and manifestations. It has come to be recognized, instead, that host and environment play equally significant roles and that the outcome of many infectious diseases, and the very nature of the characteristic pathologic changes that mark them, can be understood only in terms of the specific responses of individual hosts within an ecological framework in which relatively minor environmental changes can have large consequences. Such a perspective is still very new in the analysis of neoplastic disease, and is far from adopted by the majority of investigators. Only a few years ago, the keynote paper at a symposium on host-neoplastic-cell interactions still had to pose the underlying question: "Does the host react against his own cancer cells?" The clinical approach to cancer is similarly still centered on the neoplastic cells alone, therapeutic procedures being directed at their removal or selective destruction from outside.

It is unlikely, however, that this approach to human malignancy will lead to general solutions. There are obvious limitations to attempts aimed at physical removal of primary and metastatic neoplastic foci, and the hopes of finding categorically effective chemotherapeutic agents are remote. Even in the case of infectious diseases, where the disease-causing organisms are phylogenetically far distant from the host, only a handful from among the very many antibiotic and chemotherapeutic agents that are active *in vitro* have proven to be sufficiently selective in their toxic action to be employed safely in therapeutic quantities. In

* This work was supported by Research Grants AI–2309 and CA–05388 from the NIH, USPHS, and by grants from the Damon Runyon Memorial Fund for Cancer Research, Inc. and the Leukemia Research Foundation, Inc., of Chicago.

neoplasia, the similarity between host and neoplastic cells is such that it is questionable whether sufficiently discerning, effective, and stable agents can be found at all.

Until recently, it was perhaps not possible to see neoplasia as an interplay between distinct living organisms, because there was insufficient information to define neoplastic variants as qualitatively different from the cells of the host. A considerable body of recent work now suggests, however, that neoplastic cells are dissimilar in fundamental metabolic, physiologic, and cytologic respects from analogous normal ones, and the qualitative nature of the divergence has been indicated strongly by the findings during the past decade that all, or at least the great majority, of the tumors of experimental animals that have been studied immunologically display new surface, cytoplasmic, or nuclear antigens.[2–5] With this demonstration of the essential distinctiveness of neoplastic variants, including those of spontaneous origin, their study as parasites in parasitic association with their hosts has become conceptually possible, and such study may be hoped to lead to an understanding of the precise environmental and host idiosyncrasies that permit a single, or a very few, newly arisen antigenic parasites to grow and establish themselves in the tissues of their host and to destroy it after a prolonged association.

A prominent role of immunological parameters in host-tumor associations is suggested not only by the demonstration that many animal cancers possess new antigens. It has also been found that most carcinogenic agents and stimuli reduce immunological ability broadly, prior to cancer onset,[6,6a] and that this occurs also as a natural consequence of aging.[7,8,8a] An inverse correlation between at least some immunological capabilities and strain susceptibility to neoplasia has been shown,[9,10] and there are numerous observations in man that point, at least circumstantially, to immunological deficiency as a precondition of progressive neoplasia, as pointed out by, e.g., Fisherman,[11] Holmgren,[12] and Fudenberg.[13] Classical immunological ability makes its appearance in phylogenetic evolution at precisely the point where true neoplasia is first seen, in the primitive fish, and it has been postulated that the antibody response evolved primarily as a surveillance mechanism against neoplastic variants.[14]

It was with these considerations in mind that we initiated several years ago an intensive investigation into the immunological interactions between one species of host, several strains of inbred mice, and one species of neoplasm, spontaneous mammary adenocarcinomas. The object of these studies, begun in the laboratories of the Department of Bacteriology and Immunology and the Cancer Research Genetics Laboratory of the University of California in Berkeley and now continued at the Hebrew University-Hadassah Medical School in Jerusalem, was to analyze the nature of the neoplastic antigens and the general and specific immunological capacities of the susceptible host animals.

A detailed description of the nature of spontaneous carcinomas of inbred mice is presented in a number of recent reviews.[15–18] The chief advantages of studying this particular model lie with the fact that the tumors arise spontaneously, as part of the "natural" life history of female mice of many inbred strains and also of outbred laboratory and wild mice, and not in consequence of artificial circumstances set by the experimenter. Moreover, there is a complex, multiple etiology to the onset of these tumors, in which a related group of viral agents plays a large, but not a sole or even a minimally essential part. Spontaneous mammary carcinomas of mice thus constitute a difficult test system in which to isolate for investigation individual parameters, but at the same time these neoplasms are more likely to provide a realistic model of human neoplasia than is afforded by most of the cancers induced artificially by chemical and physical carcinogens and by laboratory-adapted strains of oncogenic viruses.

The purpose of the present communication is to present new data that points to the existence of several different categories of tumor antigens of mammary carcinomas and to present the results of recent experiments on the general immunological activation that is brought about by a tumor-protective fraction of mycobacteria. The possible relevance of these observations to psychophysiological parameters of human neoplasia will be discussed.

The Antigenicity of Spontaneous Mammary Carcinomas of Mice

It has been shown in previous communications from our laboratories that a first experience with a spontaneous mammary carcinoma bestows on isogenic and autochthonous mice a state of heightened reactivity towards a further challenge and that this heightened reactivity is immunological in nature;[5,19,20] these findings have been corroborated by other investigators.[21–25]

Subsequent investigations revealed that the mammary tumor virus (MTV) participates largely in the antigenicity of these tumors: (1) Isogenic hosts can be immunized more effectively in many instances against virus-infected tumor cells of the same genotype if they themselves are free of the agent, i.e., had been derived from a female that lost the MTV spontaneously or as a result of foster nursing from birth on a virus-free mother,[26–28] and (2) reinfection of such agent-free animals by foster nursing back on an infected mother abrogates or reduces their responsiveness.[27] These findings were interpreted as revealing the existence of antigens on the surface of the tumor cells that are controlled by the presence or activities of the MTV and against which host animals infected early in life are specifically unresponsive. This interpretation was supported by the observation that preneoplastic and normal mammary tissue from MTV-infected mice, as well as their red blood cells, which have been shown to carry MTV biological activity,[29] already have expressed at least one of the antitumor protective antigens,[26,30,31] and it was also supported by the high degree of cross-immunogenicity among all MTV-infected mammary carcinomas in MTV-free hosts.[30,32]

On the other hand, it was found that spontaneous mammary carcinomas *could*, at least in some instances and in some strains, induce heightened resistance of immunological nature in isogenic and autochthonous hosts despite the identical viral status of the immunizing and challenging neoplastic tissues and the test animals.[19,33,34] This finding could be explained in terms of an incomplete degree of specific immunological tolerance toward MTV-controlled antigens experienced in early life and thereafter or of a "breaking" of such tolerance in the process of specific immunization and challenge.[35,36] On the other hand, however, these observations could reflect the existence of a second class of protective antigens, independent of the presence or activities of the MTV.

Studies have now been undertaken to accrue additional information on the existence and nature of MTV-associated antigens, to provide further evidence of the occurrence of tumor-specific antigens independent of the MTV and to determine whether there is a competition for the expression of different categories of antigens on the surface of infected neoplastic and preneoplastic cells.

Cell-Surface Antigens Associated with the MTV

Much of our work that incriminated the MTV as a determinant of mammary tumor antigenicity was carried out with tumors originating in MTV-infected

C3H/Crgl mice, tested in the reciprocally isogenic MTV-free C3Hf/Crgl (derived by foster nursing) subline. In order to establish beyond doubt that the results of these experiments do, in fact, point to the MTV as a controller of at least one class of tumor antigens and that they are not the manifestations of some unrecognized immunological or nonimmunological peculiarity in the relationship of C3H to C3Hf mice not related to the MTV infection of only the former, further experiments were conducted in another C3H-genotype system: C3H tumors were tested for immunogenicity in another isogenic subline free of the MTV, C3H/2/Crgl, which lost the virus spontaneously some generations earlier. These experiments were begun in our laboratories at the University of California in collaboration with Dr. David Lavrin, and they have been continued by Dr. Lavrin at the University of Illinois in Chicago.[37]

The results of Dr. Lavrin's experiments with MTV-positive C3H tumors in MTV-negative C3H/2 hosts were in the same direction as those of the earlier studies in which C3H tumors were tested in C3Hf hosts,[26,27] and they also showed once again that older, and hence immunologically less reactive animals, are generally less responsive to the infected tumor isografts than are young adult mice in their immunological prime.

Although second-set reciprocal skin graft tests were performed in all these experiments to assure the continued reciprocal isogenicity of the parental C3H animals and the C3Hf and C3H/2 sublines, the slight possibility remained that a minor heterozygosis of normal transplantation antigens may have gone undetected in tests involving normal-tissue grafts but have become manifest when neoplastic cells were employed, conceivably because there could be a greater expression of such antigens on their surface.[5] To rule out this possibility with certainty, and thus to be able to ascribe unreservedly to the MTV infection of the donor tissue or to the presence of other, tumor-specific antigens the responsibility for the immunogenicity here demonstrated, the following further experiment was conducted by Dr. Lavrin.

Fragments of a spontaneous mammary carcinoma newly arisen in a C3H/2 multiparous female that had been foster-nursed on a C3H mother (therefore termed C3H/2f.C3H) were implanted into the right rear feet of male and female mice of the C3H/2, C3H, and C3H/2f.C3H lines. Animals of different ages were employed. Other mice of these lines were subjected to the implantation procedure, but were given no implants ("sham-operated"). Forty-two days later, the right rear feet of all the animals were amputated under Nembutal® anesthesia.† A week thereafter, all animals were challenged with the same tumor, now in its first transplant generation, by subcutaneous trocar implantation into the inguinal area of a fragment of healthy-appearing tumor tissue approximately 0.05 to 0.1 cu mm in size. The animals were then observed at weekly intervals for eight weeks for the development of palpable tumors at the site of implantation. The results of this experiment are presented in TABLE 1 and FIGURE 1.

It is evident from TABLE 1 and FIGURE 1 that normal, unimmunized MTV-free C3H/2 hosts offered appreciable resistance to the take and growth of isografts of an MTV-infected C3H/2f.C3H mammary tumor, that previous immunization of such hosts heightened this refractoriness, and that MTV-infected mice, whether of the C3H/2f.C3H or the C3H line, accepted the neoplastic isografts, even after immunization, to an identical extent. The results of this experiment, together with those previously reported, can leave no doubt that the MTV is responsible for

† Abbott Laboratories, North Chicago, Ill.

TABLE 1

DEVELOPMENT OF ISOGRAFTS OF A MTV-POSITIVE C3H/2F.C3H MAMMARY TUMOR IN TUMOR-IMMUNIZED AND NONIMMUNIZED HOSTS OF THE C3H/2, C3H/2f.C3H, AND C3H LINES

Host Animals						Number of Animals with Tumors 8 Weeks after Challenge
Strain	MTV Status	Pretreatment	Sex	Age* (Months)	Number	
C3H/2	(−)	Immunized†	Male	13–20	4	1
C3H/2	(−)	Immunized†	Male	7–10	4	0
C3H/2	(−)	Immunized†	Male	2	6	0
C3H/2	(−)	Immunized†	Female	12	3	0
C3H/2	(−)	Immunized†	Female	2	3	0
					20	1
C3H/2	(−)	Sham‡	Male	7–15	8	6
C3H/2	(−)	Sham‡	Male	2	4	2
C3H/2	(−)	Sham‡	Female	12	3	3
C3H/2	(−)	Sham‡	Female	2	3	0
					18	11
C3H/2f.C3H	(+)	Immunized	Male	6–8	3	2
C3H/2f.C3H	(+)	Immunized	Male	2–5	13	13
					16	15
C3H/2f.C3H	(+)	Sham	Male	6–8	4	4
C3H/2f.C3H	(+)	Sham	Male	2–4	5	5
					9	9
C3H	(+)	Immunized	Male	3–5	10	10
C3H	(+)	Sham	Male	3–6	12	12

* Age of the animals at the time of implantation of the immunizing tumor isograft or of the sham surgical procedure.

† See text for details.

‡ The same surgical procedures at the time of immunization, without implantation of tissues.

at least some of the protective antigenicity that marks these murine cancers. Because such antigens are already expressed in preneoplastic nodular tissue and in normal mammary parenchyma of MTV-infected animals, they cannot be referred to as "tumor-specific" in the strict sense of the word and are instead designated "tumor-associated."

An oncogenic virus can conceivably control the expression of antigens associated with its presence in several different ways; for one, the virion *per se,* or some of its components, could bestow antigenicity on infected cells. In most of our studies, antigenicity is revealed by resistance against neoplastic isografts and autografts and must therefore involve immune reactions against cell surface components. The MTV is an RNA virus, maturing at the surface of host cells,[38] and it is not difficult to visualize the conferring of specific antigenicity to host cells by MTV fragments or whole virions on the cytoplasmic membranes. An oncogenic agent can also, however, confer antigenicity on cells by causing the synthesis of new constituents, other than components of the virion itself, under the control of its own genome or under the control of the host-cell genome with the virus acting as a derepressing agent.[39] Experiments have accordingly been initiated to investigate the means by which the MTV induces tumor-associated protective antigens on normal and neoplastic mammary cells.

The first approach was to determine whether the MTV virion itself acts as

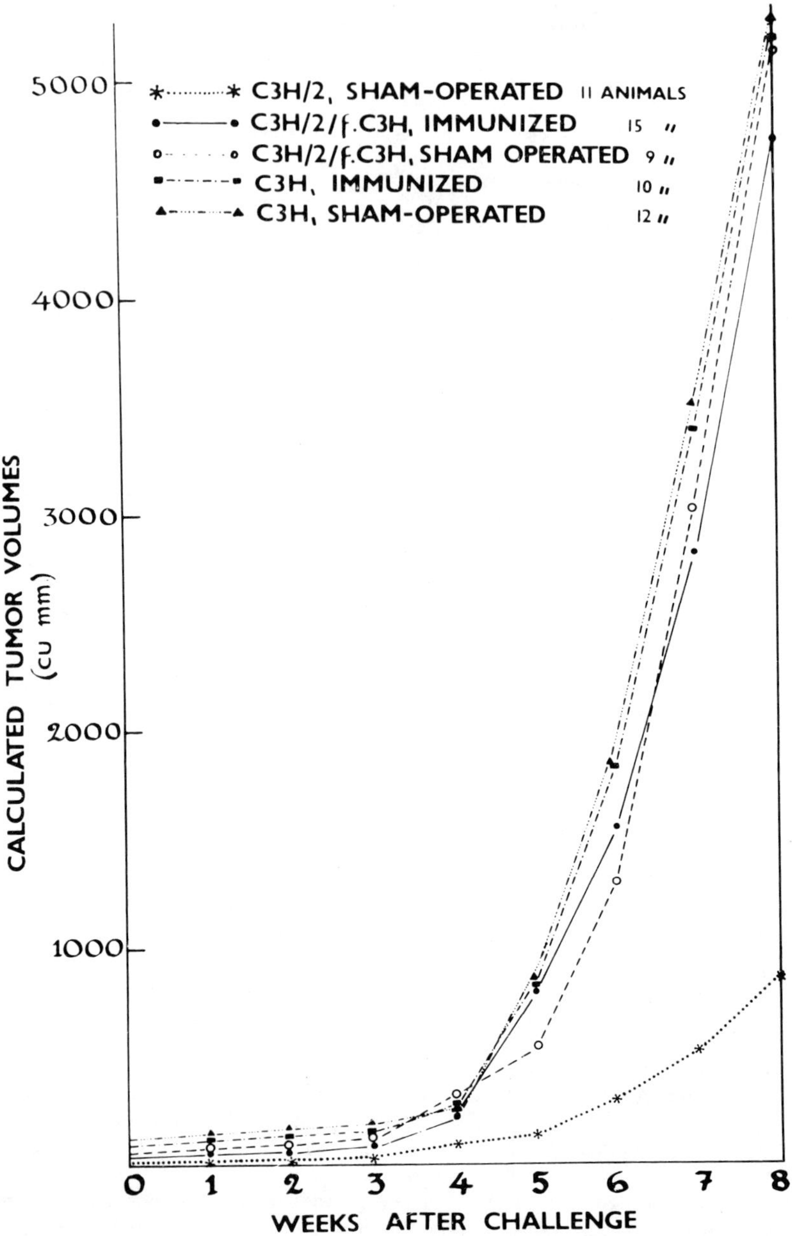

FIGURE 1. Growth rates of tumors developing in nonimmunized C3H/2 hosts and in immunized and normal C3H/2f.C3H and C3H hosts from implants of a spontaneous C3H/2f.C3H mammary carcinoma. Each point on the curves represents the arithmetic means of the tumor volumes, calculated as described previously[34] from periodic measurements of the two diameters evenly bisecting the tumors.

one of these antigens. At first sight, this seems a not unlikely possibility. One of my former associates, Dr. Phyllis Blair, had already shown some years ago that the MTV induces the formation of neutralizing antibodies in rabbits,[40,41] and more recently we have demonstrated that the mouse as well can make precipitating and neutralizing antibodies against MTV, some of which appear to react directly with the mature B-particles commonly identified as representing at least one form of this agent.[42-45] It remained to be shown that antivirion antibodies, or immunologically reactive cells directed at the same target antigens, are in fact capable of protecting against challenge with mammary tumor cells. These experiments are still in progress, but the results of an initial study suggest that the MTV B-particles may, indeed, act as tumor protective antigens. This is illustrated by the following experiment.

Purified preparations of MTV B-particles were prepared by sucrose density gradient centrifugation (SDGC) of infected milk derived from young mice of the BALB/cfC3H strain in lactation after their first or second pregnancy; the details of this procedure have been described elsewhere.[46] The appearance of a typical purified preparation is illustrated in FIGURE 2. Although the SDGC preparations were found to still contain small quantities of casein, detectable in immunodiffusion tests, and were perhaps also contaminated with small amounts of other milk products, their derivation from the milk of young, tumor-free mice makes it very unlikely that they included immunogenically active quantities of virus-induced cellular antigens.

The SDGC preparations were inactivated with 1.2×10^{-2}M formalin for three to five days at 4° C; effective inactivation was evident from the failure of the formalinized MTV to induce preneoplastic nodules in susceptible animals, in the usual noduligenic assay procedure for MTV.[47] The inactivated preparations were then employed as vaccines against tumor challenge.

Groups of young adult (10-weeks-old) BALB/c female mice were immunized with one of the following preparations: formalin-inactivated MTV in incomplete Freund's adjuvant or in saline only, living MTV derived similarly from infected BALB/cfC3H milk, or a living preparation of an unrelated RNA virus, the Rous Sarcoma Virus (RSV), employed as a control. The vaccines were administered in a series of four i.p. injections over a 22-day period; when adjuvant was used, it was employed only with the first injection. The total amount of MTV given was equivalent to 0.1 cc of whole milk; the total quantity of RSV was 2 cc of a supernatant of a chick embryo cell culture infected with the Bryan strain of RSV. One week after the last immunization, the animals were challenged by subcutaneous injection in the left hip of 1×10^4 or 5×10^4 living cells of a first-transplant-generation spontaneous mammary carcinoma derived from a multiparous female of the reciprocally isogenic BALB/cfC3H line. The test animals were observed for eight weeks for the appearance of palpable tumors. The results of this experiment are presented in TABLE 2. They show that immunization with formalinized MTV in Freund's adjuvant can afford strong protection against challenge with a number of isogenic tumor cells sufficient to establish progressively growing tumors in all animals immunized with an unrelated virus (the RSV control group) and that a degree of protection, as indicated by a slowed rate of tumor development, is bestowed even against the larger challenge. The formalinized MTV preparation without adjuvant, and living MTV, provided a lesser degree of resistance.

In a similar experiment, peritoneal-washing cells from animals immunized with formalin-inactivated MTV plus adjuvant were found to be considerably

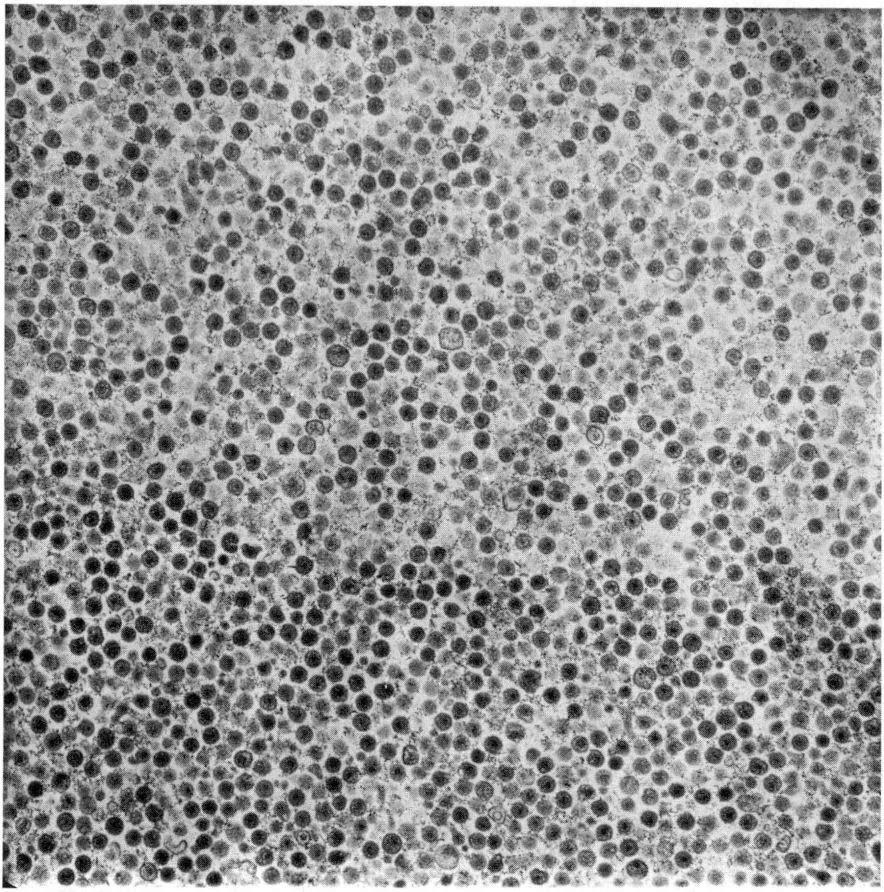

FIGURE 2. Electron microphotograph of a sucrose density gradient centrifugation preparation of mammary tumor virus derived from infected milk. Appearance of a typical SDGC preparation of MTV derived from BALB/cfC3H milk (× 18,000; orig. × 30,000). This picture, taken by Dr. Robert Cardiff of our laboratory at the University of California in Berkeley, shows a highly concentrated preparation of the viral particles commonly identified as the mammary tumor agent. The granular debris represents either viral fragments or impurities or a mixture of these.

more active in destroying mammary tumor target cells *in vitro* than were peritoneal cells from mice treated with RSV.

These findings do not yet show categorically that the protective antigen(s) in the formalinized MTV preparations lie with the virion itself. In addition to the rather remote possibility that contaminating cellular products in the SDGC concentrates are the effective immunogens, it is also just conceivable that "inactivated" MTV might still possess the ability of directing the synthesis of new, protective antigens in host cells despite the loss of its noduligenic potential. Protection experiments are now under way with still further purified preparations of formalin-treated MTV, and the mammary tissues of mice of strains free of

TABLE 2

DEVELOPMENT OF ISOGRAFTS OF A SPONTANEOUS BALB/cfC3H MAMMARY TUMOR IN BALB/c FEMALE HOSTS IMMUNIZED WITH LIVING OR INACTIVATED MTV OR WITH LIVING RSV

Immunization*	Proportion of Animals with Palpable Tumors and Tumor Size 8 Weeks after Challenge with Following Numbers of Tumor Cells			
	1×10^4		5×10^4	
	Tumor Incidence	Mean Tumor Size (cu mm)†	Tumor Incidence	Mean Tumor Size (cu mm)
Formalinized MTV in adjuvant	0/10	–	6/8	40
Formalinized MTV, no adjuvant	6/10	120	6/7	120
Living MTV	2/10	20	7/10	290
Living RSV	9/9	520	7/8	560

* See text for details.
† Tumor volumes calculated as described by Attia and Weiss.[34]

the MTV are being examined for the presence of any MTV-associated antigens after the animals are exposed to the formalinized virus.

It must also be clear that the demonstration of virion-dependent protective antigens does not rule out the simultaneous existence of antigens produced in infected host cells under control of the viral genome or of those produced as a result of a derepressing interaction of the virus with the genome of the host cell.

Cell-Surface Antigens Independent of the MTV

New evidence for the existence of MTV-independent, tumor-specific antigens on the surface of MTV-infected tumor cells has recently come from the excellent doctoral thesis experiments of Dr. Jan Vaage of our laboratory at the University of California in Berkeley. Dr. Vaage studied the immunogenicity of 23 newly arisen MTV-infected C3H mammary carcinomas in C3H and in MTV-free isogenic C3Hf hosts, following for up to 10 transplant generations the ability of living isografts of these tumors to induce states of heightened resistance against a second implantation. The experimental design was to implant the immunizing tumor grafts subcutaneously in the right flank of young adult test animals, to remove them surgically when they had reached a size of approximately 15 × 15 mm, and to immediately reinject 10^5 living tumor cells of the same or of another tumor subcutaneously in the left flank. The incidence and rates of growth of palpable tumors were then checked at periodic intervals. Challenge immediately upon termination of an immunizing experience is not the most favorable circumstance for the demonstration of heightened tumor resistance, and thus it provides a severe test for the presence of such reactivity, while at the same time assuring a close similarity between the immunizing and challenge tumor tissues.

The following findings were made:

1. Five of the 23 tumors tested were strongly immunogenic in the C3H hosts. Their immunogenicity was of the same order after repeated animal passage as it was in the first or second transplant generation, and the tumors not immunogenic upon first testing failed to show such property even after 10 passages. The five tumors immunogenic in the C3H animals were also immunogenic, as was expected, in the MTV-free C3Hf mice.

2. Massive round-cell infiltration was seen more frequently around and within challenge isografts of the immunogenic C3H tumors in C3H hosts that had been

immunized than in such hosts that had experienced no prior contact with the tumors.

3. The heightened resistance conferred on C3Hf hosts by immunization with tumors also reactive in C3H mice could be transferred by means of spleen and lymph node cells to normal C3H animals.

4. The tumors found immunogenic in C3H mice were completely cross-reactive in C3Hf test animals, but in the majority of cases they were *not* cross-reactive in the C3H hosts.

The results of the experiments showing the immunogenicity of five C3H tumors in C3H hosts, and several of the tests for cross-reactivity of four of these tumors, are depicted in TABLES 3 and 4, respectively; more detailed reports of these studies will appear elsewhere in the near future.

Experiments were also conducted in collaboration with Dr. Vaage to test the immunogenicity of spontaneous C3H mammary carcinomas in the autochthonous host. In some instances, fragments of a primary tumor were removed surgically without excision of the entire neoplasm and were used to hyperimmunize the animal, with or without adjuvants, after disruption into cell suspensions and inactivation by x-irradiation. Other animals received parallel series of immunizations with normal irradiated autochthonous tissue preparations, including liver cell suspensions, or adjuvants only. It was found that autoimmunization with irradiated liver tissue retarded development of the original tumor *in situ*. In further experiments in isogenic C3H hosts, this unexpected liver effect was confirmed, and it was found that only livers from tumor-bearing donors possessed immunogenic capacity, a phenomenon currently under further investigation. It was also found that immunization with either autochthonous liver or tumor vaccine preparations conferred appreciable resistance on the autochthonous host against the development of metastatic tumor foci following complete removal of the primary growth and intravenous reinjection of a suspension of the tumor cells.

It thus appears that at least some MTV-infected mammary tumors are capable under certain experimental circumstances of eliciting significant degrees of heightened resistance against a subsequent tumor challenge, even in MTV-infected hosts of a genotype not rated as immunologically very reactive.[9] The fact that there is infrequent cross-immunogenicity of such tumors in MTV-positive hosts, whereas cross-reactivity is total in isogenic uninfected mice, suggests strongly the presence of surface antigens not related to the presence of activities of the MTV. These antigens will be referred to in the future as "tumor-specific."

The immunogenicity of the reactive C3H tumors was found to be a stable property, manifested despite the opportunity inherent in repeated animal passage for the selection of nonantigenic variants. It may well be, therefore, that virus-independent tumor immunogenicity reflects the presence of new components on the surface of tumor cells that constitute an irreducible property of their neoplastic state. However, an alternative explanation cannot be ruled out entirely—that this immunogenicity arises from infection of some tumors by incidental microbial agents that initiate long-lasting parasitic interactions with the host cells.‡

An investigation is now in progress to assay mammary tumors and preneoplastic nodules directly for tumor-specific immunogenicity by subjecting such tissues from virus-free BALB/c mice to immunization-challenge tests in similar

‡ This possibility now seems very remote, in view of the recent findings of Dr. Vaage that different primary mammary carcinomas appearing in the same host vary with regard to the presence of tumor-specific antigens.

animals. At the same time, studies are under way to determine whether superinfection with the MTV abrogates or somehow masks preexisting tumor-specific antigens on the cell surface. The detection of any interference phenomena in the expression of tumor-associated and tumor-specific antigens on neoplastic cells would have considerable clinical implication.

Studies of the Mode of Action of a Tumor-Protective Fraction of Tubercle Bacilli

It has been reported from our laboratories that a methanol-insoluble fraction of phenol-killed attenuated tubercle bacilli of the BCG strain is capable of

TABLE 3

DEVELOPMENT OF ISOGRAFTS AND C3H MAMMARY TUMORS IN SPECIFICALLY IMMUNIZED AND UNIMMUNIZED C3H HOSTS

Tested in Transplant Generations	Immunizing Implants of Tumor	Number of Test Animals*	Number of Animals with Palpable Tumors	Percent of Animals with Palpable Tumors
2–10	#9,118	67	17	25.4
	None	70	67	95.7
2–7	#5,410	89	18	20.2
	None	58	37	63.7
2–8	#2,794	34	10	29.4
	None	64	49	76.5
2–6	#4,849	29	6	20.6
	None	27	20	74.0
2	#5,122	14	2	14.2
	None	6	5	83.3

* The numbers represent the cumulative totals of the animals in all the experiments conducted in the different transplant generations.

TABLE 4

EFFECT OF IMMUNIZATION WITH ONE IMMUNOGENIC C3H MAMMARY TUMOR ON THE DEVELOPMENT OF ANOTHER IN MTV-INFECTED C3H HOSTS

Tested in Transplant Generations	Immunizing Implants of Tumor	Challenge: Number with Tumors/Total Number Mice*	
		Tumor #5,410	Tumor #4,849
5–7	#5,410	2/16	13/16
	None	16/22	17/22
	#4,849	10/12	2/12
	None	4/6	4/6
		Tumor #9,118	Tumor #4,849
3–10	#9,118	7/27	22/27
	None	25/25	16/18
		Tumor #2,794	Tumor #5,410
5–8	#2,794	2/20	5/20
	None	12/30	23/30
	#5,410	10/36	10/36
	None	12/16	13/16

* The numbers represent the cumulative totals of the animals in all the experiments conducted in the different transplant generations.

heightening the resistance of mice and guinea pigs vis-a-vis tuberculous infection, infection with unrelated microbial pathogens, and the development of tumor isografts and of autochthonous spontaneous neoplasms.[5,48–51] Many other investigators have also noted a nonspecific protective activity by various mycobacterial organisms and bacillary fractions, and similar heterologous protective effects have been demonstrated for Gram-negative bacteria, *Corynebacteria,* and *Hemophilus* organisms.[52]

One explanation for the nonspecific immunogenic action of certain bacterial species lies with the possibility that some bacterial products may stimulate general immunological reactivity. The well-known adjuvant effects of many of the same bacterial moities when administered together with unrelated antigens could, in fact, be one manifestation of their nonspecific stimulation of immunological function. Experiments were therefore undertaken by Miss Constance Steinkuller of our laboratories to test the effects of our methanol-insoluble tubercle bacillus fraction (MER) on the immune response to a number of subsequently administered unrelated antigens and on the phagocytic activity of the reticuloendothelial system (RES).

The results of a number of completed experiments in mice have already been communicated.[52–54] It was found that MER very rapidly elevated phagocytic function, as measured by the rates of clearance of intravenously injected colloidal carbon, and that treated animals responded with a greater and more prolonged antibody response to later injections of sheep red blood cells and allogenic red and white blood cells. The immune response to the sheep red blood cells (SRBC) was measured by the Jerne technique for the quantitative estimation of lymphoid cells producing specific 19S hemolysins.[55] In these experiments, very large numbers of SRBC were employed for specific immunization of the MER-treated and saline control mice, and although the differences in the response between the two groups were statistically significant, they were not very large. Accordingly, further studies were initiated by Miss Constance Steinkuller with smaller antigenic stimuli, to determine whether MER treatment could evoke a more pronounced immunological stimulation than was evident from the first experiments. The results of one representative experiment are presented here.

Groups of 15-week-old BALB/c females were given two i.p. administration of 0.5 mg (dry weight) each of MER, 14 and 3 days, respectively, before they received an i.p. injection of 5×10^7 SRBC or of saline only. At intervals thereafter, subgroups of the animals were sacrificed, and determinations were made of the total numbers of nucleated spleen cells and of the numbers of cells producing anti-SRBC antibodies (plaque-forming cells, or PFC) on Jerne plates. The findings are shown in TABLE 5.

It is seen from TABLE 5 that pretreatment with MER increased somewhat the numbers of nucleated spleen cells, PFC/10^8 nucleated spleen cells, and PFC/spleen even in animals not injected with the specific antigen, SRBC. The differences were not statistically significant, but they have been noted consistently in other experiments as well. In animals which *were* immunized with SRBC, prior treatment with MER elicited increases in the total and specifically reactive spleen cell numbers throughout the test period, which ranged from 6 to 21 days after SRBC immunization; the differences between the MER-treated and control groups became large, and were highly significant, after the first 24 hr following the specific immunization.

MER and SRBC are, presumably, antigenically unrelated substances, and in many other experiments in which the immunological response of mice to SRBC

TABLE 5

EFFECT OF PRETREATMENT WITH MER ON NUMBERS OF TOTAL AND SPECIFICALLY REACTIVE CELLS IN THE SPLEENS OF BALB/c MICE FOLLOWING IMMUNIZATION WITH SRBC

Pretreatment	Immunization	Time of Spleen Examination After Immunization	Number of Mice	Means of Total Spleen Cell Number† (× 10^8)	P	Means			
						PFC*/10^8	P	PFC/Spleen	P
Saline	Saline	< 1 hr	8	2.64	> 0.05	87	> 0.05	232	> 0.05
MER	Saline	< 1 hr	8	3.32		149		467	
Saline	SRBC	6 hr	8	2.15	> 0.05	96	> 0.05	208	> 0.05
MER	SRBC	6 hr	7	2.74		214		524	
Saline	SRBC	12 hr	7	2.07	< 0.05	226	0.05	487	> 0.05
MER	SRBC	12 hr	7	3.27		235		764	
Saline	SRBC	24 hr	6	2.64	< 0.01	109	< 0.01	289	< 0.01
MER	SRBC	24 hr	6	3.49		287		999	
Saline	SRBC	5 days	5	2.47	< 0.05	5,850	< 0.05	15,900	< 0.01
MER	SRBC	5 days	5	6.14		37,200		260,000	
Saline	SRBC	21 days	5	2.13	< 0.05	94	< 0.05	201	< 0.01
MER	SRBC	21 days	4	3.06		489		1,585	

*** PFC: Plaque-forming cells, i.e., cells producing 19S anti-SRBC hemolysins.**
† Total number of nucleated spleen cells.

was measured by tube hemagglutination tests, animals treated with MER alone had no detectable circulating antibodies. The present observation that MER may by itself increase the numbers of spleen cells specifically reactive against SRBC could conceivably indicate a slight degree of cross-reactivity between a MER and an SRBC component. Alternatively and more likely, pretreatment with MER could have acted in the animals not given SRBC immunization by stimulating in one manner or another the immune response against whatever occult antigen in the environment is responsible for the commonly observed, low response of "normal" laboratory mice to SRBC or by facilitating the multiplication of all clones of lymphoid cells that are already responding to small antigenic stimuli in the animal's environment. In any event, it is clear from these experiments that prior treatment with MER heightens very markedly the ability of mice to respond immunologically to later administration of a heterologous antigenic substance. These studies thus support the hypothesis that the nonspecific immunogenic effects of MER, vis-a-vis both microbial and neoplastic cell challenge, may be based on a stimulation of the ability to respond immunologically to foreign compounds.

Discussion

The studies summarized in this communication present further evidence for a multiple antigenicity of cells of spontaneously arising mammary carcinomas of mice, including antigens apparently specific for, and inherent in, the neoplastic nature of the tissues. The demonstration that autochthonous as well as isogenic hosts respond to these antigens considerably raises the probability that immune reactions play a role in the natural history of these neoplasms, as indeed they play a role in the pathogenesis and immunogenesis of all chronic host-parasite interactions. Such participation by the immunological apparatus is further underscored by the present findings that the tumor-protective MER fraction of tubercle bacilli, which elicits heightened resistance against tumor development, is capable of stimulating broadly the immunological function of mice, under the same parameters of administration and testing that reveal its tumor-protective capacities.

The provocative and scholarly communication of Dr. Prehn at this symposium[56] provides further evidence for the importance of immunological factors in the onset and progression of neoplastic disease. It would be premature to state at this time that immunological dyscrasia is the single most important circumstance in permitting a neoplastic variant to grow, multiply, and colonize its host or to suggest that immunological defense mechanisms are the primary determinants of the further course of an established neoplastic process. On the other hand, there can no longer be serious doubt as to the occurrence of immunological reactions in host-tumor relationships or as to their considerable significance under at least some conditions.

The central questions before this conference are whether certain psychodynamic states stand in causal relationship to the onset and/or progression of neoplasia and whether, if this is in fact the case, the psychological parameters function via effects on the immunological apparatus. Both questions are exceedingly difficult, because they encompass a wide range of interactions between the morphological and physiological characteristics and potentials of host and neoplastic parasite and the multifaceted influences of environment. The difficulty is further compounded by the imprecisions and subjectivity that still mark current attempts at defining emotional states and functions in man. Yet the questions must be posed, because health and disease clearly cannot be understood in terms of isolated events, and enough is known today about the interactions between "physical" and "psychological" aspects of disease to make reductionist attempts at conceptually separate treatment of these facets of life wholly unscientific. What, then, are the facts available at this moment toward a more precise formulation of these questions, if not yet toward an attempt at their solution?

Many of the communications presented in this and in the preceding New York Academy of Sciences symposium on psychophysiological aspects of cancer (Vol. 125, Art. 3) and in the general literature[57] attempt to ascribe a causal relationship between certain defined personality characteristics–for example, inability successfully to express hostile feelings and emotions, or unresolved tensions regarding a parent[58]–and heightened susceptibility to neoplastic disease. There are, however, formidable problems to the ready acceptance of this evidence. Do many of these studies include appropriate controls (for that matter, can there really be such controls?) and do the observations stand up to statistical analysis? How possible is it to distinguish between cause and effect and between causal and coincidental manifestations, and how reliable are retrospective analyses of personality traits? The cumulative evidence appears to suggest an association between some psychodynamic and neoplastic processes, but very careful study seems still to be necessary both to corroborate and to define the nature of this association.

Assuming that such further study *will* incriminate specific emotional factors in the causation of human neoplastic disease, what can be said at this point of immunological affects as vehicles of this association? The possibility of an immunological pathway between certain emotional states and altered susceptibility to neoplastic disease is, a priori, an attractive one. The immunological apparatus of animals, encompassing phagocytosis and the elaboration of antibodies and sensitized cells, is manifested over the entire vertebrate kingdom, and phagocytic activity with varying degrees of specific recognition is already seen in primitive animals. At the same time, this ubiquitously expressed function is a very labile one. Relatively minor changes in a great number of extrinsic and intrinsic environmental factors can affect the immune response. Thus, the outcome of a given antigenic stimulus can be a marked or a minimal immune response, resistance or enhancement, immunity or tolerance, beneficial or pathogenetic, depending on what may be subtle changes in the total environment pertaining during the period of sensitization and reaction. An opportunity for the translation of psychic factors into altered susceptibility to cancer could thus be readily envisaged within the area of immunological function.

Some years ago, Solomon and Moos[57] presented a lucid discussion of the possible modes of interaction among emotions, immunity, and neoplastic as well as other diseases. At this conference, considerable emphasis has again been given to hormonal changes induced by emotional effects, and such changes can be envisaged quite readily as influencing a neoplastic process or even of triggering it, directly, or, in turn, via the immunological apparatus. Different effects by the same hormone on the immunological reactivity of animals of different genetic background have been known for some time,[59] and genotype may thus be an important determinant in the interaction of hormonal with immunological factors as a significant parameter in resistance to neoplasia. The demonstration that the elaboration of catechol amines is markedly influenced in some experimental animals by certain "stress" conditions may be of special interest. It has been suggested recently by Fine[60] that the mysterious death of humans who experience extreme and unremitting psychic tension for some days, as appears to be the case in self-imposed fear of bewitchment and spells in certain primitive societies, and the analogous phenomenon of animals dying after continuous threat, but no physical injury, from a superior enemy may arise from peripheral vascular collapse in the splanchnic viscera. This collapse, it is suggested, is brought about by the synergistic action on small blood vessels of minute quantities of bacterial endotoxin in the tissues and excess amounts of catechol amines released by the prolonged and unrelenting sympathetic activity. Circumstances can readily be envisaged in which even less dramatic vasodynamic changes could impinge strongly on the immune response, afferently and efferently.

Seen in the context of host-parasite relationships in general, neoplastic disease may well be subject to immunological influence at all levels, from infection to ultimate pathologic manifestation, and it may be as pertinent for neoplasia as for infectious diseases that the ultimate fate of a host-parasite interaction may be decided in the first minutes or hours after contact.[61]

It must be emphasized, nonetheless, that there still is no proof for a pathway leading from emotional state via immunological mechanisms to an effect on neoplasia, and even much stronger evidence than is currently available on the impairment of immune function under certain psychodynamic conditions that also favor neoplasia would still not prove categorically that the relationship is causal and not coincidental. It is clear that we still find ourselves in the area of circumstantial and suggestive, rather than direct, evidence and are dealing more with intriguing possibilities and frames of reference than with hard data. There is nothing wrong with such a state of affairs, as long as there occurs no misreading of ideas for facts. Many of the possible interactions discussed at this conference are subject to experiments or at least to careful clinical observation, and the design of new and better studies is, after all, a major function of all scientific discussion.

References

1. Kidd, J. G. 1961. Does the host react against his own cancer cells? Cancer Res. **21:** 1170.
2. Southam, C. M. 1960. Relationships of immunology to cancer: A review. Cancer Res. **20:** 271.
3. Old, L. J. & E. A. Boyse. 1964. Immunology of experimental tumors. Ann. Rev. Med. **15:** 167.
4. Klein, G. 1966. Tumor antigens. Ann. Rev. Microbiol. **20:** 223.
5. Weiss, D. W. 1967. Immunology of spontaneous tumors. *In* Proceedings of the Fifth Berkeley Symposium on Mathematical Statistics and Probability. L. Lecam & J. Neyman, Eds. : 657–706. University of California Press. Berkeley, Calif.
6. Berenbaum, M. C. 1964. Effects of carcinogens on immune processes. Brit. Med. Bull. **20:** 159.
6a. Stjernswärd, J. 1966. Age-dependent tumor-host barrier and effect of carcinogen-induced immunodepression on rejection of isografted methylcholanthrene-induced sarcoma cells. J. Nat. Cancer Inst. **37:** 505.
7. Aoki, T. & M. N. Teller. 1966. Aging and cancerigenesis. III. Effect of age on isoantibody formation. Cancer Res. **26:** 1648.
8. Stern, K. 1960. The reticuloendothelial system and neoplasia. *In* Reticuloendothelial Structure and Function. J. H. Heller, Ed. : 233–258. The Ronald Press Company. New York, N. Y.
8a. Stern, K. & C. A. Joyce. 1964. Reticuloendothelial phagocytosis in mice with spontaneous tumors. Proc. Amer. Assn. Cancer Res. **5:** 61.
9. Davidsohn, I. & K. Stern. 1954. Heterohemoantibodies in inbred strains of mice. II. Immune agglutinins and hemolysins for sheep and chicken red cells. J. Immun. **72:** 216.
10. Klein, E. & O. Linder. 1961. Factorial analysis of the reactivity of C57B1 females against isologous male skin grafts. Transpl. Bull. **27:** 457.
11. Fisherman, E. 1960. Does the allergic diathesis influence malignancy? J. Allerg. **31:** 74.
12. Holmgren, I. 1917. Försök och iakttagelser över kancerjukas förhallande till tuberkulin. Hygiea **79:** 218.
13. Fudenberg, H. H. 1966. Immunologic deficiency, lymphoma, and autoimmune disease: Observations, implications, speculations. Arthritis Rheum. **9:** 464.

14. THOMAS, L. 1959. Discussion. *In* Cellular and Humoral Aspects of the Hypersensitive States. H. S. Lawrence, Ed. : 529–532. Hoeber Medical Division. Harper & Row, Publishers. New York, N. Y.
15. DEOME, K. B. 1963. The role of the mammary tumor virus in mouse mammary noduligenesis and tumorigenesis. *In* Viruses, Nucleic Acids, and Cancer. 17th Annual Symposium on Fundamental Cancer Research at the University of Texas M.D. Anderson Hospital and Tumor Institute : 498–507. The Williams & Wilkins Co. Baltimore, Md.
16. NANDI, S. 1964. Interactions among hormonal, viral, and genetic factors in mouse mammary tumorigenesis. *In* Proceedings of the Sixth Canadian Cancer Conference : 69–81. Pergamon Press, Inc. New York, N. Y.
17. DEOME, K. B. & S. NANDI. 1966. The mammary-tumor system in mice, a brief review. *In* Viruses Inducing Cancer. W. J. Burdette, Ed. : 127–137. Utah University Press. Salt Lake City, Utah.
18. NANDI, S. 1966. Host-virus interactions in the mouse mammary tumor system. *In* Carcinogenesis–A Broad Critique. Twentieth Annual Symposium on Fundamental Cancer Research at the University of Texas M.D. Anderson Hospital and Tumor Institute : 295–314. The Williams & Wilkins Co. Baltimore, Md.
19. WEISS, D. W., L. J. FAULKIN, JR. & K. B. DEOME. 1964. Acquisition of heightened resistance and susceptibility to spontaneous mouse mammary carcinomas in the original host. Cancer Res. **24**: 732.
20. ATTIA, M. A., K. B. DEOME & D. W. WEISS. 1965. Immunology of spontaneous mammary carcinomas in mice. II. Resistance to a rapidly and a slowly developing tumor. Cancer Res. **25**: 451.
21. MORTON, D. L. 1962. Successful immunization against a spontaneous mammary tumor in C3H/HEN mice. Proc. Amer. Assn. Cancer Res. **3**: 346.
22. MORTON, D. L., L. GOLDMAN & D. A. WOOD. 1965. Immunological tolerance to spontaneous mammary adenocarcinomas (SMC). Proc. Amer. Assn. Cancer Res. **6**: 47.
23. RIGGINS, R. S. & Y. H. PILCH. 1964. Immunity to spontaneous and methylcholanthrene-induced tumors in inbred mice. Cancer Res. **24**: 1994.
24. MÜLLER, M. & E. R. WELCKER. 1965. Akzeleration von Mammakarzinomtransplantaten bei CBA/Bln-Mäusen durch Vorbehandlung mit kleinen Dosen vitaler isologer Tumorzellen. Acta Biol. Med. German **15**: 147.
25. PREHN, R. 1967. Personal communication.
26. LAVRIN, D. H., P. B. BLAIR & D. W. WEISS. 1966. Immunology of spontaneous mammary carcinomas in mice. III. Immunogenicity of C3H preneoplastic hyperplastic alveolar nodules in C3Hf hosts. Cancer Res. **26**: 293.
27. LAVRIN, D. H., P. B. BLAIR & D. W. WEISS. 1966. Immunology of spontaneous mammary carcinomas in mice. IV. Association of the mammary tumor virus with the immunogenicity of C3H nodules and tumors. Cancer Res. **26**: 929.
28. MORTON, D. L. 1964. Acquired immunological tolerance to spontaneous mammary adenocarcinomas following neonatal infection with mammary tumor agent (MTA). Proc. Amer. Assn. Cancer Res. **5**: 46.
29. NANDI, S., D. KNOX, K. B. DEOME, M. HANDIN, V. V. FINSTER & P. B. PICKETT. 1966. Mammary tumor virus activity in red blood cells of BALB/c f.C3H mice. J. Nat. Cancer Inst. **36**: 809.
30. DEZFULIAN, M., D. H. LAVRIN, A. SHEN, P. B. BLAIR & D. W. WEISS. 1966. Immunology of spontaneous mammary carcinomas in mice. Studies on the nature of the protective antigens. *In* Carcinogenesis–A Broad Critique. Twentieth Annual Symposium on Fundamental Cancer Research at the University of Texas M.D. Anderson Hospital and Tumor Institute. : 365–388. The Williams & Wilkins Co. Baltimore, Md.
31. DEZFULIAN, M., T. ZEE, K. B. DEOME, P. B. BLAIR & D. W. WEISS. 1968. Role of the mammary tumor virus in the immunogenicity of spontaneous mammary carcinomas of mice and in the responsiveness of the hosts–studies in BALB/c animals. Cancer Res. **28**: 1759.
32. WEISS, D. W. & A. SHEN. 1966. Immunology of spontaneous mammary tumors in mice. Cross-reacting immunogenicity of C3H tumors in C3Hf and C3H/2 mice. Proc. Amer. Assn. Cancer Res. **7**: 75.
33. VAAGE, J., R. BONHAG & D. W. WEISS. 1966. Immunological prophylaxis and therapy of spontaneous mammary tumors. Exp. Hematol. **9**: 24.
34. ATTIA, M. A. M. & D. W. WEISS. 1966. Immunology of spontaneous mammary carcinomas of mice. V. Acquired tumor resistance and enhancement in strain A mice infected with mammary tumor virus. Cancer Res. **26**: 1787.
35. CINADER, B. 1962. Acquired tolerance, autoantibodies and cancer. J. Canad. Med. Assn. **86**: 1161.

36. Nachtigal, D., R. Eshel-Zussman & M. Feldman. 1965. Restoration of the specific immunological reactivity of tolerant rabbits by conjugated antigens. Immunology **9:** 543.
37. Lavrin, D. H. To be published.
38. Duesberg, P. H. & P. B. Blair. 1966. Isolation of the nucleic acid of mouse mammary tumor virus (MTV). Proc. Nat. Acad. Sci. USA **55:** 1490.
39. Joklik, W. K. 1964. The intracellular uncoating of poxvirus DNA. II. The molecular basis of the uncoating process. J. Molec. Biol. **8:** 277.
40. Blair, P. B. 1960. Serologic comparison of mammary tumor viruses from 3 strains of mice. Proc. Soc. Exp. Biol. Med. **103:** 188.
41. Blair, P. B. 1966. Immunology of the murine mammary-tumor virus (MTV): Development of methods of assay. *In* Viruses Inducing Cancer. W. J. Burdette, Ed. : 288–304. Utah University Press. Salt Lake City, Utah.
42. Blair, P. B. & D. W. Weiss. 1966. Immunology of the mouse mammary tumor virus: Comparison of mammary tumor virus with the agent found in C3Hf/Crgl mice. J. Nat. Cancer Inst. **36:** 423.
43. Blair, P. B., D. H. Lavrin, M. Dezfulian & D. W. Weiss. 1966. Immunology of the mouse mammary tumor virus (MTV): Identification *in vitro* of mouse antibodies against MTV. Cancer Res. **26:** 647.
44. Blair, P. B., D. W. Weiss & D. R. Pitelka. 1966. Immunology of the mouse mammary tumor virus: Correlation of the immunodiffusion precipitate line with type-B virus particles. J. Nat. Cancer Instit. **37:** 261.
45. Blair, P. B., C. Smoller, R. S. Bonhag & D. W. Weiss. 1968. Immunology of the mouse mammary tumor virus (MTV). Electron microscopic studies of the interaction between MTV and specific antibody in immunodiffusion. J. Nat. Cancer Instit. **40:** 1325.
46. Blair, P. B. 1965. Immunology of the mouse mammary tumor virus (MTV): A qualitative *in vitro* assay for MTV. Nature **208:** 165.
47. Nandi, S. 1963. New method for detection of mouse mammary tumor virus. 2. Effect of administration of lactating mammary tissue extracts on incidence of hyperplastic mammary nodules in BALB/cCrgl mice. J. Nat. Cancer Instit. **31:** 75.
48. Weiss, D. W. & A. Q. Wells. 1960. Vaccination against tuberculosis with nonliving vaccines. III. Vaccination of guinea pigs with fractions of phenol-killed tubercle bacilli. Amer. Rev. Resp. Dis. **82:** 339.
49. Weiss, D. W., R. S. Bonhag & K. B. DeOme. 1961. Protective activity of fractions of tubercle bacilli against isologous tumors in mice. Nature **190:** 889.
50. Weiss, D. W., R. S. Bonhag & J. A. Parks. 1964. Studies on the heterologous immunogenicity of a methanol-insoluble fraction of attenuated tubercle bacilli (BCG). I. Antimicrobial protection. J. Exp. Med. **119:** 53.
51. Weiss, D. W., R. S. Bonhag & P. Leslie. 1966. Studies on the heterologous immunogenicity of a methanol-insoluble fraction of attenuated tubercle bacilli (BCG). II. Protection against tumor isografts. J. Exp. Med. **124:** 1039.
52. Steinkuller, C., L. G. Krigbaum & D. W. Weiss. Studies on the mode of action of the heterologous immunogenicity of a methanol-insoluble fraction of attenuated tubercle bacilli (BCG). Immunology **16:** 255.
53. Steinkuller, C. & D. Burton. 1966. Immunology of spontaneous mammary tumors in mice. Mode of action of a tumor protective fraction of tubercle bacilli (MER). Proc. Amer. Assn. Cancer Res. **7:** 68.
54. Weiss, D. W., C. Steinkuller & L. Greetham. 1967. Immunology of spontaneous mammary tumors in mice. Further studies on the mode of action of a tumor-protective fraction of tubercle bacilli. Proc. Amer. Assn. Cancer Res. **8:** 72.
55. Jerne, N. K., A. A. Nordin & C. Henry. 1963. The agar plaque technique for recognizing antibody producing cells. *In* Cell-Bound Antibodies. B. Amos & H. Koprowski, Eds. : 109–122. Wistar Institute Press. Philadelphia, Pa.
56. Prehn, R. T. The relationship of immunology to carcinogenesis. Ann. N. Y. Acad. Sci. This monograph.
57. Solomon, G. F. & R. H. Moos. 1964. Emotions, immunity, and disease. Arch. Gen. Psychiat. **11:** 657.
58. LeShan, L. L. & R. E. Worthington. 1956. Personality as factor in pathogenesis of cancer: Review of literature. Brit. J. Med. Psychol. **29:** 49.
59. Stern, K. & I. Davidsohn. 1955. Effect of estrogen and cortisone on immune hemoantibodies in mice of inbred strains. J. Immun. **74:** 479.
60. Fine, J. On the mechanisms of defense against massive injury. Amer. Sci. In press.
61. Miles, A. A. 1964. The acute reactions of injury as an antimicrobial defense. *In* Injury, Inflammation, and Immunity. L. Thomas, J. W. Uhr & L. Grant, Eds. : 162–177. The Williams & Wilkins Co. Baltimore, Md.

THE RELATIONSHIP OF IMMUNOLOGY TO CARCINOGENESIS*

Richmond T. Prehn
The Institute for Cancer Research
Philadelphia, Pa.

Since psychophysiologic factors, particularly various forms of stress, have been repeatedly implicated as modifiers of immunologic reactions, it is logical to consider this pathway when evaluating possible effects of the psyche upon carcinogenesis. That immunologic reactions play an important role in carcinogenesis seems to have been established in a variety of animal experiments. In this paper I will review some of the more pertinent evidence for this role, and particularly more recent data from my laboratory.

There is no doubt that many animal tumors are directly due to the actions of viruses. It will indeed be surprising if a similar situation does not exist in man, although definite evidence is still lacking. The oncogenic viruses are antigenic and can arouse strong immune responses; their immunology is similar to that of the better known and supposedly non-oncogenic viral agents. Thus, the immunology of the viral agents does not require special discussion in regard to oncology, except to point out that many of the oncologic viruses in lower animals are transmitted "vertically" from parent to offspring. This transmission may be via the ovum, the placenta, or, sometimes, immediately after birth. The important features of these modes of transmission are that ordinary isolation procedures are ineffective in the control of viral spread, and that the immune reactions of the host are markedly affected by the early age at which the animal is first exposed. The fetus and the very young of most species are immunologically deficient. If "imprinted" at this critical early time with a viral antigen, they may remain deficient throughout life with respect to that antigen.[1] The immunology of the oncogenic viruses has been extensively reviewed.[2–4]

In addition to viruses, many other types of carcinogenic agents have been identified, including hundreds of chemicals, various radiations, and physical (i.e., smooth surface) factors. Tumor cells of whatever varied etiology, viral included, appear to possess antigens capable of arousing a defensive cytologic immunity.[2–4] It is the role of this antitumor-cell immunity, as distinct from antiviral immunity, that will constitute the principal substance of this paper.

There is no need to recount the extensive researches that have established the existence of these apparently tumor-specific histocompatibility antigens. This has been the subject of numerous reviews.[2–4] Instead, I will discuss some of the evidence concerning their role in carcinogenesis and the possible implications for psychophysiologic mechanisms.

I believe that some of the most impressive indirect evidence concerning the importance of these antigens in carcinogenesis comes from a consideration of the interrelationships of latent period, antigenicity, and tumor incidence. Very early in the study of these antigens it was found that the apparent antigenic titre, especially in the case of the chemically induced tumors, varied markedly from tumor to tumor.[5] Some tumors appeared to be very antigenic and others only weakly so, if indeed they were antigenic at all. There appeared to be a marked relationship between the latent period, after application of a particular dosage of carcinogen,

* Supported by USPHS grants CA–08856, CA–06927, and FR–05539 from the National Cancer Institutes, and an appropriation from the Commonwealth of Pennsylvania.

and the antigenicity of the resulting tumors.[6,7] This area has recently been reinvestigated by my associate, Dr. Gerald Bartlett.[8] The relationship found is shown in FIGURE 1. It can be seen that all of the tumors of high antigenicity, as measured by their ability to illicit marked immunization against the growth of a challenge tumor implant, were tumors of relatively short or moderate latent periods. In no case was a tumor of long latency markedly antigenic. It should be noted, however, that not all early arising tumors were highly antigenic – they might or might not be so. Additionally, there may have been a deficiency of highly antigenic tumors among the very first to arise; i.e., before the third month. There were no apparent relationships between degree of malignancy, rate of growth after tumor appearance, and antigenicity. To me, one of the most striking aspects of this distribution is that it is, to a large extent, simultaneously a measure of antigenic distribution and tumor frequency. Also noteworthy is the fact that the distribution also suggests the known relationship between time and the depression of immune responses by the carcinogen.[9] All carcinogens interfere with immune reactions, and the one used in these experiments, 3-methylcholanthrene, depresses them to a marked degree.[9] A plot of this depression against time would substantially reproduce the curve produced by plotting antigenicity against time in FIGURE 1. Thus, no depression of the homograft reaction is seen in response to 3-methylcholanthrene, as used in these experiments (a paraffin, 1% carcinogen

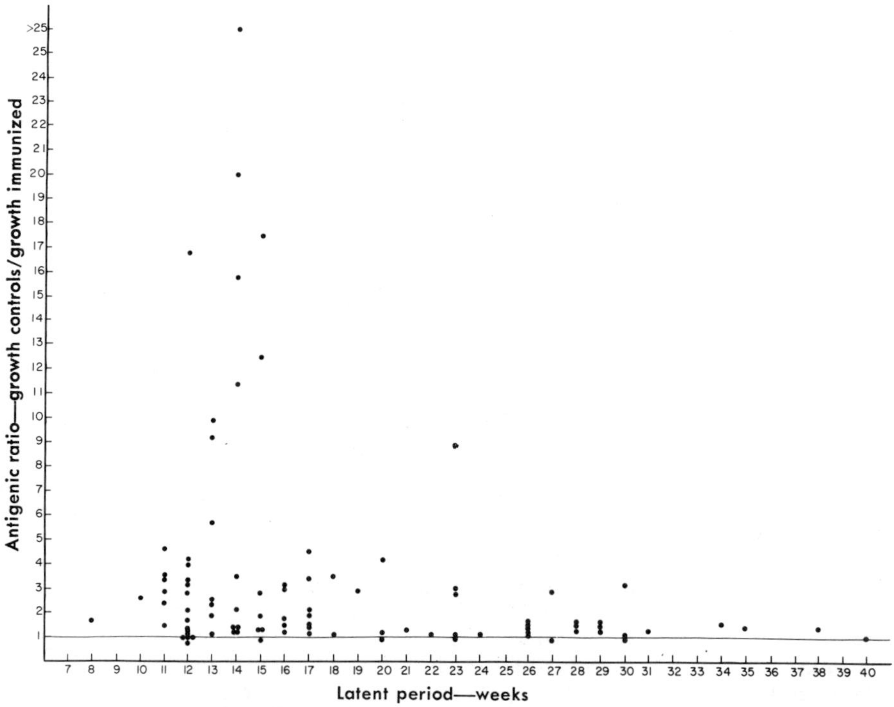

FIGURE 1. Relationship between latent period and antigenicity. Abscissa (y axis): Antigenic ratio, average size in controls/average size in immunized. Ordinate (x axis): Time in weeks after carcinogen implantation.

pellet subcutaneously) until about a month after administration. Then depression increases rapidly to a maximum, followed by a slow decline over a period of many months.[10] Thus, both the points of maximum tumor inception and tumor antigenicity reach a peak at approximately the time of maximum depression of the homograft reaction. It seems to me that this coincidence is more than fortuitous, and has a number of interesting implications.

The first implication is that a necessary, if not sufficient, activity of the carcinogen appears to be immunosuppression. Tumors appeared in direct proportion to the degree of immunodepression, and their antigenicity was also related. This evidence, combined with other data yet to be discussed, suggest that immunodepression is a very important aspect of experimental carcinogenesis.

The distribution of antigenicities in FIGURE 1 further suggests that the titre of antigenicity was a random variable and was not entirely due to the dosage of carcinogen or to the latent period. When immune reactions were near normal, those tumors that were highly antigenic were apparently suppressed before their gross appearance and only relatively nonantigenic tumors were seen. At those times when the carcinogen had produced immunodepression, highly antigenic tumors were seen in addition to more weakly antigenic ones. Experiments currently under way will tell whether or not highly antigenic tumors will be found throughout the distribution if the animals are kept immunologically crippled throughout the entire study.

Not all investigators have reached identical conclusions. In the case of polyoma viral-induced tumors, the tumor-cell antigenicity also decreased with increasing latent period, but only one tumor of little antigenicity and short latency was found.[4] However, the sample examined was not large. Recently, a study with chemically induced tumors also failed to show the early arising tumors of relatively little antigenicity that are so evident in our work.[11] The reason for this apparent disparity has not yet been determined.

Other types of experiments also suggest that the immune mechanism normally acts to suppress a large number of tumors that would otherwise be fatal. Studies of chemical carcinogenesis in immunologically crippled animals have given highly suggestive, but not dramatic, results. The usual experiment has been to produce immunologic cripples by thymectomy performed shortly after birth. Later exposure to carcinogen resulted in a somewhat shorter latency of tumor formation than that seen in sham-thymectomized controls.[11–14] That these experiments have not been more dramatically successful is not surprising. Application of the carcinogen results in immunologic crippling in both experimental and control animals, a situation to which the newborn thymectomy can be expected to add relatively little.

To overcome this inherent deficiency, one of my students, Mr. Marc Lappe, has recently published an account of a modified procedure for studying the role of immunologic surveillance.[15] The procedure used was to treat the mouse skin with what was ordinarily a subcarcinogenic dosage of 3-methylcholanthrene. The skin was then transplanted to isogenic animals of varying immunologic competence: increased by treatment with BCG, normal, or decreased by radiation. It was found that the act of transplantation was an added stimulus sufficient to elicit numerous papillomas in a short time. The incidence and latent period, however, were markedly affected by the immunologic status of the new host. Both the number of papillomas and the time to appearance were decreased in radiated recipients and lengthened in the immunologically stimulated. Additionally, regression occurred earlier and with greater frequency in the latter. The number of lesions that progressed to malignancy was greater in the immunologically crippled recipients but appeared to be, in any particular time interval, a constant percentage of the papillomas at risk. Immunologic surveillance apparently worked during the early benign stages of the lesions to decrease the numbers of papillomas, but did not appear to affect directly the further progression to malignancy.

Thus, it seems to me that the evidence that the immune mechanism, by acting against tumor-specific histocompatibility antigens, acts as a surveillance mechanism, is very strong. The probability that carcinogenesis could be affected by psychic factors working via the immune response is thus very good.

The question why certain tumors, despite at least some degree of antigenicity, survive and grow becomes largely a matter of a balance of forces between the immune reaction and the growth potential of the particular tumor. Similarly, the antigenicity of the pneumococcus does not prevent all, but only most, cases of potential pneumonia. Anything tending to lessen or delay the immune response (psychophysiologic effects?) will increase the chance of a tumor-cell clone escaping immunologic control.

The apparent importance of the immunologic mechanism in tumor surveillance raises interesting phylogenetic and evolutionary questions. The capacity to mount an immunologic defense against foreign or altered cells arises in evolution at or about the stage of the hagfish, a primitive cyclostome.[16] In ontogeny, the immune capability begins to develop in the last quarter of gestation, and in most mammals does not reach full effectiveness until after birth.[16] Curiously, it is the general concensus that neoplasms, in the true sense of the word as used in mammalian pathology, are rare or absent in animals of the lower end of the phylogenetic scale. Indeed, direct attempts to produce tumors with chemical carcinogens have proved very difficult in amphibia, and especially in their larvae before metamorphosis.[17] Attempts to produce tumors by injection of 3-methylcholanthrene into the newt produced only two sarcomas, but numerous accessory limbs![18] It appears that there is a general inverse correlation between the ability of an animal to regenerate an amputated limb and its susceptibility to chemical carcinogenesis.[17] Furthermore, it seems that the gradual loss of regenerative capacity as one ascends the phylogenetic scale corresponds in at least a rough way with the development of the immune mechanism. These relationships suggest to me the possibility that the development of the immune reaction, as a surveillance mechanism against cancer, may have been necessitated by the evolutionary loss of a control mechanism associated with regenerative ability. Indeed, a malignant tumor produced in a mammal in response to 3-methylcholanthrene may represent merely a perverted and pathological attempt to form the blastema of regeneration that would have been the result of carcinogen treatment in a more primitive beast.

If psychophysiologic mechanisms alter tumor biology via an affect on the immune response, it is not surprising that the results of animal experimentation have yielded inconsistent and, at times, contradictory results.[19,20] We have already seen how varying are the antigenicities of various tumors. A further factor that I have not touched upon is the important question of immunologic enhancement.[2] Sufficient to say that humoral immunity, rather than being inimical to tumor growth, may actually aid some tumors to survive. When one considers these varying responses of different tumors to immunologic factors and the probably differing effects of various types of psychophysiologic stresses on the type of the immune response, it is small wonder that reproducible and predictable results are difficult to obtain in experimental work. Further, it is possible that psychic factors also influence tumors by pathways other than the immune response. The complexities of the experimental situation are not an argument against the importance of psychophysiologic factors; the complexities do suggest to me that in this important area most of the useful observations, in the immediate future as in the past, will come from the clinic, rather than from animal experimentation.

In summary, I have presented several lines of evidence to suggest that antitumor-cell immunity plays a role in carcinogenesis and that the immune mechanism serves as a surveillance mechanism to prevent carcinogenesis. One of these lines of evidence concerned the interrelationships between immune depression by a carcinogen, the latent period between carcinogen application and tumor appearance, and the antigenicities of the tumors. Other evidence concerned various types of carcinogenic studies in immunologically crippled or stimulated animals. The variability of tumor-cell antigenicity makes a prediction of the influence of psychic factors in a particular case difficult. Finally, I speculated that the immune reaction may have arisen as an evolutionary replacement for a cell-control mechanism associated with the regenerative ability of lower animals, an ability lost at that time on the phylogenetic scale when the immune reaction first became prominent.

References

1. Miller, J. F. A. P. & D. Osoba. 1967. Current concepts of the immunological function of the thymus. Physiol. Rev. **47:** 437.
2. Hattler, B., Jr. & B. Amos. 1966. The immunobiology of cancer: tumor antigens and the responsiveness of the host. Monogr. Surg. Sci. **3:** 1–34.
3. Klein, G. 1966. Tumor antigens. Ann. Rev. Microbiol. **20:** 223–252.
4. Sjogren, H. O. 1965. Transplantation methods as a tool for detection of tumor specific antigens. Progr. Exp. Tumor Res. **6:** 289–322.
5. Prehn, R. T. 1957. Immunity to methylcholanthrene-induced sarcomas. J. Nat. Cancer Inst. **18:** 769–778.
6. Prehn, R. T. 1962. Role of immune mechanisms in the biology of chemically and physically induced tumors. M. D. Anderson Hospital Symposium on Fundamental Cancer Research **16:** 475–485.
7. Old, L. J., E. A. Boyse, E. Carswell & D. A. Clarke. 1962. Immunologic studies on chemically induced tumors. Ann. N. Y. Acad. Sci. **101:** 80–106.
8. Bartlett, G. 1968. Unpublished observations.
9. Prehn, R. T. 1963. Function of depressed immunologic reactivity during carcinogenesis. J. Nat. Cancer Inst. **31:** 791–805.
10. Stjernsward, J. 1966. Age-dependent tumor-host barrier and effect of carcinogen-induced immunodepression or rejection of isografted methylcholanthrene-induced sarcoma cells. J. Nat. Cancer Inst. **37:** 505–512.
11. Johnson, S. 1968. The effect of thymectomy and of the dose of 3-methylcholanthrene on the induction and antigenic properties of sarcomas in C57BL mice. Brit. J. Cancer **22:** 93–104.
12. Balner, H. & H. Dersjant. 1966. Neonatal thymectomy and tumor induction with methylcholanthrene in mice. J. Nat. Cancer Inst. **36:** 513–521.
13. Miller, J. F. A. P., G. A. Grant & F. J. C. Roe. 1963. Effect of thymectomy on the induction of skin tumors by 3,4,benzopyrene. Nature **199:** 920–922.
14. Grant, G., F. J. C. Roe & M. C. Pike. 1966. Effect of neonatal thymectomy on the induction of papillomata and carcinomata by 3,4,benzopyrene in mice. Nature **210:** 603–604.
15. Lappe, M. A. 1968. Evidence for the antigenicity of papillomas induced by 3-methylcholanthrene. J. Nat. Cancer Inst. **40:** 823–846.
16. Good, R. A. & B. W. Papermaster. 1964. Ontogeny and phylogeny of adaptive immunity. Advances Immun. **4:** 1.
17. Seilern-Aspang, F. & K. Kratochwil. 1962. Induction and differentiation of an epithelial tumor in the newt. J. Embryol. Exp. Morph. **10:** 337–356.
18. Breedis, C. 1952. Induction of accessory limbs and of sarcoma in the newt (*Triturus viridenscens*), with carcinogenic substances. Cancer Res. **12:** 861–866.

19. OLENOV, Y. M. 1955. On induced cancer in mice with experimental neurosis. Vop. Onkol. **8**: 26–32.
20. GOTTFRIED, G. & H. MOLOMUT. 1963. Effect of surgical trauma and other external stress agents on tumor growth and healing of cancer. Proc. 8th Anti-Cancer Congress **3**: 473.

DISCUSSION OF THE PAPER

DR. BENNETTE: The last comments about the newt interested me, considering the work of Seilern-Aspang and Kratochwil, who found that injection of methylcholanthrene produced tumors, although other workers have shown that they produced additional limbs. In this case, the tumors, I believe, were claimed to undergo a redifferentiation or maturation, which seems to me to be very relevant to the question of the possibility that the immune mechanisms, in their great diversity, include the possibility of morphostatic control systems as well as surveillance mechanisms. I wondered whether you would be willing to comment on that thought?

DR. PREHN: I agree that this is a most interesting area of speculation, and it is one of the things that excites us so much about the mammary tumor system.

Here we have a system where one interpretation, at least, is that the neoplastic cells have gone back to normal. This is overtly what seems to happen; that we put in what are neoplastic tissues, and we get out what appear to be normal tissues. This is, as you point out not completely without precedent in biology.

We think that is the unlikely explanation in our system, but it is certainly one that we have to rule out, and one that we cannot completely ignore at this point. It will be another year or two before we can settle this problem.

DR. BENNETTE: May I ask why it seems to be necessary to rule out something that seems to be so relevant to the question of spontaneous regression of tumors, now so well documented?

DR. PREHN: Well, I am one of those workers who thinks that most progress in research is made by ruling out hypotheses; that is the only reason I spoke in that fashion. I must also say that my personal intuition, as well as a little bit of evidence suggests that this is not the explanation in our system.

DR. SOLOMON: Is there evidence that physiologic levels of corticosteroids would be sufficiently immunosuppressant to affect tumor immunity?

DR. PREHN: I do not think that we can answer this question, especially as regards the human. In the human, we are very "stuck"; we have not even demonstrated in the human that any of these things I said about the mouse is definitely true. We can infer that they are, I think, because I am much more impressed with the likenesses between man and mouse than with the differences. But this is all speculation at this point, and I am afraid that I can not go any further than that.

UNIDENTIFIED SPEAKER: Sir, in regard to high levels of corticosteroids, or ACTH stimulation, would that affect any of the systems you studied?

DR. PREHN: Certainly; there is no question but that high levels of corticosteroids can indeed affect the homeograft reaction, and the systems that I have talked about.

DR. SOLOMON: I know that massive doses can, but high physiologic levels that can be obtained with ACTH may not be immunosuppressive.

DR. PREHN: Yes, I think that with high levels of ACTH, similar things might be observed.

DR. SOLOMON: I was wondering if you might comment on the differentiation between the concept of specific tolerance as related to carcinogenesis, and the concept of more generalized immune depression. Presumably, the approaches dealing with these two issues as related to etiology would be different. One would be an attempt to break tolerance, and the other would be an attempt, presumably, to enhance the generalized immunological responsivity, especially the cellular response. Could you talk about that?

DR. PREHN: I think that one point that needs to be made is that as far as I am aware, immunologic tolerance is not an absolute affair. It is not an all-or-none response. When we say an animal is tolerant, we mean that he is relatively tolerant, and consequently I think that, in some systems at least, the breaking of tolerance is no different than is the raising of the immunologic reactivity against the antigen for which there already is some activity.

What role tolerance plays in tumorogenesis, I do not know. Dr. Klein and Dr. Weiss both presented evidence that tolerance can be very important in some systems, especially in the viral systems. In these cases there is immunologic tolerance to the virus and to the antigens produced by it, and presumably very little immune reaction against the tumors. While Dr. Weiss elegantly has shown that the spontaneous tumors (i.e., virally induced tumors) are antigenic, they certainly are only weakly so in the animal that harbors the virus. If most tumors turn out to be virally induced and we harbor the viruses and are tolerant to them, we will not be able to contribute much, immunologically. However, I think I should leave further comments about that to Dr. Klein's discussion. There is one thing I should like to say before I lose the opportunity. I think Dr. Bennette yesterday raised the question about the alienation of cells, and about what this has to do with the production of tumors—alienation, I gather, being an elegant way of saying that the cells become separated and their communications disturbed. Somehow or other, this would lead to carcinogenesis.

This is an excellent idea, for which there is considerable experimental evidence. But I suggest that one of the examples he cited is not a good one. He mentioned the plastic film type of carcinogenesis. Here you have a barrier between cells, and you get tumors. And if you punch holes in the barrier, you no longer get the tumors, because now the cells can communicate, and as Dr. Kaplan pointed out, the function of connective-tissue cells is to connect, and if they cannot connect, they feel frustrated and therefore become tumors.

Unfortunately, my former colleague, Dr. Bates, published a paper several years ago, showing quite nicely that one did not have to punch holes in the film. If one merely made the surface rough, or scratched the surface, one no longer got tumors. And this, I think, effectively rules out the connection hypothesis, or the alienation aspects, in this particular system. It is not a direct interference with connection; it is a smooth surface that is important for carcinogenesis.

DR. MARGOLIN: I am fascinated by some of the suggestions made by Dr. Prehn and I should like to ask two questions about the hyperplastic nodule that was transplanted into your *in vivo* preparation.

First, what was the histologic state of the implanted tissue? Was it preneoplastic or neoplastic? If it is preneoplastic and therefore capable of generating normal tissue, does it act as an organizer in the sense of classical experimental embryology by converting some *Anlage* in the host animal?

DR. PREHN: Can I take it right from there?

DR. MARGOLIN: I have a related second part to this question. Since this process is controlled by estrogenic factors, is it not appropriate to ask whether these hyperplastic nodules have been assayed for estrogenic potential or estrogen content? Do you wish to answer my multiple first question before I ask my second one?

DR. PREHN: In the first place, the cleared fat pad has no *Anlage* for breast tissue. The breast grows in from outside the fat pad; i.e., it develops from the nipple and grows into the fad pad. There is little or no possibility that fat-pad tissue itself is converted into breast tissue.

As to whether this is neoplastic or premalignant tissue, or whether you want to consider this as being preneoplastic tissue, is a matter of definition. The people at Berkeley customarily call this preneoplastic tissue. I think they are far off base in this, because it certainly has a heritable alteration—a heritable defect—because it is transplantable serially. It grows like any other benign tumor.

I regard benign tumors as neoplasms; i.e., premalignant neoplasms. And I so regard these. Now, as far as hormonal relationships are concerned, these are indeed responsive to the hormonal environment. A certain hormonal milieu is necessary for their production, and they remain dependent on hormonal factors, at least much more so than the resultant malignancy that arises in them.

DR. WEISS: Just one question regarding Dr. Bates' experiment: Did he find more of an inflammatory response around rough than around smooth films?

DR. PREHN: I do not believe he said, but in our own work I can pretty well assure you that there is indeed a much greater chronic inflammatory reaction around the rough films than around the smooth, so much so that we have entertained the hypothesis that the primary reason one did not get tumors was this inflammatory response. But I think this is a hypothesis that has to be proved, and we have not yet succeeded in doing so.

DR. WEISS: One might consider the fact that at some stages of the inflammatory response there is a much-increased communication between the local area and surrounding tissues. This greater degree of intercommunication must be juxtaposed against the mechanical walling-off of an area of inflammation at later stages of the inflammatory process.

DR. PREHN: That is true.

DR. BAHNSON: Dr. Prehn, aside from all the technical aspects that I cannot appreciate sufficiently, I was very gratified and struck by your speculation.

Lang Stevenson in England and Jonas in this country have been speculating that neoplasias may represent phylogenetically old regeneration attempts in an organism that now is geared to a different defense or operational system. One of your thoughts was that the old regeneration mechanism had been replaced, or had faded out at the same time in phylogeny that the immune response took over. Now, there is not a direct relationship between your observations and speculations and Jonas' and Stevenson's, but there certainly is enough evidence at hand to start a somewhat speculative discussion tomorrow about this very point.

DR. SALK: I do not want to preempt any of the discussion that we will have when we pull together some of the splendid thoughts that came from the paper by Dr. Klein yesterday, and Dr. Weiss and Dr. Prehn today. I think you have been treated to a feast of highly delectable facts, and you have seen how minds work that are willing to encompass a complex problem and look at it from a variety of points of view.

The presentations this morning reveal how enormous advances can occur in a field that just a few years ago was really in a realm of speculation, and many of the speculations that were made at that time have now been demonstrated to have validity, including some of the historical references to which Dr. Weiss referred.

Dr. Prehn has pointed to spontaneous regression in precancerous lesions where the cancerous cells seem to have disappeared. Does this not have its counterpart in a clinical situation in which there is the suggestion that a neoplasm that is surrounded by lymphocytes has a far better prognosis than a neoplasm in which there is no lymphocytic reaction? That is the first question that I would ask.

The second question: When you talk about your tumors, being antigenic, I detected that you were talking only about inducing resistance. I should like to know if you have any data on human antibody response.

The third point concerns the role of endocrinologic factors, and here alone a great deal of speculation is possible. I am sure the data will be developed in time. Very subtle differences in hormonal balance are sufficient to produce very striking effects, as one sees in the diabetic, for example, and as one sees in pregnancy; pregnancy predisposes a woman to the development of paralytic polio when exposed, and this is not evident either before or after pregnancy. Hormonal balance has a marked effect on the acceleration of certain tumors, as seen in a woman who has a tumor and becomes pregnant. Therefore, it would appear that, within the physiological range, endocrinologic factors do play a role.

To what extent do physiological factors play a role with changing age, or with a difference in the aging of the two different components of the immunologic system, tending to favor one over the other? I am speculating now that with advancing age, the rejecting mechanism may age sooner than that component of the immunologic mechanism that is responsible for tumor enhancement, which may age more slowly. This, too, could shift the balance.

It is easy to see how hormonal factors may operate differently on each component of the immunologic system, the corticosteroids acting on delayed hypersensitivity, perhaps, and the adrenalin acting on the other components. I know that in some laboratories, studies are now being done on the effect of very slight differences in epineprine concentration on humoral antibody response.

The reason I bring these few points out at this moment, before we try to pull all this together, is to indicate that the field is pregnant with all kinds of possibilities of interest to those who are concerned with the problem of neoplasia and its possible control. I could not agree more with Dr. Weiss when he indicated that this seems, at the moment, to be the most fruitful area of investigation.

DR. PREHN: I agree. As far as lymphocytic infiltration is concerned, we feel very strongly that this is a good indicator of immunologic resistance. And, in fact, in the experiments I cited in the papilloma system, in which the immune mechanism was crippled by one means or another, or stimulated, the morphologic response was very obvious: clouds of lymphocytes around the regressing lesions in the one system, absolute lack of this around the progressing lesions in the other system.

As far as the humoral antibody situation is concerned, I have not really pressed this in my own laboratory, but the general experience has been that humoral antibody in the methylcolanthrene-induced sarcoma system has been difficult to detect. However, when it has been detected, it has again, as in other systems, shown no correlation with resistance to the growth of the tumor. So we feel quite confident that this is a cellular immunity that we are dealing with. This is the part of the immune response that is doing the business. And as far as your third comments are concerned, I agree entirely.

EMOTIONS AND IMMUNITY

A. F. Rasmussen, Jr.

Department of Medical Microbiology and Immunology and Brain Research Institute
University of California, Los Angeles, School of Medicine
Los Angeles, Calif.

This paper will present a summary of the work that has gone on in our laboratory in the Brain Research Institute at UCLA over the last several years.

Some readers may have a legitimate objection to the use of the term "emotion." Our experimental work was largely based on the mouse, and there must indeed be some question as to how one appraises emotionality in that species. The choice of the term, however, is my own, and it comes from the initial motivation for these studies, which goes back to discussions with Dr. Norman Brill, Professor of Psychiatry at UCLA, and especially Dr. James Marsh, an experimental psychologist who participated actively in the development of this program. My own interest stemmed from a general interest in nonspecific factors and resistance, Dr. Brill's from his personal experience in psychiatric practice, and Dr. Marsh's from interest in developing experimental systems that might simulate conditions associated with emotional stress in man. I shall (1) present a very brief summary of our earlier work, (2) discuss these results briefly in general terms as they may relate to changes in immunity following stress, and (3) describe in greater detail our experience with two experimental systems particularly pertinent to this conference, polyoma and Rauscher leukemia virus infections. These latter studies were largely conducted by K. K. Chang (polyoma) and Marcus M. Jensen (Rauscher leukemia).

After preliminary experiments with various systems, Dr. James Marsh adopted a modified Miller shuttle box as our main stressor.[1] "Stress" and "stressor" are used interchangeably, as defined by Dr. Friedman and his associates elsewhere in this monograph. Later, because of possible influences of physical activity induced by the stressful situation and of the occasional acceptance of an electrical stimulus by the animals, we used two other systems, constraint[1] and noise,[2] for comparison. Responses were similar, although the avoidance-learning situation appeared to be more continuously effective over longer periods. Sound stress consisted of daily three-hour exposures to an 800-cps sine wave sound at about 120 db intensity. Avoidance-learning stress was produced by a shuttle box apparatus automatically programmed to require the mice to jump a barrier to the opposite side of a compartment once every five minutes on the presentation of a warning buzzer and light. Mice failing to jump received an electric shock. Mice soon learned to avoid the electric shock and were thus exposed primarily to the stress of anticipation of pain and fear. Daily six-hour periods of this stressor were used.

The readily observable bodily changes induced by repeated applications of the avoidance-learning situation were hypertrophy of the adrenals,[1] leukopenia,[1] primarily due to reduction in lymphocytes,[1] hypotrophy of the spleen,[1] hypotrophy of the thymus,[1] persistent pseudoestrous without ovulation in females,[3] and suppression of granuloma formation.[4] The responses to experimental infections in mice exposed repeatedly to this stressful situation were an increased susceptibility to herpes simplex,[5] poliomyelitis,[6] Coxsackie B,[7] and polyoma virus infections.[8] No changes were seen in resistance to influenza and related respiratory viruses,[9] and only a slight suppression of the progression of Rauscher leukemia was observed.[10] Detectable changes in immunological mechanisms were a decreased clearance of foreign particles from the blood,[11] a delay in the rejection of skin grafts,[12] absence of any detectable influence on antibody response as measured by the response of hemagglutinating antibodies to influenza virus vaccine,[13] and response in neutralizing antibody to vesicular stomatitis virus infection.[14]

One of the most pronounced and readily demonstrable changes was a decrease in susceptibility to acute passive anaphylaxis induced by the intravenous administration of antigen-antibody complexes.[15,16] An important change, which might not fall in the category of immunity as precisely defined, was the fall in interferon levels in stressed, as compared with control, mice.[17] Both the decrease in susceptibility to anaphylaxis and the fall in interferon levels were found to be transitory and to be related to immediate responses to stress, even though they were first observed in chronically stressed animals.[16,18]

I cannot explain the discrepancy between our experience with antibody response and those reported by Dr. Friedman's group and elsewhere in this monograph by Dr. Solomon. I suspect that a number of variables in this kind of experiment may be responsible. In the first place, influenza virus and vesicular stomatitis virus (VSV) make good vaccines because the surface antigens of these viruses are very effective in inducing an immune response. Thus, a relatively severe impairment of immunologic capacity might be necessary before any changes would be observable. A second possible explanation is that we were measuring largely gamma G antibody. There is increasing evidence that gamma A and gamma M antibodies are important in resistance, particularly in the early stages of infection, and we have made no attempt to measure these antibodies in our system. A third possibility is that both influenza and VSV are mediumsized viruses and do not present anything like the number and complexity of antigens that cholera vaccine presents. Thus, the individual subject's immunologic capacity is not pressed as it might be when confronted with a large number of diverse antigens, as in cholera vaccine.

Turning to Rauscher leukemia virus infection in chronically stressed mice, there is a slight but definite suppression of the progression of the Rauscher leukemia in stressed, as compared with control, mice. This increased resistance is not seen in adrenalectomized mice and can, I believe, be related to the fact that the Rauscher-virus-transformed cells are cells of the lymphatic system that are sensitive to the modulating influence of adrenalcorticoid hormones.

In contrast, stress has an adverse influence on the course of polyoma virus infection in experimentally infected mice. This adverse influence is more pronounced in younger than it is in older animals.[8,19] Further, there are distinct differences in the response of the highly susceptible AKR strain and a resistant strain, C57 black. Early in the course of the infectious process, the influence of stress is most pronounced on the AKR's with an accelleration of the development of malignant disease. However, the net outcome is essentially the same in stressed and control mice, with 100% of both dying with disseminated tumors. On the other hand, in the resistant AKR mice and in the AKR X C57 hybrids or the naturally intermediately susceptible strain of Webster Swiss mice, stress becomes the determining factor, e.g., determining that more stressed than control mice will die.

Thus, it is in the heterozygous animal of intermediate susceptibility that we see the greatest influence of stress on the host-virus-tumor relationship. This observation has special relevance to the question before us.

The mechanisms responsible for the differences in the interactions of stress and resistance in these two virus tumors are not known. In the polyoma system, there are two distinctly different virus-host cell relationships: first, a virulent cycle of viral infection with replication of virus and destruction of infected cells; second; infection of different host cells without replication of virus and without destruction of cells but with malignant conversion of some infected cells. The first is accomplished with high efficiency early in the course of infection and is not associated with overt disease. The second, which results in tumors, is a relatively rare event requiring as much as a million or more times as many infectious units of virus per cell as does the virulent cycle. That phase of polyoma virus infection based on virulent cycles is responsive to specific AB, probably gamma G, directed at the surface antigens of the virus which could prevent infection of new targets and thus reduce the amounts of virus available for malignant conversion. Our failure to relate the increased susceptibility following stress to impaired antibody production argues against, but does not rule out, such a mechanism. On the other hand, even a transitory suppression of interferon production could play an important role in determining the amounts of virus replicated and available either to infect new cells in virulent cycles or to accomplish malignant conversion. The probability of malignant conversion would depend on the absolute numbers of polyoma virions in the blood and tissue fluids and on the time over which these virions were present. In the Rauscher leukemia, each target cell also produces virus and, for this reason, may be less susceptible to stress-modified influences. However, one should be cautious in generalizing from our limited observations because, in avian leucosis, maturation of immunologic responsiveness has been shown by Peterson and his associates[20,21] and by Baluda[22] to be a determining factor in the outcome of infection. Stress effects on maturation of immunologic competence may very well play a role in the pathogenesis of other leukemias.

In summary, we have shown that under these rather artificial, but still not completely irrelevant, experimental situations there is an early involution of the thymus and the spleen. There is a decreased blood clearance, and others have shown suppression of antibody response. We have shown that there is a delay in rejection of homeografts and a possible influence on the production of interferon in stressed, as compared with control, mice. Only further work with more sophisticated approaches will give us the true picture–for example, the kinds of work to which Dr. Weiss and Dr. Salk have referred, a definitive study of the effect of stress on the whole category of antibodies and cellular immune mechanisms. The role of interferon has to be looked into more carefully.

Acknowledgments

I wish to acknowledge with thanks the active collaboration of my colleagues, particularly N. Q. Brill, J. T. Marsh, Torsten Johnsson, K. K. Chang, W. H. Hildemann, and M. I. Sellers, and of pre- and postdoctoral students in our laboratory, Marcus Jensen, Perry Treadwell, John Lavender, Richard Wistar, Edwin Spencer, Melvin Shapiro, Glen Funk, and A. Yamada.

References

1. MARSH, J. T. & A. F. RASMUSSEN, JR. 1960. Response of adrenals, thymus, spleen and leucocytes to shuttle box and confinement stress. Proc. Soc. Exp. Biol. Med. **104:** 180.
2. JENSEN, M. M. & A. F. RASMUSSEN, JR. 1963. Stress and susceptibility to viral infection. II. Sound stress and susceptibility to vesicular stomatitis virus. J. Immun. **90:** 21.
3. FUNK, G. A. & M. M. JENSEN. 1967. Influence of stress on granuloma formation. Proc. Soc. Exp. Biol. Med. **124:** 653.
4. SHAPIRO, M., J. T. MARSH & A. F. RASMUSSEN, JR. Unpublished data.
5. RASMUSSEN, A. F., JR., J. T. MARSH & N. Q. BRILL. 1957. Increased susceptibility to herpes simplex in mice subjected to avoidance-learning stress or restraint. Proc. Soc. Exp. Biol. Med. **96:** 183.
6. JOHNSSON, T. & A. F. RASMUSSEN, JR. 1965. Emotional stress and susceptibility to poliomyelitis virus infection in mice. Arch. Ges. Virusforsch. **18:** 392.

7. JOHNSSON, T., J. F. LAVENDER, E. HULLIN & A. F. RASMUSSEN, JR. 1963. The influence of avoidance-learning stress on resistance to Coxsackie B cirus in mice. J. Immun. **91:** 569.
8. CHANG, K. K. & A. F. RASMUSSEN, JR. Unpublished data.
9. LAVENDER, J. F., M. M. JENSEN & A. F. RASMUSSEN, JR. Unpublished data.
10. JENSEN, M. M. 1968. The influence of stress on murine leukemia virus infection. Proc. Soc. Exp. Biol. Med. **127:** 610.
11. WISTAR, R. T. & A. F. RASMUSSEN, JR. Unpublished data.
12. WISTAR, R. T. & W. H. HILDEMANN. 1960. Effect of stress on skin transplantation immunity in mice. Science **131:** 159.
13. RASMUSSEN, A. F., JR. Unpublished data.
14. YAMADA, A., M. M. JENSEN & A. F. RASMUSSEN, JR. 1964. Stress and susceptibility to viral infections. III. Antibody response and viral retention during avoidance-learning stress. Proc. Soc. Exp. Biol Med. **116:** 677.
15. RASMUSSEN, A. F., JR., E. T. SPENCER & J. T. MARSH. 1959. Decrease in susceptibility of mice to passive anaphylaxis following avoidance-learning stress. Proc. Soc. Exp. Biol. Med. **100:** 878.
16. TREADWELL, P. E. & A. F. RASMUSSEN, JR. 1961. Role of the adrenals in stress-induced resistance to anaphylactic shock. J. Immun. **87:** 492.
17. CHANG, S. S. & A. F. RASMUSSEN, JR. 1965. Stress-induced suppression of interferon production in virus infected mice. Nature **205:** 623.
18. JENSEN, M. M. 1968. Transitory impairment of interferon production on stressed mice. Proc. Soc. Exp. Biol. Med. **128:** 174.
19. RASMUSSEN, A. F., JR., W. H. HILDEMAN & M. I. SELLERS. 1963. Malignancy of polyoma virus in relation to stress. J. Nat. Cancer Inst. **30:** 101.
20. PETERSON, R. D., B. R. BURMESTER, T. N. FREDERICKSON, H. G. PURCHASE & R. A. GOOD. 1964. Effect of bursectomy and thymectomy on the development of visceral lymphomatosis in the chicken. J. Nat. Cancer Inst. **32:** 1343.
21. PETERSON, R. D., H. G. PURCHASE, B. R. BURMESTER, M. D. COOPER & R. A. GOOD. 1966. Relationships among visceral lymphomatosis, bursa of fabricius, and bursa-dependent lymphoid tissue of the chicken. J. Nat. Cancer Inst. **36:** 585.
22. BALUDA, M. A. 1967. The role of the bursa-dependent lymphoid tissue in oncogenesis by avian myeloblastosis virus. Virology **32:** 428.

DISCUSSION OF THE PAPER

UNIDENTIFIED SPEAKER: Did you investigate the levels of catecholamines and the corticosteroids in these stressed animals?

DR. RASMUSSEN: We did not; Dr. Solomon has looked at the catecholamines and the steroids.

DR. SOLOMON: I think that is an important point because of the question of what is a stress and what is not. We did steroid correlations in the interferon work, but it has not been done in all work. I think it probably would be a good idea if it is, although I do not necessarily feel that the only mediation of stress effects on the immune system is through adrenal hormones.

DR. AMKRAUT: I am a bit puzzled by the fact that you stated that clearance is decreased by stress. As I mentioned yesterday, we have done some experiments of clearance of red cells, and this is in fact enhanced in stressed rats. I want to add that subsequent to the first experiment, in which rats had been shock- and noise-stressed for five or six days prior to the experiment, we did a second one, in which we took rats that had not been handled for a long time off the shelf and repeated the experiment. Both stressed and control groups acted as though they had been stressed. Now, this experiment involved removal of tagged mouse red cells from the peritonium and clearance from the blood. Looking back into the literature about hormonal effects on phagocytosis, it seems to be clear that the levels of steroids are very significant, in that one can get both enhancement and depression. I wonder whether you would like to comment on the importance of the type of stress that you apply and the length of application.

I think that in general it might probably be a good idea to correlate some second parameter, like steroid levels, with stress effects. Also, I should like to add that regarding hemagglutination, which probably tests mainly for 19S antibody, there seems to be no stress effect. I have done some Jerne plaque experiments, which so far have shown no effect of stress.

DR. RASMUSSEN: I will start at the end and then go backward. Dr. Chang also tried to show differences in immunologic capacity by Jerne plaque assays, and lymphocytes from stressed and from normal animals seem to have comparable capacity.

However, I point out, and this answers the first question, that these changes in clearance were seen in animals in which the spleens were so much smaller that it was dramatic. Thus it was surprising to us that there was not more impairment of clearance, in view of the obvious atrophy of one of the major filtering organs.

In considering the acute changes another factor must be considered, and that is the rate of blood flow through the filtering organs, as Benacéraff and Halpern showed very early in their classical studies on clearance. To a degree, then, clearance is simply a measure of blood flow through the liver and the spleen, and one has to take this factor into account, as well.

DR. SOLOMON: I wish to say, too, that steroids may themselves have different effects at different levels. In *in vitro* systems, for example, an absence of adrenal hormones will result in immunosuppression, adding a small amount of steroids will enhance immune response, and adding a large amount will suppress it. These biphasic responses are very common in hormonally-receptive biologic systems.

DR. ELIAS COHEN (*Roswell Park Memorial Institute, Buffalo, N. Y.*): I gather from the discussion that antibody titer levels have not been evaluated in animals under stress. But since hyperproteinemia or nutritional deficiencies might affect levels of antibodies, I raise the question whether the stress itself may affect the feeding of animals, and whether in your studies pair feeding was ever used in experimental versus control groups?

DR. RASMUSSEN: No, there was some impairment of nutrition and some general evidence of impairment of overall endocrine balance. Most of our experiments were conducted in females, because we seemed to see the greatest difference between the stressed and controls using females, and such females do not gain weight as rapidly as do controls, so that at six weeks of age their average weight was about 20 grams, rather than 22. Otherwise, they were sleek, and appeared well nourished.

But they did have a persistent pseudoestrus, and there was some general nutritional impairment. Food was withheld from the controls for the same six-hour period each day, they were placed in the same kinds of boxes, and both stressed and control animals were fed *ad libitum* at other times of the day.

We did not try to force-feed the animals to make up for that increment-failure to gain, which is less than 10% of the animal's normal weight at that age.

DR. PAPAY: If I may make a comment, I think it is important to point out that not all of the organ changes that accompany chronic stress, in the eyes of an immunologist, read out as equaling immune depression. I think that the most important change that occurs, and that I was not aware of, and that may explain some of your paradoxical findings, is this spleenic hypotrophy, or involution.

In studies done by Prehn, and by our own group, we found that removing the spleen significantly increases the delayed hypersensitivity, the delayed allergy end of the immune responsiveness. This might explain some of the "flip-flop" effects you have.

REMARKS ON DR. KORNEVA'S WORK

George F. Solomon

Stanford University School of Medicine, Stanford, Calif.

The paper on "The Role of the Central Nervous System in the Regulation of Immunogenesis" was to be given by Dr. E. A. Korneva of the Institute of Experimental Medicine in Leningrad. Unfortunately, to her disappointment and to ours, she was unable to obtain the necessary clearances for her to visit us today, and, again unfortunately, her paper likewise has not arrived.

I will, instead, say a few words about Dr. Korneva's work, which I think may be very significant, although it is somewhat difficult to evaluate adequately.

In work early in the sixties, she ablated areas in the dorsal hypothalamus and claimed that these lesions led to a marked suppression, and in some cases elimination, of immune response. She used rather crude antigens of foreign sera and found that antigens had prolonged retention in the blood, without elimination, under such circumstances. Since that time, she has done work in which she implanted pairs of electrodes in the same region of the brain, passed electric current through them, and found stimulation and enhancement of antibody response.

Apparently this region is a very delicate one. If the electrodes were so placed that they did not straddle the area but rather entered it, an immune suppression occurred as a result of damage to the region. Only if they were in exactly the right area was this stimulation obtained.

I hope very much that Dr. Stein will be able to comment on this type of work, since I am rather confused, because in the area of the hypothalamus that Dr. Korneva found to influence immune responses was the dorsal hypothalamus, while Dr. Fessel and Dr. Forsyth in earlier work had found that stimulation of the lateral hypothalamus affects gammaglobulin levels. Their work showed that stimulation of this area would either lead to elevation in some animals or to depression of gamma globulin in others. I believe that Dr. Stein's work relates to the anterior hypothalamus, which is closely allied with endocrine function.

THE HYPOTHALAMUS AND IMMUNE PROCESS*

Marvin Stein, Raul C. Schiavi, and Thomas J. Luparello

Department of Psychiatry
State University of New York
Downstate Medical Center
College of Medicine
Brooklyn, N. Y.

There is considerable clinical evidence suggesting that emotional factors modify some types of allergic and immune mechanisms; however, until recently there have been few experimental studies that have considered the effect of psychosocial phenomena on immunological processes. Rasmussen and his coworkers have demonstrated that mice subjected to a standardized avoidance-conditioning stress show an increased susceptibility to herpes simplex virus,[1] as well as decreased susceptibility to passive anaphylaxis.[2] Chronic avoidance conditioning was also found by Wistar and Hildeman[3] to depress the immune reaction responsible for the rejection of skin homografts. A decrease in susceptibility to Type 1 polio virus has been observed in monkeys following an acute avoidance-conditioning procedure.[4] A number of reports in the Russian literature have considered the effect of psychological mechanisms on antibody titers.[5–8] Petrovski,[9] for example, studied changes in agglutinin titers associated with behavioral disturbances induced in immunized dogs and baboons by stressful stimuli or by conflict-conditioning techniques. He observed a parallelism between the intensity and duration of the behavioral disturbances and the fall in circulating antibody titers. It has also been reported that mice housed in groups have a significantly lower level of circulating antibodies than mice housed individually.[10]

Recently the neurophysiological mechanisms that might mediate the psychosocial influences on immunological reactions have been experimentally studied. There is a growing body of literature indicating that central nervous system (CNS) processes may modify hypersensitive mechanisms, and specifically anaphylaxis. The effect of midbrain lesions on the course of anaphylaxis in the guinea pig has been investigated by Freedman and Fenichel.[11] Bilateral electrolytic lesions at the level of the superior colliculus involving the reticulothalamic tracts and deep tegmental nucleus inhibited anaphylactic death. Szentivanyi and Filipp[12–14] were among the first to study the role of the hypothalamus on anaphylaxis. They demonstrated that lethal anaphylactic shock in the guinea pig can be prevented by bilateral local lesions in the tuberal region of the hypothalamus.

In our laboratories, Luparello and colleagues[15] investigated the effect of hypothalamic lesions on rat anaphylaxis in an effort to determine if the effect of an alteration of hypothalamic processes were species-specific and related to a modification in the guinea pig of the responsivity of the shock tissue; i.e., the bronchioles. In order to investigate this question, the effect of hypothalamic lesions on a species with a different major shock organ in anaphylaxis was also studied. The albino rat was chosen, since in this species anaphylactic shock is accompanied by congestion and hemorrhage of the small intestine without major

* Supported in part by grant MH 13,408 from the National Institute of Mental Health and by Research Scientist Development Award 5–K03–MH 15,620 from the National Institute of Mental Health.

pulmonary changes. In the study,[15] three groups of animals – control, posterior hypothalamic-lesioned, and anterior hypothalamic-lesioned – were sensitized to ovalbumin, and subsequently challenged with various doses of the antigen. Dose-mortality curves were plotted for the control and two experimental groups. FIGURE 1 shows that ovalbumin was less potent in the animals with anterior hypothalamic lesions than in both the control rats and those with posterior lesions. The decrease in potency was significant at the <0.001 level.

Little is known about the mechanisms involved in the antianaphylactic effect of hypothalamic lesions. We have been studying the effect of lesions on circulating antibodies in the guinea pig as measured by a passive hemagglutination technique. At present, two studies have been completed. The first study investigated the effect of hypothalamic lesions on circulating antibodies following one sensitizing dose of 1.0 mg of ovalbumin administered intraperitoneally. The results can be seen in FIGURE 2. The animals with anterior hypothalamic lesions made ten days prior to sensitization has significantly ($p < 0.05$) lower antibody titers by the seventh week following sensitization than the posterior hypothalamic-lesioned guinea pigs or the controls. There were no significant differences between the titers of the control and experimental groups by the eleventh week after sensitization. The second study was undertaken with hypothalamic-lesioned and control animals hyperimmunized by means of three intraperitoneal injections of ovalbumin. There were no significant differences in circulating antibodies between

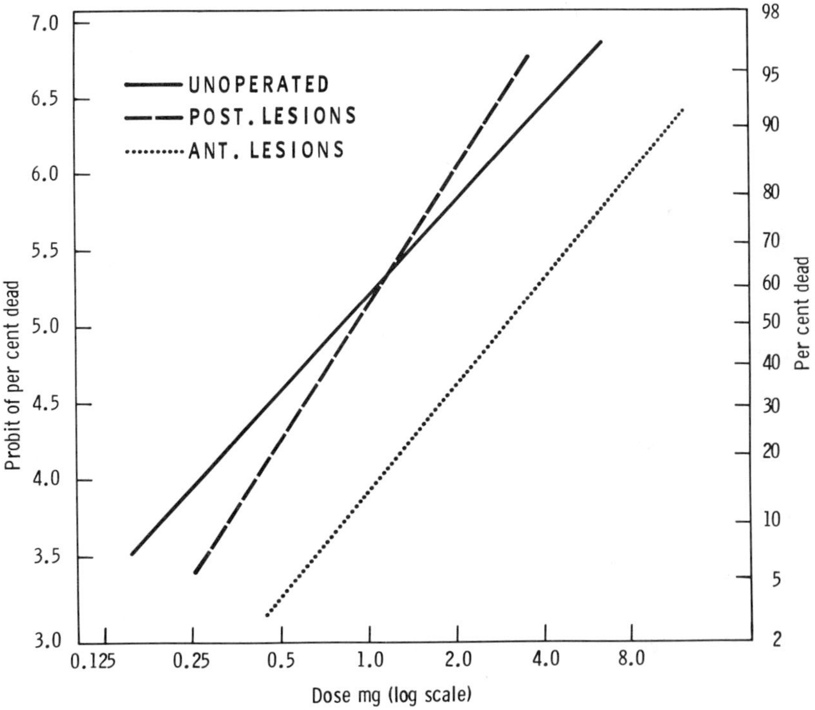

FIGURE 1. Dose-effect curve illustrating the effect of anterior hypothalamic lesions on rat anaphylaxis.

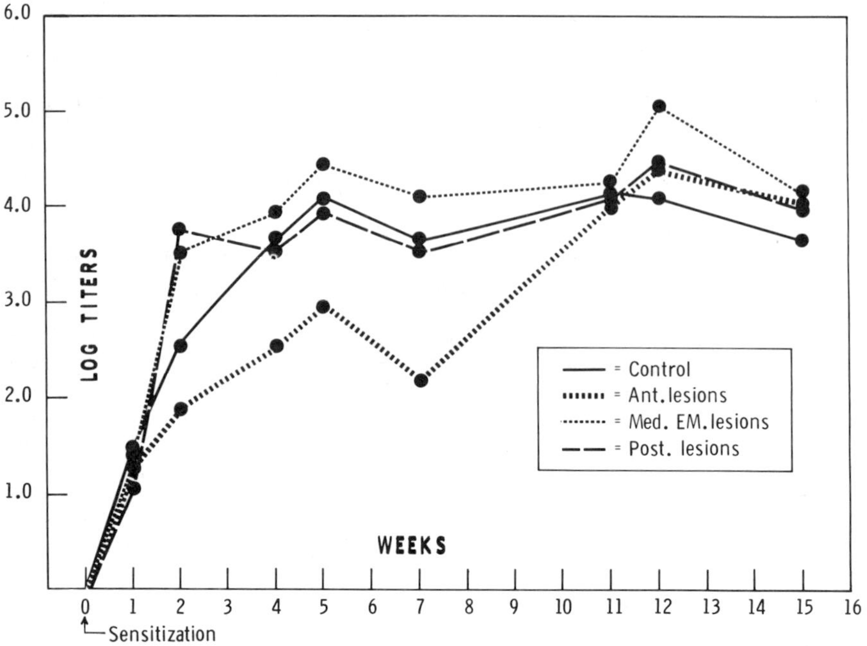

FIGURE 2. Effect of hypothalamic lesions on circulating antibodies in guinea pigs as measured by a passive hemagglutination technique. Each value represents the mean of the group.

the control and experimental groups of guinea pigs over a period of one month following the first sensitizing injection. Further investigation including a larger sample of animals is currently in progress.

Flipp and Szentivanyi[13] have reported that circulating as well as tissue-fixed antibodies were markedly reduced in tuber-injured guinea pigs. Low precipitin levels were observed in sensitized animals following hypothalamic lesions, as evidenced by the Ring test. Korneva and Khai[16] also found that lesions in the posterior ventral hypothalamus of rabbits induced a complete suppression of the production of complement-fixing antibodies and a prolonged retention of the antigen in the blood. In cases where the areas of destruction were localized in other parts of the hypothalamus, the thalamic structures, the caudate nucleus, and the posterior commisure, the course of immune processes was similar to that in control animals. The antianaphylactic effect of hypothalamic lesions, however, cannot be explained solely by an inhibition of antibody production, since guinea pigs passively sensitized with homologous as well as with heterologous (rabbit) serum are also protected by lesions.[12]

It is possible that anterior hypothalamic lesions, in addition to their effect on circulating antibodies, may modify the reactivity of the organism to histamine and other substances liberated during the antigen-antibody reaction. Several studies have reported that the central nervous system modifies the susceptibility of animals to exogenous histamine. Whittier and Orr[17] found that bilateral lesions of the caudate nuclei of rats were associated with a significant increase in survival time following the intraperitoneal administration of histamine phosphate; sham operatons and lesions in the cerebral cortex did not modify the time of survival.

Przybylski[18] investigated the effect of the removal of the region of the quadrigeminal bodies and of the cerebral cortex on histamine toxicity in guinea pigs. The animals in which the quadrigeminal bodies were removed showed a decreased susceptibility to histamine when administered either intravenously or by inhalation of an aerosal. Removal of the cerebral cortex did not modify the reactivity of the animals. Schiavi and co-workers,[19] in our laboratory, recently studied the effect of bilateral electrolytic lesions in the anterior and posterior medial hypothalamus on histamine toxicity in the guinea pig, as measured by dose-mortality curves. Histamine was significantly less potent in the animals with anterior lesions than in both the control and posterior-lesioned guinea pigs.

The mechanism by which anterior hypothalamic lesions modify the susceptibility of the animals to exogenous histamine is not apparent from the above studies. Maslinski and Karczewski[20–22] extensively investigated the effect of electrical stimulation of the brain of guinea pigs with current intensities above and below the seizure threshold on the susceptibility of the animals to histamine. They found that electrical stimulation of guinea pigs through temporal electrodes with a 50–100 cycles/sec current at levels between 5 and 10 ma has a marked protective effect against lethal histamine shock. These investigators demonstrated that the decrease in histamine susceptibility was transitory and was associated with a marked decrease in the bronchospastic effect of histamine. Karczewski[23] found that the parameters of electrical stimulation effective against lethal histamine shock also induced a marked depression of the electrical activity of the afferent and efferent fibers of the vagus. This and other observations led to the conclusion that the modified histamine susceptibility following brain stimulation could be due to a reduced physiological tone of the airway leading to a reduced response to the constricting stimuli.

Austen and associates[24] are investigating in our laboratories the effect of anterior and posterior hypothalamic lesions on inspiratory and expiratory airway resistance and the ventilatory response of guinea pigs exposed to an aerosol of histamine. Although no significant differences in airway resistance have been found between groups prior to the exposure to histamine, there are significant differences in the ventilatory response. As can be seen in FIGURE 3, the minute volume of the control animals increases markedly after 30 seconds of exposure to the aerosol of histamine. No change in the minute volume of the hypothalamic-lesioned guinea pigs was observed during the histamine exposure. These differences in the response of the control and experimental groups were significant at the <0.01 level. A study is in progress investigating airway-resistance measures during the exposure to a histamine aerosol. These preliminary findings suggest that hypothalamic lesions may modify the physiological reactivity of the bronchiolar tree to bronchoconstricting agents.

What are the other possible mechanisms mediating the effect of hypothalamic lesions on immune processes? It is possible that the alteration of immune mechanisms may be due, at least in part, to changes in neuroendocrine function induced by the destruction of specific hypothalamic structures. It has been shown[25,26] that the anterior medial hypothalamus is involved in the regulation of the secretion of thyroid-stimulating hormone (TSH) by the hypophysis. Electrolytic lesions in this area induce low plasma levels of TSH and decreased thyroid function. A number of investigators have demonstrated in the rat and guinea pig a relationship between thyroid physiology and immune processes. It has been noted[27] that the resistance to the anaphylactic reaction is increased in thyroidectomized rats. Similar findings were observed by Nilzen[28–30] in the guinea pig

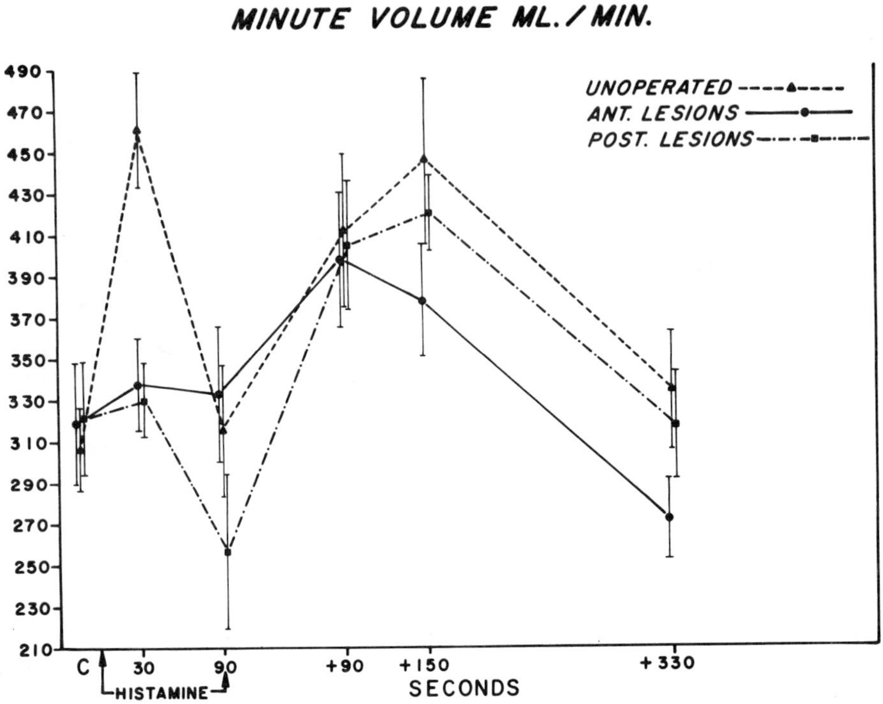

FIGURE 3. Effect of hypothalamic lesions on the minute volume of guinea pigs exposed to an aerosol of histamine. Each value represents the mean ± the standard error.

following thyroidectomy or administration of ^{131}I. Suppression of thyroid activity inhibits local and systemic anaphylaxis, abolishes circulatng precipitins, and decreases the susceptibility of the animals to exogenous histamine. Hypothalmic lesions can also modify ACTH secretion and blood-corticoid levels. Adrenal steroids have been found to have a protective effect against anaphylactic shock in the rat and an inhibitory effect on antibody formation in rats and guinea pigs.[31,32] Adrenocortical hormones also have a profound action on the metabolism and effects of histamine. They have inhibitory effects on histidine-decarboxylase activity,[33] on the tissue-binding of newly formed histamine,[34] and on the amount of histamine released by the tissues.[35] Although adrenal steroids have a protective effect against histamine toxicity in mice and rats, they do not appear to modify significantly the susceptibility of guinea pigs to anaphylaxis and to exogenous histamine.

The effect of hypothalamic lesions on immune processes may also be mediated by a modification of the tonic autonomic activity in the sympathetic-parasympathetic nervous system. Many studies have demonstrated that the hypothalamus is intimately involved with autonomic nervous activity. Electric stimulation of the posterior hypothalamus, for instance, causes a sympathetic discharge with a demonstrable release of adrenalin and noradrenalin by the adrenal medulla, while lesions in the posterior hypothalamus decrease sympathetic activity.[36] Very few studies have evaluated the effect of lesions and electrical stimulation of the brain on immune processes in terms of autonomic activity. Tjabbes and associates[37] reported that lesions in the posterior hypothalamus completely prevents the eosinophilia induced by the injection of pertussis vaccine or by the administration of protamine sulphate. Similar effects were observed following the transection of the spinal cord between C_7 and T_1, interrupting the nervous connection between the brain and the spinal part of the sympathetic nervous system and the sympathetic ganglia. As mentioned earlier, susceptibility to histamine may also be associated with changes in parasympathetic activity.

In summary, this presentation has suggested that psychosocial phenomena may modify immune processes by way of CNS mechanisms (FIGURE 4). The review of experimental work indicates that the CNS is intimately involved in immune processes. The hypothalamus, probably through its control of neuroendocrine and autonomic activity, plays an important role in immune and allergic phenomena. This observation, in view of the close relationship between the hypothalamus and central mechanisms concerned with emotions, provides a basis for the understanding of the physiology and chemistry involved in the mediation of the influence of psychosocial phenomena on immune and allergic processes.

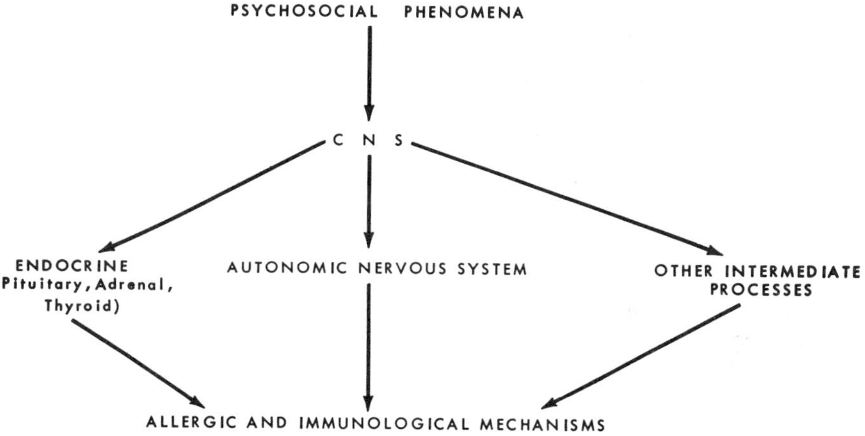

FIGURE 4. Schematic representation of the effect of psychosocial phenomena on immune processes by way of the central nervous system.

References

1. RASMUSSEN, A. F., J. T. MARSH & N. Q. BRILL. 1957. Increased susceptibility to Herpes simplex in mice subjected to avoidance-learning stress or restraint. Proc. Soc. Exp. Biol. Med. **96:** 183.
2. RASMUSSEN, A. F., E. S. SPENCER & J. T. MARSH. 1959. Decrease in susceptibility of mice to passive anaphylaxis following avoidance-learning stress. Proc. Soc. Exp. Biol. Med. **100:** 878.
3. WISTAR, R., JR. & W. H. HILDEMANN. 1960. Effect of stress on skin transplantation immunity in mice. Science **131:** 159.
4. MARSH, J. T., J. F. LAVENDER, CHANG SHVEH-SHEN & A. F. RASMUSSEN. 1963. Poliomyelitis in monkeys: decreased susceptibility after avoidence stress. Science **140:** 1414.
5. SAVCHUK, O. Y. 1958. The reflex mechanism of the formation of antibodies. Zh. Mikrobiol. **29:** 131.

6. Dzhumkhade, A. P. 1960. Role of conditioned reflexes in production of antibodies. Zh. Vyssh. Nerv. Deiat Pavlov **10:** 599.
7. Monaenov, A. M. 1956. The influence of changes in the activtiy of the cerebral hemispheres in immunological reactions. Zh. Mikrobiol. **12:** 88.
8. Gordienko, A. N. 1956. Reflex reactions from skin receptors in the mechanism of antibody formation. Sborn. Nauch. Leprol. Dermatol. **7:** 451.
9. Petrovskii, I. N. 1961. Problems of nervous control in immunity reactions. II. The influence of experimental neurosis on immunity reactions. Zh. Mikrobiol. **32:** 1451.
10. Vessey, S. H. 1964. Effects of grouping on levels of circulating antibodies in mice. Proc. Soc. Exp. Biol. Med. **115:** 252.
11. Freedman, D. X. & G. Fenichel. 1958. Effect of midbrain lesions in experimental allergy. Arch. Neurol. Psychiat. **79:** 164.
12. Szentivanyi, A. & G. Filipp. 1958. Anaphylaxis and the nervous system. Part II. Ann. Allerg. **16:** 143.
13. Filipp, G. & A. Szentivanyi. 1958. Anaphylaxis and the nervous system. Part III. Ann. Allerg. **16:** 306.
14. Szentivanyi, A. & J. Szekely. 1958. Anaphylaxis and the nervous system. Part IV. Ann. Allerg. **16:** 389.
15. Luparello, T. J., M. Stein & C. D. Park. 1964. Effect of hypothalamic lesions on rat anaphylaxis. Amer. J. Physiol. **207:** 911.
16. Korneva, E. A. & L. M. Khai. 1963. Influence of hypothalamic lesions on antibody production. Fiziol. Zh. SSSR **49** (1): 42.
17. Whittier, J. R. & A. Orr. 1962. Hyperkinesia and other physiologic effects of caudate deficit in the adult albino rat. Neurology (Minneap.) **12:** 529.
18. Przybylski, A. 1962. Effect of the removal of the cortex cerebri and the quadrigeminal bodies region on histamine susceptibility of guinea pigs. Acta Physiol. Pol. **13:** 535.
19. Schiavi, R. C., J. Adams & M. Stein. 1966. Effect of hypothalamic lesions on histamine toxicity in the guinea pig. Amer. J. Physiol. **211:** 1269.
20. Maslinski, C. 1959. L'action protectrice de currant élèctrique transcerebral sur les choc histaminique et anaphylactique. J. Physiol. (Paris) **51:** 639.
21. Maslinski, C. & W. Karczewski. 1955. Prevention of so-called histamine shock by stimulation of the brain with electric current; preliminary communication. Acta Physiol. Pol. **6:** 373.
22. Maslinski, C. & W. Karczewski. 1957. The protective influence of brain stimulation by electric current on histamine shock in guinea pigs. Bull. Acad. Pol. Sci. **5:** 57.
23. Karczewski, W. 1964. The electrical activity of the vagus nerve on "antianaphylactic" stimulation of the brain. Acta Allerg. (Bobenhavn) **19:** 229.
24. Austen, B., R. C. Schiavi & M. Stein. (In preparation.)
25. Florsheim, N. H. 1958. The effect of anterior hypothalamic lesions on thyroid function and goiter development in the rat. Endocrinology **62:** 783.
26. De Jong, W. & J. Moll. 1965. Differential effects of hypothalamic lesions on pituitary-thyroid activity in the rat. Acta Endocrinol. **48:** 522.
27. Leger, J. & G. Masson. 1947. Factors influencing an anaphylactic reaction in the rat. Fed. Proc. **6:** 150.
28. Nilzén, Å. 1954. The influence of the thyroid gland on hypersensitivity reactions in animals. I. Acta Allerg. (Kobenhavn) **7:** 231.
29. Nilzén, Å. 1955. The influence of the thyroid gland on hypersensitivity reactions in animals. II. Acta Allerg. (Kobenhavn) **8:** 57.
30. Nilzén, Å. 1955. The influence of the thyroid gland on hypersensitivity reactions in animals. III. Acta Allerg. (Kobenhavn) **8:** 103.
31. Dews, P. B. & C. F. Code. 1951. Effect of cortisone on anaphylactic shock in adrenalectomized rats. J. Pharmacol. Exp. Ther. **101:** 9.
32. Rose, B. 1959. Hormones and allergic responses. International Symposium on Mechanisms of Hypersensitivity. J. H. Shaffer, G. A. LoGrippo & M. W. Chase, Eds. : 599. Churchill. London, England.
33. Parrot, J. L. & C. Laborde. 1961. Inhibition d'histidine—decarboxylase par la cortisone et par le salicylate de sodium. J. Physiol. (Paris) **53:** 441.
34. Shayer, R. W., J. K. Davis & R. L. Smiley. 1955. Binding of histamine *in vitro* and its inhibition by cortisone. Amer. J. Physiol. **182:** 54.
35. Yamasaki, H. & T. Yamamoto. 1963. Inhibitory effect of adrenal glucocorticoids on histamine release. J. Pharmacol. Soc. Japan. **13:** 223.

36. Gelhorn, E., H. Nakao & E. S. Redgate. 1956. The influence of lesions in the anterior and posterior hypothalamus on tonic and phasic autonomic reactions. J. Physiol. (London) **131**: 402
37. Tjabbes, T., P. G. Smelik & D. De Wied. 1962. Protamine sulphate induced eosinophilia in rats. Influence of the hypothalamus on the spinal cord. Arch. Int. Pharmacodyn. **135**: 207.

DISCUSSION OF THE PAPER

Dr. Weiss: This is in the nature of a speculative comment, but one that may not be entirely out of place here. I was most interested to hear Dr. Stein refer to neurohormones as playing a possible role in the translation of psychodynamic circumstances and affects to neoplastic events, and I should like to elaborate on this thought for a moment.

It was shown years ago by A. A. Miles of London, and since then by other investigators as well, that the events of the first hours, and perhaps even minutes, that follow the initial contact between a host and a microbial parasite may determine the ultimate fate of this contact: whether progressive disease will occur or not, whether this will be severe or mild. There are many reasons why neoplastic cells should be viewed as representing a kind of microbial parasite and therefore to consider the first minutes or hours after appearance of a neoplastic variant as crucial.

Let us now plug in the possible role of neurohormones in the psychophysiology of cancer into this consideration, within an immunological frame of reference. I have mentioned earlier the synergistic effect between ubiquitously present traces of bacterial endotoxins in animal tissues and the catecholamines in bringing about vasodynamic changes. It would not stretch the imagination too far to conceive of significant immunological consequences resulting from sudden alteration in small-vessel tone and function at a moment when a neoplastic cell makes its appearance—certainly, the translocation of antigens to the nearest site of immunological reactivity and the ingress of circulating or cellular immune factors are a direct function of blood and lymphatic transport, and sudden constriction, stasis, and other vasodynamic changes must effect directly both the afferent and efferent prongs of the immune response.

Systemic and local concentrations of catecholamines might thus be decisive as to whether a newly arisen antigenic neoplastic cell will live, and be able to propagate, and perhaps soon come to be surrounded by protective sheaths of connective tissue that can interfere with later immunological attack.

This comment is purely in the realm of conjecture, but it is subject to test; and it does at least provide a kind of model for visualizing how a psychic circumstance may translate itself, via a hormonal mechanism, into an immunological effect, and thereby, eventually, to susceptibility or resistance toward a hostile cell.

Dr. Stein: I have little to add to that, other than that I agree. It seems to me that if psychological factors play a role, and I prefer to use the concept of psychosocial phenomena, it seems that this must be mediated by way of the central nervous system, and the place most likely to look is in the hypothalamus, also involving catecholamines, and adrenal and thyroid function. I think that to speculate that there is a specific center (for example, in the hypothalamus) that is concerned with immune processes, would get us nowhere. But in terms of trying to understand some of this, as in the last schematic presentation, I would agree very much with Dr. Weiss.

Dr. Solomon: I might just add that Soviet work that has to do with stimulation or ablations in regard to innervations of the site of antigen deposition and consequent alteration of immune response may provide some evidence along the lines about which Dr. Weiss was speculating.

Dr. Amkraut: I should like to interject a note of caution here, which I hope might be helpful. With the current degree of sophistication in terms of the multifaceted aspects of the immune response that have been brought out here and with the increasing number of identifiable immunoglobulins, I do not think we are justified any longer in talking about the "immune response" in terms of what you are measuring with any single technique, whether it is precipitation measuring total antibody levels or whether it is hemaglutination, where you are probably measuring preferentially lg M. We know very well, for example, that there is 1 μg or less of 1g E in 100 ml of serum of allergic patients, but when you transfer a minute portion of this, you can still get profound physiological effects; and there is recent evidence that steroid hormones can change, in the guinea pig, the complexion of the gammaglobulins from a preferential gamma-two to a preferential gamma-one response, and the gamma-one response, as you know, is that which is significant in autologous biological response.

I should like to ask you whether you immunize your guinea pigs with adjuvant, and whether you have looked at a gamma 2/gamma 1 ratio?

Dr. Stein: Let me do this. In terms of the sophistication of the techniques, I think you have hit upon a very important point, and, as our work has gone on, we are adding more and more in terms of some, I think, of the current methodologies that are available.

We have not used adjuvant with our guinea pigs, and we have not looked at the gamma one and gamma two, but we are in the process of exploring this situation at the present time.

Dr. Stern: Many things go on in the hypothalamus, and I wondered whether, in your lesions of the anterior hypothalamus, you were interfering with the region of the ventromedial nucleus, and if you were, whether you were causing some atrophy of the ovaries, and whether if that were the case, this would have some relationship to your findings?

Dr. Stein: It is very difficult to know exactly what you are doing in placing a lesion. The argument has always been about whether you are ablating the specific area or whether you are stimulating an adjacent area. And it is hard to be clear about that. All we can say is that, operationally, we know that we have ablated this area.

We have not taken any look at the ovaries of these animals, since they were all males, and I cannot answer this question.

DISCUSSION

EMOTIONS, IMMUNOLOGY, AND CANCER: HOW MIGHT THE PSYCHE INFLUENCE NEOPLASIA?*

Chester M. Southam

Medical Oncology Service of Memorial Hospital and the Sloan-Kettering Institute for Cancer Research
New York, N. Y.

As a clinician, I have been impressed by the marked influence of cancer on the psyche and by cases that appear to show an influence of the psyche on the clinical course of cancer and perhaps even on its onset. I am most pleased to know that these interesting associations are receiving serious study. That the psyche might exert a significant influence on the etiology or the pathogenesis of malignant neoplastic disease seems entirely reasonable to me; in fact, it seems probable. But I know of no solid evidence for the existence of such effect. In fact, if such a relationship were proved we would not be having this symposium, for our objective here is to consider this question, not to propound a gospel.

As a laboratory investigator in the area of experimental pathology, I feel uncomfortable in the foreign land of psychology. I feel a need to recognize tangible mechanisms to explain biological effects. I need to perceive biological mechanisms through which the psychologic state might exert an influence on neoplastic disease. Until reasonable mechanisms for such an influence are elucidated, or until influence of the psyche or neoplasia is more certainly demonstrated, I prefer to remain sceptical but not negativistic.

In view of these personal attitudes and my concept of the discussant's role, I would like to consider some possible mechanisms by which psychic factors might affect cancer. I cannot comprehend such concepts as extrasensory perception (ESP), and certainly I cannot conceive any ESP-like mechanism that could influence cancer. Rather, I must seek humoral, cellular, or neural mechanisms that are activated by emotional stress or at least influenced by the psychological state. Several such mechanisms have been identified.

Release of adrenalin and adrenal corticosteroids is increased by emotional as well as by physical stress. Release of the sex steroid hormones is at least in part under hypothalamic control, and through this or other mechanisms it is influenced by the psychologic state in humans. The influence of emotional states on the autonomic nervous system and the end organs that it controls are well known to all of us from personal experience. And certainly these are not the only physiologic responses that are responsive to psychic stimuli. Now let us consider whether any of these recognized factors might influence neoplastic disease.

The process of metastasis is dependent upon the escape of malignant cells from the primary tumor site, their dissemination through vascular channe's or other body fluids, and eventual implantation and growth in a new site. We recognize that manipulation of a tumor mass during surgery or physical examination may increase the dissemination of tumor cells, and it is easy to conceive that smooth muscle contraction, controlled by adrenalin and autonomic nerves but initiated by psychic stresses, might also influence tumor cell dissemination–particularly

* The author's research work is supported by grants from the National Cancer Institute (CY–3215) and the American Cancer Society (T–229).

from gastrointestinal neoplasms. The diameter of precapillary arterioles is the major determinant of blood flow through capillary networks, and where the flow of blood (or lymph) is slow the possibility is increased that embolic tumor cells will pass through the vascular endothelium and grow in the interstitial tissues. Adrenal corticosteroids and sex steroids affect clotting mechanisms. The hypercoagulable state, especially if it results in intravascular deposition of fibrin, increases the probability that circulating tumor cells will adhere to and penetrate through capillary walls. These possibilities may seem esoteric, but each step that I have mentioned is well documented. All that is lacking is the demonstration that the entire chain of events–psychic stress, hormone release, cardiovascular and coagulation responses, and effect on tumor cell dissemination and implantation–will actually go to completion. Although proof is lacking, it is entirely reasonable that such a sequence of reactions may in fact have a major influence on cancer as a disease process. Let me remind you that circulating cancer cells present no problem. Trouble begins only when the circulating cells implant and grow.

The survival and growth of the cancer cell might also be affected by mechanisms that are influenced by emotional stimuli. Dr. Rasmussen (this monograph) reports studies that suggest that stress may depress specific immunologic reactions such as homograft rejection. Homograft rejection is mediated primarily, perhaps entirely, by cellular mechanisms of specific immune reaction–the same mechanisms that appeared to be important in immunologic reactions against tumors in the experimental systems discussed by Doctors Klein, Prehn, and Weiss in this monograph. It seems probable that these immune mechanisms maintain a constant surveillance of the body's cells, recognizing as abnormal those cells that undergo neoplastic transformation from whatever cause and destroying them before they can develop into tumors. There is some evidence that even when these surveillance mechanisms fail to eliminate neoplastic cells, they may slow their propagation. These mechanisms are markedly depressed by corticosteroid hormones, and therefore it should not surprise us that they may be depressed by emotional stress that results in elevated levels of corticosteroids.

Specific immunologic mechanisms are not the only forms of host defense against disease. Nonspecific mechanisms–that is, mechanisms such as fibrosis and phagocytosis that are not tailor-made to react with a specific antigenic structure–are of great importance in the control of infectious disease, and perhaps they also influence the growth of neoplastic tissue. Fibroblastic activity, phagocytosis by neutrophilic leukocytes, and the acute inflammatory reaction to tissue damage are all inhibited by such steroids as cortisone and desoxycorticosterone.

So far I have considered only the pathogenesis of cancer–the growth and spread of cancer cells. Is it conceivable that mechanisms influenced by psychic stimuli might influence the origin of cancer–the cellular phenomenon of neoplastic transformation? Specific immune mechanisms influence oncogenic virus infections. In fact, in experimental animals, the efficacy of immunologic reactions determines whether or not infection by an oncogenic virus will eventuate in neoplastic disease. Many oncogenic viruses cause tumors only if they infect during the neonatal period when the host is immunologically immature. Some studies suggest that immunosuppression also increases the frequency of tumor production by chemical carcinogens such as methylcholanthrene.

Neoplasia can arise only from propagating cells. Therefore factors that bring about the maturation and differentiation of specialized cells, and consequently decrease or stop their multiplication, also decrease the probability that a neoplastic transformation will arise or be perpetuated. A clinical example that probably illustrates this phenomenon is the effect of estrogen and progesterone on the endometrium. Continuous estrogen stimulation, which occurs in certain anovulatory conditions, causes sustained proliferation of the endometrium and is associated with an increased incidence of endometrial edenocarcinoma. In contrast, steroids with high progestational activity often cause regression of endometrial adenocarcinoma, presumably by forcing the carcinoma cells to differentiate into the nonpropagating secretory phase. Recent investigations have revealed that excretion of these ovarian hormones is controlled in large part by the hypothalamus via the anterior pituitary, and there is ample clinical evidence to indicate that psychic influences may alter the secretion of these hormones, presumably through this hypothalamic pathway.

Other factors that influence carcinogenesis are the metabolic processes of excretion and detoxification. For example, the carcinogenic effect of analine and phenanthrene compounds is dependent upon the way in which they are processed by kidney and liver. I know of no evidence that such metabolic processes are affected by the psyche, but the possibility is not unreasonable.

To conclude: Though an influence of the psyche on cancer is not proved, it is not unlikely. Even in our present state of ignorance concerning the factors that affect the initiation, propagation, and spread of cancer, we can suggest several mechanisms by which psychologic stimuli might influence cancer. The problem certainly merits our interest and serious investigation.

DR. B. B. KAMRIN (*The Museum of Natural History, New York, N. Y.*): I should like to comment on Dr. Southam's skepticism about the relationship of responsiveness and immunological state. I have a pilot experiment that I reported in the literature last year,† in which I obtained immune tolerant chicks, and determined their responsiveness to set situations, and I found that the immune tolerance, as measured by the prolonged retention of homografts, permitted them to change entirely in their characteristics.

There are classical methods of imprinting, which occur between zero, the first day of hatching, and the fifth day, in which chicks do or do not imprint or follow an object. There are also classical methods of determining escape mechanisms when a chick is placed in a closed enclosure.

In both these instances, all immune tolerant chicks had nondiscriminatory behavior to the extent of imprinting easily and readily, and all of them had a greater degree of activity than normal controlled chicks of the same age, the same sex, and the same strain.

† 1967. Anim. Behav. **15:** 217–222. 1968. Physiolog. Bohemoslov. **17:** 521–525.

PART IV. THE NERVOUS SYSTEM, HORMONES, AND CANCER

STEROID EXCRETION PATTERNS AND PERSONALITY IN LUNG CANCER

David M. Kissen* and L. G. S. Rao

Psychosomatic Research Unit
Southern General Hospital
Glasgow, Scotland

Our psychophysiological studies on lung cancer started with the clinical impression, gained by the late Dr. Kissen over a long period of time, of the personality of lung-cancer patients. Dr. Kissen described it as a poor outlet for emotional discharge (Kissen, 1966). This statement implies that lung-cancer patients have an increased ability to contain and absorb emotional conflicts without any apparent overt or covert effective response.

To begin with, psychosocial and psychological measures were designed to investigate the clinical impression of the role of emotional factors in lung cancer. These studies produced results that are consistent with the clinical impression. It was possible to include some physiological measures in our investigations into lung cancer. This multidisciplinary approach has proved to be very useful as a psychophysiological study of lung cancer and has given more information than separate studies with either psychological or physiological methods.

The obvious physiological parameter to include in the psychological study of emotional factors would be some physiological measure that is known to be closely related and influenced by emotional factors. The endocrine system would be the obvious choice, since it is now well known that it is influenced by emotional factors, through the hypothalamus and the hypophysis and the autonomic nervous system. Therefore, it was considered desirable to include adrenal function, which is shown to be almost directly correlated with emotional activity, as one of the measures used in the investigation of the role of emotional factors in the understanding of lung cancer. The results of the present study show that lung-cancer patients have some abnormalities in adrenal function, compared with control patients, and these abnormalities are related to certain psychological measures that are characteristic of lung-cancer patients.

Methods and Materials

Adrenal function was investigated by the measurement of the excretion of 17-ketosteroids (17-KS) and 17-hydroxycorticosteroids (17-OHCS) in seven consecutive 24-hour urine collections as soon as possible after admission to the hospital. It is appreciated that more sophisticated methods for the investigation of adrenal function are now available, but these methods were chosen because of their simplicity and reliability (Medical Research Council, 1963). These criteria are of great value, particularly if a large number of patients are to be investigated. The steroid values are expressed on a creatinine basis to correct for any possible incompleteness of the 24-hour urine collection.

The subjects for this study were all male patients mainly between 45 and 65 years of age, admitted to the hospital with chest complaints for investigations for

* Dr. David Kissen died on February 23, 1968, prior to this conference.

diagnosis and treatment. Our studies were carried out without the knowledge of diagnosis and before any intensive treatment had started. Those patients who were later diagnosed as not having lung cancer, but having some other chest disorder such as bronchitis, served as controls for lung-cancer patients in the statistical analysis of the results. Subdivision of the lung-cancer patients into groups according to histology of their tumors has not been done in this study.

Results and Discussion

The hypothesis to be investigated was that lung-cancer patients have poor outlets for emotional discharge and therefore show a lowered response to the stress of hospital admission, compared to the control patients. FIGURES 1 and 2 show the mean daily excretion of 17-KS and 17-OHCS and the total and ratio of these two groups of 48 cancer and 48 control patients over a period of seven days after admission to hospital. There is an increase in the mean excretion from day 1 to day 2 in the controls and a gradual fall over the next five days. The cancer patients do not show so large an increase from day 1 to day 2, and also do not show so large a decrease over the next five days as do the controls. These results can be interpreted as evidence supporting the hypothesis that lung-cancer pa-

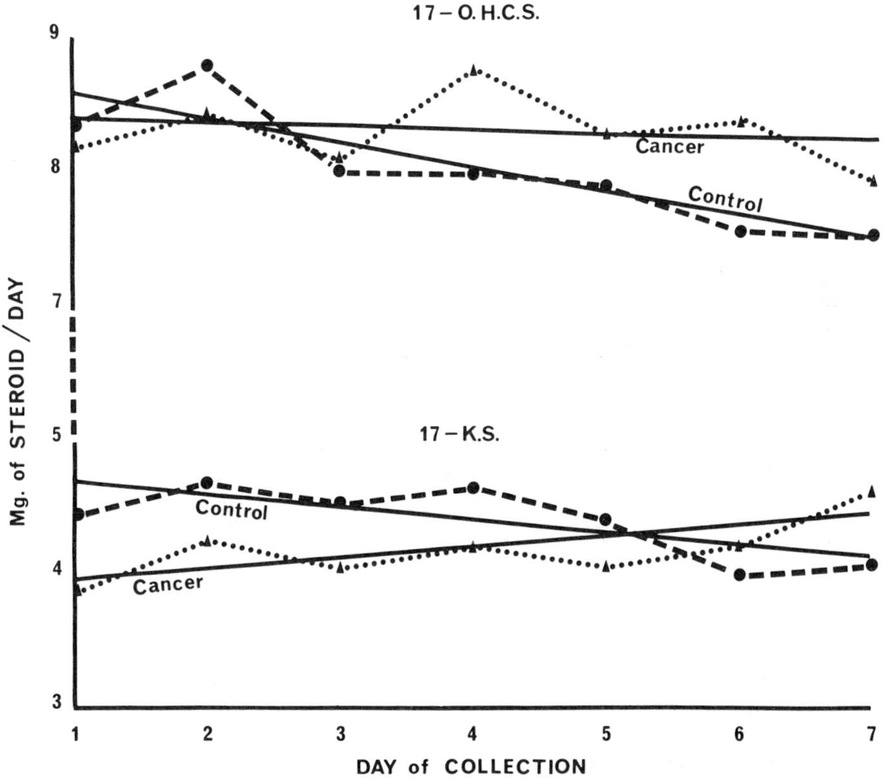

FIGURE 1. Mean excretion of 17-ketosteroids and 17-hydroxycorticosteroids/gm of creatinine/day of 48 cancer and 48 control patients.

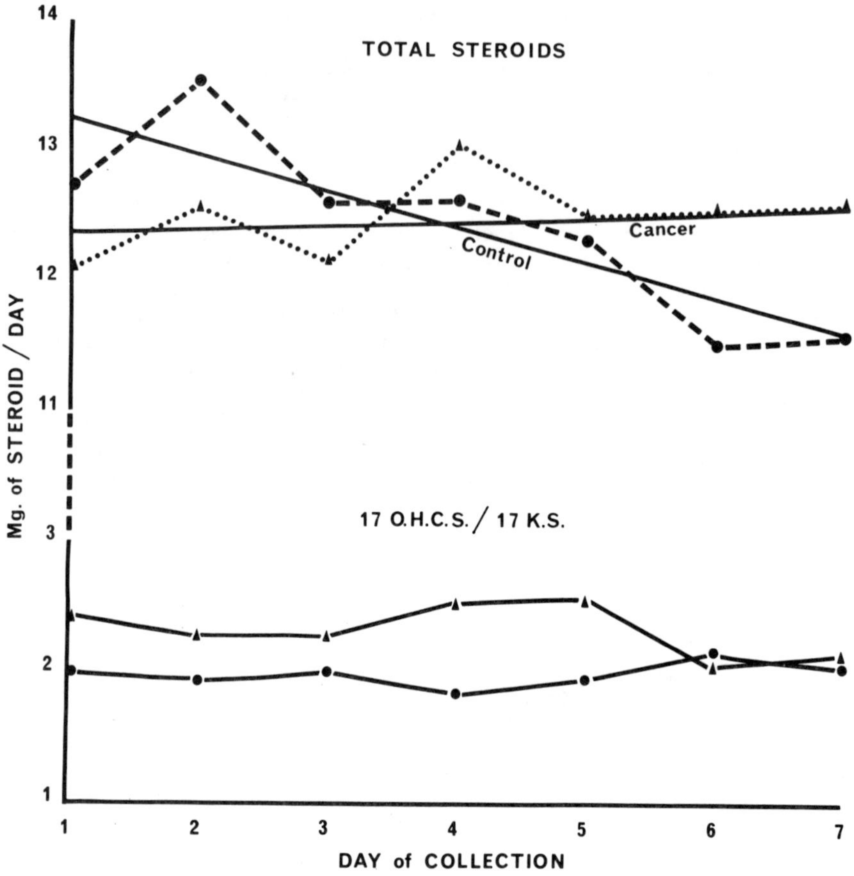

FIGURE 2. Mean excretion of total of 17-ketosteroids and 17-hydroxycorticosteroids and the ratio of these two groups of steroids on the same patients as in FIGURE 1.

tients show a lowered adrenal response to the stress of hospital admission than that of controls. However, the stress of admission may not be of the same magnitude for all patients, and it is difficult to measure the amount of stress experienced by each patient. Therefore, we consider these results as only suggestive evidence for the above hypothesis.

On the other hand, these results revealed an unusual characteristic of lung-cancer patients regarding the patterns of excretion of adrenocortical steroids. This feature is an increased fluctuation in the amounts of steroids excreted from day to day over a period of seven days in the lung-cancer patients, compared to the controls. This day-to-day variation was found in the excretion of the 17-KS, as well as of the 17-OHCS, both the sum of these two and the ratio of these two groups of steroids. TABLE 1 shows that this variation has been found to be significantly higher by the method of the analysis of variance for all the steroid measures used. This increased variation in the cancer patients was found to be independent of age or smoking habits.

TABLE 1

DIFFERENCES BETWEEN CANCERS AND CONTROLS IN THE VARIANCE OVER SEVEN DAYS

	p value
17-KS	0.01
17-OHCS	0.05
Ratio	0.01
Total	0.01

An analysis of variance was carried out on the day-to-day fluctuation over five days, and the significance of differences in the variance of the 17-KS and the ratio was not decreased, but the variance of the 17-OHCS and that of the total steroids decreased to insignificant levels.

Before trying to find explanations for this difference between cancer and controls, in these measures, it was considered desirable to confirm that this finding was not due to chance (although the probability of this being so was very slight—less than one percent). Hence, these investigations were repeated on another batch of patients. The results of the second batch, comprised of 64 controls and 36 cancer patients, were in agreement with those of the first batch. Cancer patients had a significantly higher day-to-day variation in the excretion of the 17-KS and the ratio of 17-OHCS/17-KS ($p = 0.01$). It therefore appears that this fluctuation in adrenal function is a characteristic of lung-cancer patients.

The significance of these findings is not clear. There are few studies on steroid excretion in men on consecutive days, either in normal or in diseased conditions. It is generally believed that steroid excretion is reasonably constant from day to day for each individual under the same experimental conditions. It is for this reason that in many clinical investigations only a single 24-hour urine collection is examined. The fact that a large fluctuation from day to day can occur even in disease states must surely be disturbing news for steroid biochemists and clinicians. It is, however, a consolation that it is the cancer patients and not the controls who show this abnormality. In the few studies done on consecutive 24-hour specimens e.g. those by Fox and co-workers (1961) and Harkness (1967), normal males do not show a great day-to-day variation in the 17-KS and 17-OHCS excretion. The only reported instances of big fluctuations from day to day is in skin disorders like hirsutism (Lloyd, 1964) or acne vulgaris (Harkness and coworkers, 1968). Androgens are implicated in the etiology of these disorders. However, the mean daily excretion of androgens is not high in all these patients and many of them have normal values, and the high levels required possibly to reach a threshold level for their actions may be obtained only infrequently but may still be enough to sustain their effects. Androgens also stimulate growth and are implicated in the etiology of some forms of cancer in human beings. Experimental tumors can be produced by single doses of androgens. Therefore, it is conceivable that androgens may be implicated in lung cancer, as well. Our finding that the increased fluctuation in the levels of the 17-KS may also be of some significance in the etiology of lung cancer.

Other clues to the possible significance of the increased day-to-day fluctuation in adrenal function in lung-cancer patients have come from the consideration of the relationships between these physiological measures and certain psychological measures of personality. A good deal of information is available on the effect of emotional factors on adrenocortical function. Since the work of Hans Selye, it has been established that the adrenal gland readily responds to any type of stress, including emotional stress, by an increased secretion of adrenocortical steroids. A positive correlation has been found between levels of anxiety and psychological defensiveness on the one hand and adrenocortical secretions on the other (see review by Persky, 1962). It was therefore considered desirable to find out if any correlations existed between the steroid-excretion patterns and the psychological measures we used on the same patients. TABLE 2 shows the correlations obtained by the Spearman Rank correlation method between the several steroid measures and the two psychological measures of personality we used: the neuroticism (N) and extraversion (E) scores of the Eysenck Personality Inventory (EPI). These correlations were carried out on 46 controls and 36 cancer patients. There is a significant positive correlation between extraversion and several steroid measures; namely, with the mean of the 17-KS in controls, the mean of the 17-OHCS in cancers, the variance of the 17-OHCS, and the variance of the total steroids of the cancers. The N scores of the EPI showed a negative correlation with the ratio variance of the controls. It is of interest that no correlation has been found to apply for both cancer and control patients. When these correlations were tried on the second batch of patients, only the correlation between the ratio variance and N scores in the controls was significant. All other correlations were not significant. It is unfortunate that this is so, but we have some reason to think that this second batch of cancer patients were unrepresentative of the rest of the cancer patients in some psychological measures.

It is interesting that these correlations are consistent with the differences observed between cancer patients and controls in the psychological and physiological measures. Control patients have high N scores and low ratio variance, and the correlation between these two measures is negative. Although extraversion is not found to be significantly greater in cancer patients in the present study, it is found to be greater in breast cancer, and also in a small, earlier study in lung cancer. Therefore, it can be said that low extraversion scores are not a cancer characteristic, unlike low N scores, and the positive correlation between the E scores and 17-OHCS variance and total steroid variance, both of which are high among cancers, becomes meaningful.

We should not forget to point out that these abnormalities in steroid excretion in cancer patients may be the result of the disease and may not be related to the cause of the disease at all. Before etiological significance is ascribed to these findings, it must be established that these abnormalities are not results of the disease. However, if these abnormalities are involved in the causation of the disease, then we have come across one or two more clues toward an understanding of the disease. The possibility of elucidating a hitherto unknown pathway will

TABLE 2

CORRELATIONS BETWEEN STEROID MEASURES AND EYSENCK PERSONALITY INVENTORY SCORES

	Cancers	Controls
Mean of Seven Days		
1. 17-KS/Extraversion	n.s.	$p = 0.05$
2. 17-OHCS/Extraversion	$p = 0.05$	n.s.
Variance over Seven Days		
3. 17-OHCS/Extraversion	$p = 0.025$	n.s.
4. Total Steroids/Extraversion	$p = 0.025$	n.s.
5. Ratio/Neuroticism	n.s.	$p = 0.05$ (–ve)

be made easier to the extent that these two landmarks are no longer entirely unconnected; there is now at least a freshly trodden track between them.

Acknowledgments

We wish to express our thanks for the skilled assistance of Mr. Gerald Lynam, the Misses Nancy Allan and Joan Ferrier, and Mrs. Maija-Liisa Rao. Our thanks are also due to the nursing staff of Hairmyres, Mearnskirk, and Ayrshire Central Hospitals for the collection of specimens. We are grateful to Doctors R. J. C. and J. Cuthbert, R. Barclay, R. McCluskey, and J. T. Boyd of these hospitals for permission and facilities to investigate the patients under their care. We are also grateful to Mr. R. A. Elton and Mr. P. A. K. Covey-Crump of the Department of Statistics for their help in the statistical analysis of the results. We gratefully acknowledge the encouragement and interest shown by Dr. J. K. Grant of the Steroid Biochemistry Department. We are extremely grateful to Professor T. Ferguson Rodger of the Department of Psychological Medicine for the laboratory facilities and interest in this work. The psychological work was carried out by Mr. R. I. F. Brown, and we are grateful to him and Miss Elizabeth Girvan for help in the calculation and statistical analysis of the results.

References

Fox, H. M., B. J. Murawski, A. F. Bartholomay & S. Gifford. 1961. Psychosom. Med. **23**(1): 33.

Harkness, A. 1967. (Personal communication.)

Harkness, R. A., A. A. A. Ismail, G. W. Beveridge & E. W. Powell. 1968. Proc. Workshop Conference on Testosterone. Tremsbüttel. J. Tamm, Ed. : 192. Georg Thieme Verlag. Stuttgart, Germany.

Kissen, D. M. 1966. Proc. N. Y. Acad. Sci. **125**: 820.

Lloyd, C. W. 1964. Proc. Second International Congress on Endocrinology. Excerpta Medica **25**: 591.

Medical Research Council. 1963. A standard method of estimating 17-oxo-steroids and total 17-oxogenic steroids by the Medical Research Council Committee on Clinical Endocrinology. Lancet **1**: 1415.

Persky, H. 1962. *In* Adrenocortical Function During Anxiety from Physiological Correlates of Psychological Disorder. R. Roessler & N. S. Greenfeld, Eds. : 171. University of Wisconsin Press. Madison, Wis.

DISCUSSION OF THE PAPER

Dr. Wilfred Abse (*University of Virginia, Charlottesville, Va.*): I wish to make a few remarks about some work we are doing at the University of Virginia, and I hope that the few statements I make may serve as a tribute to Dr. Kissen from our University, because he came there not long ago as a visiting professor, and spent several months with us.

What I have to talk about relates to Dr. Rao's work on the significance of the personality of lung cancer patients. Following Dr. Kissen's visit, I took out some time myself to make arrangements with the people in surgery to see post-lobectomy patients, patients who had had bronchogenic carcinoma. Over a period of a few months, I saw seven patients, and I was impressed by the fact that these particular patients were so similar in type, and in so many ways.

All of them, it so happens (and this may not be generally a regular feature, but I saw one after the other, all men in their 50's), had reached an attitude of some degree of futility. It seemed as though, whatever basis they had started on, they had reached a certain plateau in their lives. They were resigned that things would continue much as they had been, and, though making good contact with reality, they were much better related to things than to people; their relationships with people were extremely poor. Now, what I tried to do after confirming Dr. Kissen's views as to type of personality, was to get a more accurate cigarette-smoking history from them. They all were much the same in this respect, and I will describe an average case. This was a man about 55, who had smoked from the age of 16 or 17, beginning with one pack of cigarettes a day and usually proceeding on to smoke at least two packs a day, certainly during his 30's. Then, about seven or eight years before the actual signs or symptoms of carcinoma, this individual had gone to bed at night communicating very poorly with people around him, feeling quite tense, and not being able to sleep. He could not get to sleep.

But then he got up and had a glass of beer, or something like that, and smoked cigarettes during the course of the night. Six out of the seven, actually, had this night smoking history. Now, in reviewing the charts of these people, I found that all that was put down in writing was that they smoked heavily.

That really sums it up: they were very inadequate cigarette-smoking histories. Now I did not find that it was always easy to get a clear smoking history from these people immediately. If one accepted their first version, this was sometimes found to be quite inaccurate.

All these people were postlobectomy patients, about seven to ten days after lobectomy. All that happened as the result of this investigation was that this set the stage for me to do something more, and, being occupied with other things myself, I arranged with one of the residents in psychiatry to do a more controlled series of interviews with these patients, together with administering a questionnaire, particularly to get a smoking history.

Now it so happened that he saw 25 patients who were lung cancer patients, and he saw 25 noncancer chest cases. His results were quite equivocal. He found only that about half the lung cancer cases (although there were many more cases of night smoking in the lung cancer group) had night smoking histories. Now, of course, we have gone on from there, too. We hope to elaborate this into a much more satisfactory research project.

What I wish to say with reference to Dr. Rao's talk in connection with biological periodicity, one index of which is that steroid metabolism is depleted during the night, is that it is a fact that many of these people smoke at night. I regard this as a factor of great importance myself, at the moment, because resistance to irritation could be greatly depleted during the night hours.

PRETREATMENT URINARY HORMONE PATTERNS AND SURVIVAL IN PATIENTS WITH BREAST CANCER, PROSTATE CANCER, OR LUNG CANCER*

Jessie Marmorston, Paul J. Geller,
and John M. Weiner
University of Southern California
School of Medicine
Los Angeles, Calif.

Previous studies of cancer of the breast, prostate, and lung have suggested associated disturbances in endocrine function. These observations have been demonstrated by clinical and laboratory methods.[1-46]

Our study was initiated to delineate the hormone excretion pattern as completely as possible in order to discover any characteristic patterns or relationships that might afford etiologic clues or serve as diagnostic aids in differentiating cancer from benign disease at the same sites.

Much of the material has been subjected to multivariate analysis, which permits the simultaneous assessment of a large number of interdependent parameters. In these multivariate studies, Fisher's linear discriminant analysis[47] was emphasized. This method is useful in deriving the combination of urinary steroids most involved in separating the cancer, benign, or normal subjects. The discriminant scores for a given comparison can be used to identify patients belonging to cancer groups as contrasted with comparable clinically normal individuals or patients with benign disease. Results of some of these studies are reported elsewhere.[48-50]

The purpose of this report is to describe the survival of patients with, respectively, cancer of the breast, prostate, or lung. These data aid in delineating an even greater need, that of developing a mode for the earlier detection of the patient with cancer. Our observations related to a system for earlier detection will be discussed.

Methods

Persons admitted to the study received a complete physical examination. A detailed medical history on each subject included a record of developmental, social, environmental, and familial data, past illnesses, food preferences, and habits such as use of medication, tobacco, and alcohol. In addition, an adjective check list was used to obtain a description of personality-related factors. Cancer patients were studied prior to onset of any therapy.

Two consecutive 24-hr specimens of urine were collected from each subject. The urinary steroids measured were androsterone, etiocholanolone, 11-oxy-17-ketosteroids, beta fraction, dehydroepiandrosterone, pregnanediol, estrone, estradiol, estriol, Porter-Silber chromogens, and 17-ketogenic steroids. In addition, biological activity of the total gonadotropin residue was assayed, and the total protein and carbohydrate content of the residue were quantitatively determined. The activities of the protein or carbohydrate in the residue were not measured. Laboratory methods are described in detail elsewhere.[51] Baseline nonendocrine measurements of physiologic state included age, height, weight, and the specific gravity and creatinine content of the urine.

* Supported by the National Cancer Institute, USPHS Contract SA–43–PH–3714, and the Bella and Andre Meyer Foundation.

All cancers were histologically verified. Diagnosis of benign disease was confirmed using appropriate clinical and laboratory criteria; normal subjects were identified clinically.

A total of 287 persons were studied. Twenty-eight of the women were breast cancer patients (seven premenopausal, 21 postmenopausal); 18 had benign breast tumor (all premenopausal); 44 were normal women (24 premenopausal, 20 postmenopausal). Twenty-one men had cancer of the prostate; 17 men had benign prostatic hypertrophy; 55 men had lung cancer (17 adenocarcinoma, 18 squamous carcinoma, and 20 anaplastic carcinoma); 45 men had pulmonary emphysema; 59 were normal men.

Findings

The cancer patients have been followed since initial detection in 1960–63. Of the 28 breast cancer patients, nine have survived (two premenopausal and seven postmenopausal). Those now dead lived an average of 21 to 22 months. The patients with cancer of the prostate lived an average of 31 months, with only one of the 21 alive at the present time. As expected, the lung cancer patients had a considerably shorter survival time, averaging seven months after detection. Only one of the 55 is still living. No marked differences in survival were observed among the three types of lung cancer studied (i.e., adenocarcinoma–four months; squamous carcinoma–seven months; and anaplastic carcinoma–seven months).

Each patient was individually treated, and no attempt was made in this survey to test the efficacy of particular treatments. In the breast cancer patients, 24 of the 28 were subjected to surgery (radical mastectomy). The majority of these cases also received x-ray, chemotherapeutic agents, and estrogens. Nine of these 24 (38%) are still living. The other four patients received x-ray, chemotherapy, and/or hormones. None survived.

In the prostrate cancer patients, the predominant treatment was diethylstilbestrol (11 of the 21). Orchiectomy alone, or in combination with diethylstilbestrol, was used in four patients. Two underwent retropubic prostatectomies. The remainder received palliative transurethral resections. The one survivor was treated by prostatectomy.

Seven of the lung-cancer patients were resected. Forty of the patients were treated with x-ray and/or chemotherapeutic agents. Eleven received no treatment. Exploratory thoracotomy was used to determine the severity of disease in 20 of the 55 patients.

These observations may be used to highlight the clinical problem in treating the patient with cancer. In lung cancer, one of the 55 survived. This patient was treated by lobectomy for grade I disease. The remaining 54 patients, although treated intensively with the accepted modalities of therapy, all succumbed. One might infer that these cases were all too far advanced for the treatments used to be of real value in influencing survival.

Similarly, the prostate-cancer cases were detected subsequent to that point in time when prostatectomy could be considered as a possible procedure. The palliative treatments suggested by Huggins and Hodges[4] were used in the majority of the cases, yielding an average of 2.5 years of survival.

The breast-cancer cases appear to be only slightly more fortunate than the other cancers. The survival time was less than two years in the 19 who died, although nine of the women are still alive. One may infer that these nine patients represent cases detected earlier or those with a more localized cancer.

The problem at this time in our understanding and management of patients with cancer of the breast, prostate, or lung is not which treatment is better, since none are yielding five-year survival in 50% or more of the patients. The essential problem is one of detecting these cancers earlier and, it is to be hoped, while they are more localized, so that the known treatments may be instituted earlier.[52-55]

With a view toward developing a scheme for the earlier detection of cancer, we reviewed our urinary steroid findings in order to determine if these measurements may be useful. We had published previously[48] a discriminant pattern using androsterone, protein in the gonadotropin residue, and estriol. The discriminant was −2.7 androsterone + 2.2 protein + 0.7 estriol. Use of this formula gives rise to significantly different mean values in the premenopausal women with breast cancer and in matched normal women. The distribution of discriminant scores showed that 100% (seven) of the breast-cancer patients had positive scores and 75% (18) of the normal women had negative scores. An average correct classification of 87% was observed.† The average urinary hormone pattern scores for this comparison are shown in FIGURE 1. The cancer patients

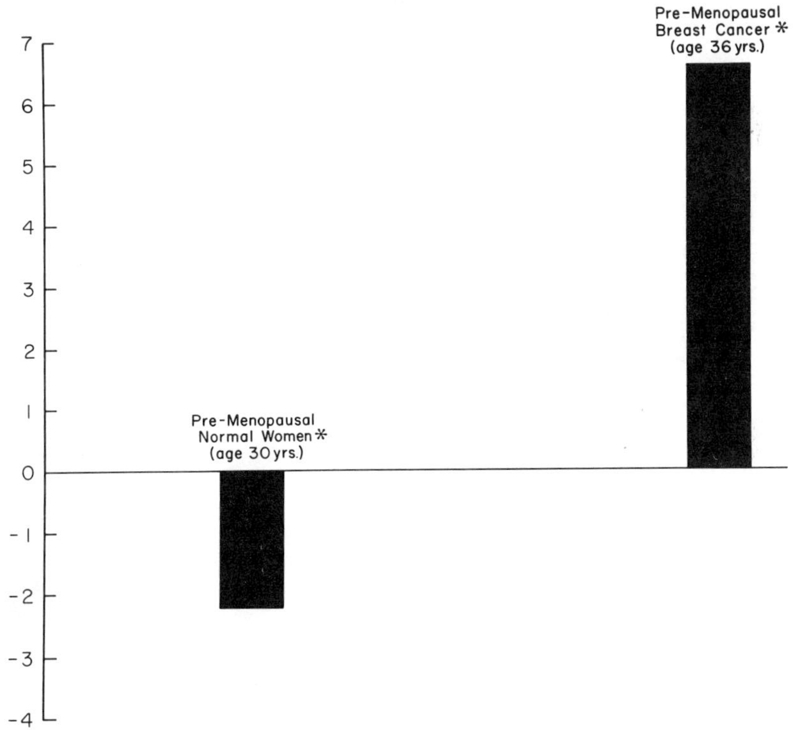

* The scale is computed using the equation: Score = −2.7 (androsterone) + 2.0 (protein in gonadotropin residue) + 0.7 (estriol).

FIGURE 1. Average urinary hormone pattern scores in premenopausal women with untreated breast cancer and premenopausal normal women.

† It is recognized that the average proportion correctly classified will be overestimated when the original samples are classified using the derived discriminant. The degree of overestimation is slight when two to five variates are used in the discriminant and particularly when they are selected using either the Student t method or stepwise discriminant function. This subject is dealt with in another report.[56]

have an average score of 6.6 and the matched normal women an average of −2.2. These urinary steroids, when analyzed by this statistical method, significantly distinguish normal women from women with breast cancer.

The real value of the discriminant is to classify new observations. When androsterone, protein, and estriol are measured in new individuals and the values used in the discriminant equation, those new discriminant scores that are positive would be classified as *cancer* and those that are negative would be classified as *normal.* If the breast-cancer-normal discriminant pattern is useful in detection of cancer, then new samples of known normal subjects and of known cancer types should be correctly identified by this combination of urinary hormones. The results of testing this breast cancer pattern—using average urinary hormone values for the normal men, normal postmenopausal women, men with lung cancer, men with prostate cancer, and postmenopausal women with breast cancer—are shown in FIGURE 2. The breast-cancer-normal average values are shown for reference. Note that each diagnostic group is classified correctly with respect to normal or cancer. Further, the average urinary hormone pattern scores give a continuum which appears to be related to the clinical classification of the groups. That is, normal men have the most "normal" score (i.e., lowest score), normal premenopausal women next, then normal postmenopausal women, lung cancer,

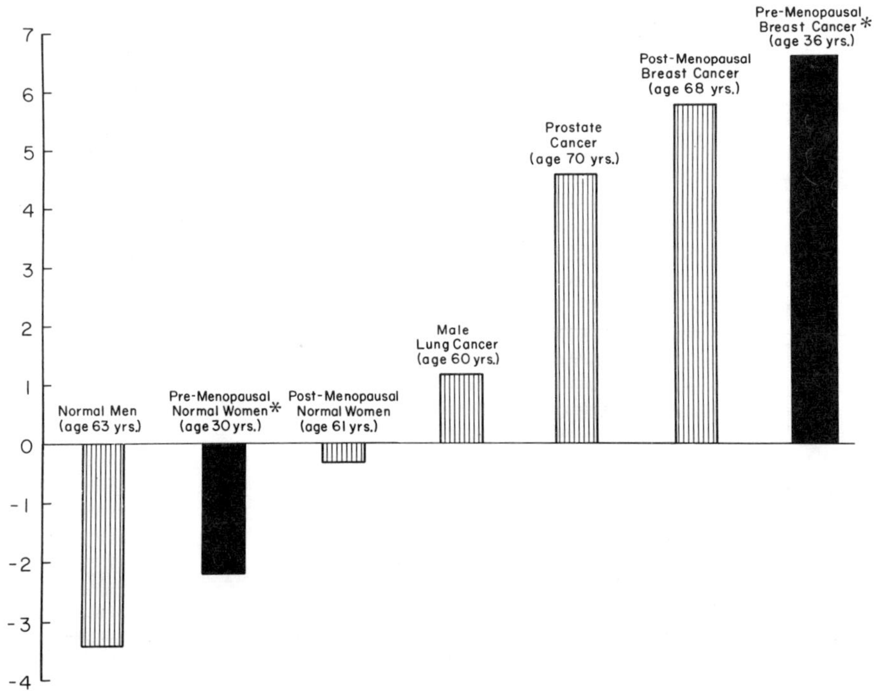

* The scale is computed using the equation: Score = −2.7 (androsterone) + 2.0 (protein in gonadotropin residue) + 0.7 (estriol).

FIGURE 2. Average urinary hormone pattern scores in other known cancer and normal groups, using the breast cancer pattern.

prostate cancer, postmenopausal breast cancer, and the highest or most-cancer score is assigned to the premenopausal breast cancer.

The next question to be investigated dealt with the breast cancer pattern classification of known sick control groups, i.e., emphysema, benign tumor of the breast, and benign prostatic hypertrophy. These results are shown in FIGURE 3. Again, the normal average value and the breast-cancer average value are included for reference. As seen in FIGURE 3, the average urinary hormone pattern score for the emphysema group is −0.8, indicating a correct classification as noncancer (more like normal than cancer). The benign breast tumor value is +0.9, and the benign prostate value is +3.1, both indicating more similarity to cancer than to normal and both being *incorrectly classified* as cancer.

If indeed the urinary hormone pattern combining androsterone, protein, and estriol is useful, then it appears to be so in differentiating, on the average, the tumor groups from the nontumor groups.

As part of this investigation, we analyzed the data to see if a urinary hormone pattern could be determined that would discriminate breast cancer from benign tumor. A pattern was observed consisting of etiocholanolone and estriol. There was also sufficient difference in the age of the two groups to suggest that this information be taken into account. Accordingly, the discriminant pattern is −3.8 etiocholanolone + 2.8 estriol + 2.4 age. The average discriminant scores for premenopausal breast cancer and for benign tumor are shown in FIGURE 4. The

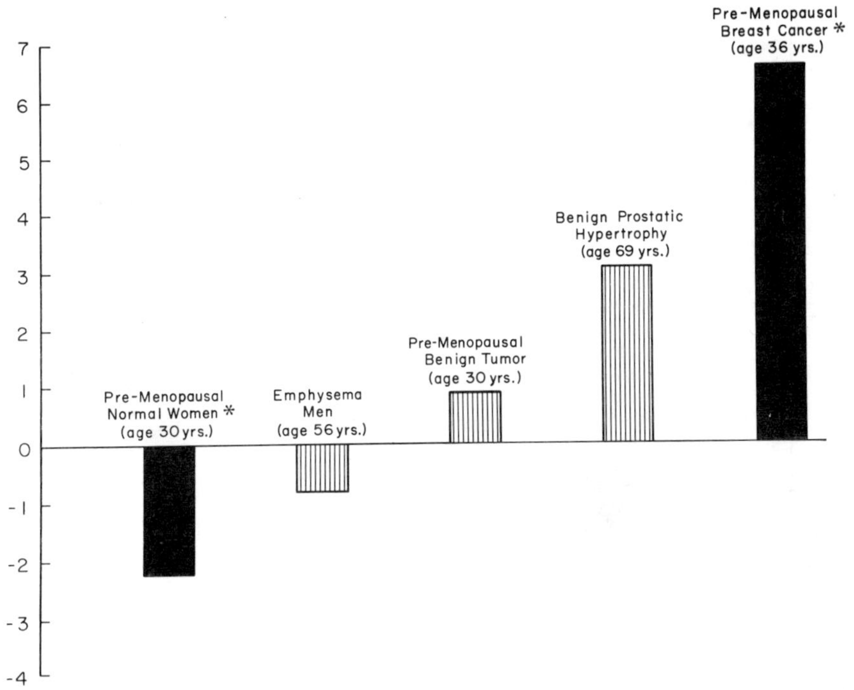

* The scale is computed using the equation: Score = −2.7 (androsterone) + 2.0 (protein in gonadotropin residue) + 0.7 (estriol).

FIGURE 3. Average urinary hormone pattern scores in known sick control groups using the breast cancer pattern.

difference in mean values is highly significant ($P < .01$). The distribution of individual scores showed that all seven of the cancer patients had positive pattern values and that 14 of the 18 benign tumor patients had negative pattern values. The average correct classification was 89%.

We had previously published a discriminant pattern comparing prostate cancer with benign hypertrophy.[50] This discriminant was as follows: 2.1 (estrone) − 3.8 (estriol) − 1.1 (17-ketogenic steroids) + 2.1 (Poter-Silber chromogens) − 1.1 (beta fraction). The average pattern values for prostate cancer and benign prostate groups are shown in FIGURE 5. Seventeen of the cancer patients (80%) and 16 of the benign (94%) were properly classified using this pattern for an average correct classification of 87%.

Discussion

This report has considered the survival picture in 28 patients with breast cancer, 21 patients with prostate cancer, and 55 patients with lung cancer. Differences in survival time are directly related to the site of cancer, with none of the groups showing five-year survival in 50% or more of the cases. The lung cancer cases were dead in seven months on the average, the breast cancer in 20 to 22 months, and the prostate cancer in 30 months. One may infer that the treatments rendered, as well as the short survival times, point up the major defect in cancer therapy, namely, failure to detect the disease early enough to alter its course.

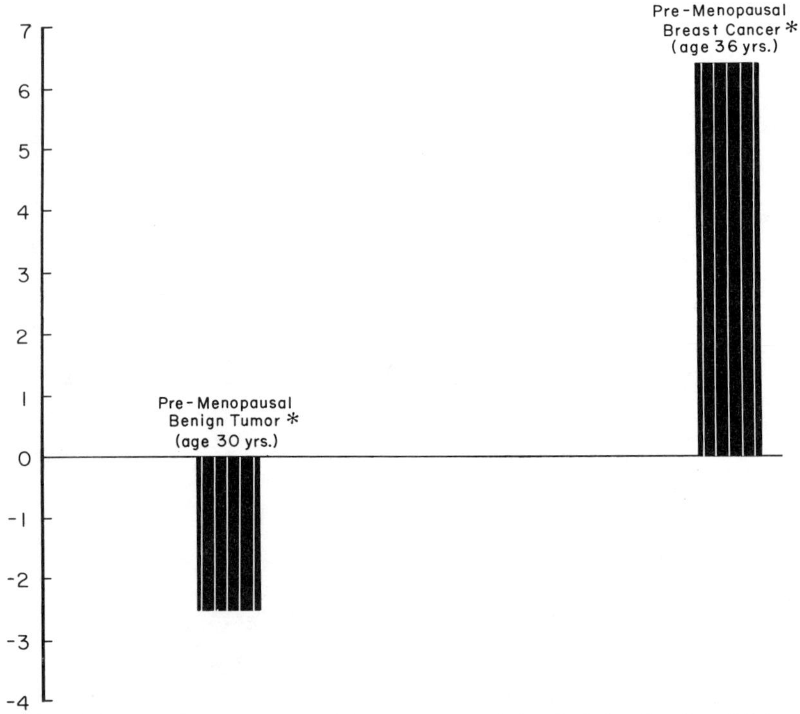

* The scale is computed using the equation: Score = −3.7 (etiocholanolone) + 2.8 (estriol) + 2.4 (age).

FIGURE 4. Average urinary hormone pattern scores in premenopausal women with untreated breast cancer and premenopausal women with benign breast tumor.

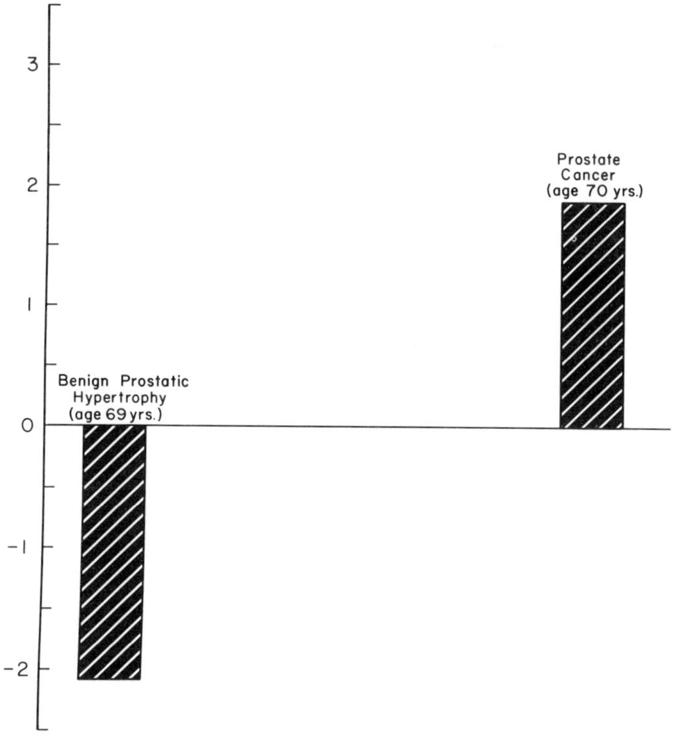

FIGURE 5. Average urinary hormone pattern scores in men with cancer of the prostate and with benign prostatic hypertrophy. The scale is computed using the equation: Score = —2.1 (estrone) + 3.8 (estriol) + 1.1 (17-ketogenic steroids) —2.1 (P-S chromogen) + 1.1 (beta-fraction of 17-ketosteroids).

In considering the urinary steroid pattern as a screening device for earlier detection of the individual with cancer, a number of factors are favorable. First, a large number of studies have linked endocrine aberrations and cancer. As one example, Bulbrook and Hayward[57] have shown a urinary steroid disturbance in women prior to the development of breast cancer. Second, hormonal therapies have been used in the treatment of cancers of endocrine target tissue with varying degrees of success. Third, hormones are known to regulate many metabolic functions, and disturbances in these functions may be reflected by changes in the regulating hormones themselves.[58] Fourth, the present-day diagnostic techniques are highly dependent upon overt manifestations of the disease. These techniques are obviously inadequate in detection of cancer at its earliest stage. That is, the recognition of a lump in the breast, a shadow on the chest x-ray, a change in consistency of the prostate on examination may represent late signs of malignancy.

One advantage of using urinary steroids in early detection of cancer is the ease of obtaining the sample. In addition, present-day methodologies[59,60] enable the rapid processing of large numbers of urine samples. It thus becomes practical to determine the effectiveness of using these steroid patterns in detecting cancer. Such a prospective study is being developed in our laboratory, using 5,000 subjects.

Review of the urinary steroids found to be important in the three patterns presented suggests that the endocrine disturbance is possibly multidimensional and reflects shifts in the pituitary-adrenal-gonadal axes. These findings can be further clarified by carefully determining the concentration of individual steroids making up the phenolic, neutral ketonic, and nonketonic fractions. In the contemplated study, the original steroids measured will be augmented by studying metabolites of cortisol and cortisone and by determining concentrations of urinary testosterone and epitestosterone.

If urinary steroids are useful in early detection of cancer suspects, the clinician then may pursue a tissue diagnosis, which is so important in today's treatment. In the case of breast cancer, mammography, for example, may be performed in search for the lesion. When found, needle biopsies may be obtained for tissue analysis. In lung cancer, the suspect may be further studied, for example, by tomography, bronchoscopy, cytological analyses of bronchial washings, and exploratory throracotomy. In prostate cancer, needle biopsies may be used to obtain samples for analysis. The cancer suspect would be examined frequently, so that early identification of the malignancy is enhanced.

Summary

Two hundred eighty-seven subjects were studied to determine whether urinary steroids were related to cancer of the breast, prostate, or lung. A urinary hormone pattern consisting of androsterone, protein in the gonadotropin residue, and estriol was found to be effective in properly differentiating tumor from nontumor groups. Two additional urinary steroid patterns were presented for distinguishing breast cancer from benign tumor and prostate cancer from benign hypertrophy. Survival data were reviewed in these patients, with the conclusion that earlier detection is the most important consideration in the effective treatment of breast, prostate, or lung cancer.

The methodologies for rapidly performing large numbers of urinary steroid analyses have been developed. However, the justification for using the urinary steroids as indicators of early cancer have only recently become available. The findings to date of Bulbrook and Hayward[57] and those presented in this report suggest that the urinary steroid pattern analysis is important in cancer detection and should be considered more intensively in future research.

Acknowledgments

The authors gratefully acknowledge the significant contributions to this research made by Lawrence G. Crowley, M.D., Ray B. Evans, Ph.D, Hyman W. Gierson, M.D., Doris L. Herman, M.D., Carl E. Hopkins, Ph.D., Louis J. Lombardo, M.D., Sara M. Myers, Ph.D., Elizabeth Stern, M.D., Mr. Jim H. Pare, and Mrs. Lucia Noll.

References

1. Altschul, A. 1938. Gynecomastia in lung tumor. New York J. Med. **38:** 637–640.
2. Moore, R. A., M. L. Miller & A. McLellan. 1940. The urinary excretion of androgens by patients with benign hypertrophy of the prostate. J. Urol. **44:** 727–737.
3. Dingemanse, E. & E. Laqueur. 1940. The content of male and female hormone in the urine of patients with prostatic hypertrophy. J. Urol. **44:** 530–540.
4. Huggins, C. & C. V. Hodges. 1941. Studies on prostatic cancer. I. The effect of castration, of estrogen and of androgen injection on serum phosphatases in metastatic carcinoma of the prostate. Cancer Res. **1:** 293–297.
5. Frame, E. G. & H. J. Jewett. 1944. The excretion of 17-ketosteroids in carcinoma of the prostate. J. Urol. **52:** 330–333.
6. Huggins, C. 1947. The etiology of benign prostatic hypertrophy. New York Acad. Med. Bull. **23:** 696–704.
7. McCullagh, E. P., R. W. Schneider, W. Bowman & M. B. Smith. 1948. Adrenal and testicular deficiency. J. Clin. Endocr. **8:** 275–294.

8. HUGGINS, C. & D. M. BERGENSTAL. 1951. Surgery of the adrenals. JAMA **147**(2): 101–106.
9. PEABODY, H. D. & A. M. OLSEN. 1951. Association of bronchogenic carcinoma and diabetes insipidus: report of cases. Proc. Mayo Clin. **26**: 107–112.
10. HUGGINS, C. 1952. Endocrine factors in cancer. J. Urol. **68**: 875–884.
11. HUGGINS, C. & D. M. BERGENSTAL. 1952. Inhibition of human mammary and prostatic cancers by adrenalectomy. Cancer Res. **12**: 134–141.
12. SOMMERS, S. C. 1955. Endocrine abnormalities in women with breast cancer. Lab. Invest. **4**: 160–174.
13. HUGGINS, C. 1956. Control of cancers of man by endocrinologic methods–A review. Cancer Res. **16**(2): 825–830.
14. SOMMERS, S. C. 1957. Endocrine changes with prostatic carcinoma. Cancer **10**: 345–358.
15. SOMMERS, S. C. & W. A. MEISSNER. 1957. Endocrine abnormalities accompanying human endometrial cancer. Cancer **10**: 516–521.
16. KOVACH, R. D. & L. H. KYLE. 1958. Cushing's syndrome and bronchogenic carcinoma. Amer. J. Med. **24**: 981–988.
17. BULBROOK, R. D., L. M. FRANKS & F. C. GREENWOOD. 1959. Hormone excretion in prostatic cancer: the early and late effects of endocrine treatment on urinary oestrogens, 17-ketosteroids and 17-ketogenic steroids. Acta Endocr. **31**: 481–499.
18. O'CONOR, V. J., JR., R. E. DESAUTELS, J. W. PRYOR, P. L. MUNSON & J. H. HARRISON 1959. Studies of hormonal changes in relation to cancer of the prostate: a progress report. J. Urol. **81**: 468–473.
19. HALL, P. F. 1959. *In* Gynaecomastia. Monographs of the Federal Council of the Brit. Med. Assn. in Australia. No. 2: 138–141.
20. VANDEWIELE, R. & S. LIEBERMAN. 1960. The metabolism of dehydroisoandrosterone. *In* Biological Activities of Steroids in Relation to Cancer. Academic Press, Inc. New York, N. Y.
21. WERK, E. E. & L. J. SHOLITON. 1960. Adrenocortical function in carcinoma of the lung. Cancer **13**: 469–481.
22. ALLOTT, E. N. & M. O. SKELTON. 1960. Increased adrenocortical activity associated with malignant disease. Lancet **2**: 278–284.
23. DIAMOND, M. T. 1961. Carcinomatous neuropathy. Ann. Intern. Med. **54**: 1259–1266.
24. WERK, E. E., L. J. SHOLITON, R. T. MARNELL & J. INCZE. 1961. Further studies of adrenocortical function in bronchogenic carcinoma. J. Lab. Clin. Med. **58**: 972–973.
25. NAKANO, K. 1961. Endocrinological study of prostate cancer: effects of anti-androgenic treatments on urinary 17-ketosteroids and its fractionation. Jap. J. Urol. **52**: 1047–1077.
26. MARKS, L. J., A. E. ANDERSON & H. LIBERMAN. 1961. Carcinoma of the lung associated with marked adrenocortical hyperplasia and adrenal hyper-responsiveness to ACTH in the absence of Cushing's syndrome. Ann. Intern. Med. **54**: 1243–1248.
27. KARTEN, I. & H. BARTFELD. 1962. Bronchogenic carcinoma simulating early rheumatoid arthritis. JAMA **179**: 162–163.
28. WILLIAMS, M. J. & S. C. SOMMERS. 1962. Endocrine and certain other changes in men with carcinoma of the lung. Cancer **13**: 559–601.
29. BELSKY, J. L. & L. J. MARKS. 1962. Plasma 17-hydroxycorticosteroid responsiveness to ACTH in patients with bronchogenic carcinoma. Metabolism **11**: 435–442.
30. HYMES, A. C. & R. P. DOE. 1962. Adrenal function in cancer of the lung, with and without Cushing's syndrome. Amer. J. Med. **33**: 398-407.
31. HUGGINS, C. & N. C. YANG. 1962. Induction and extinction of mammary cancer. Science **137**: 257–262.
32. BULBROOK, R. D., J. H. HAYWARD, C. C. SPICER & B. S. THOMAS. 1962. A comparison between the urinary steroid excretion of normal women and women with advanced breast cancer. Lancet **2**: 1235–1237.
33. BULBROOK, R. D., J. H. HAYWARD, C. C. SPICER & B. S. THOMAS. 1962. Abnormal excretion of urinary steroids by women with early breast cancer. Lancet **2**: 1238–1240.
34. WILLIAMS, M. J. & S. C. SOMMERS. 1962. Endocrine and certain other changes in men with carcinoma of the lung. Cancer **15**: 109–117.
35. PRUNTY, F. T. G., R. V. BROOKS, J. DUPRE, T. M. D. GIMLETTE, J. S. M. HUTCHINSON, R. R. MCSWINEY & I. H. MILLS. 1963. Adrenocortical hyperfunction and potassium metabolism in patients with "non-endocrine" tumors and Cushing's syndrome. J. Clin. Endocr. **23**: 737–746.
36. MARMORSTON, J., L. G. CROWLEY, S. M. MYERS, E. STERN & C. E. HOPKINS. 1965. Urinary excretion of neutral 17-ketosteroids and pregnanediol by patients with breast cancer and benign breast disease. Amer. J. Obstet. Gynec. **92**: 447–459.

37. MARMORSTON, J., L. G. CROWLEY, S. M. MYERS, E. STERN & C. E. HOPKINS. 1965. Urinary excretion of estrone, estradiol, and estriol by patients with breast cancer and benign breast disease. Amer. J. Obstet. Gynec. **92:** 460–467.
38. MARMORSTON, J., L. J. LOMBARDO, S. M. MYERS, H. W. GIERSON, E. STERN & C. E. HOPKINS. 1965. Urinary excretion of neutral 17-ketosteroids and pregnanediol by patients with prostatic cancer and benign prostatic hypertrophy. J. Urol. **93:** 276–286.
39. MARMORSTON, J., L. J. LOMBARDO, S. M. MYERS, H. W. GIERSON, E. STERN & C. E. HOPKINS. 1965. Urinary excretion of estrone, estradiol, and estriol by patients with prostatic cancer and benign prostatic hypertrophy. J. Urol. **93:** 287–295.
40. MARMORSTON, J., H. W. GIERSON, S. M. MYERS & E. STERN. 1965. Urinary excretion of neutral 17-ketosteroids and pregnanediol by patients with lung cancer and emphysema. Amer. Rev. Resp. Dis. **92:** 404–416.
41. MARMORSTON, J., H. W. GIERSON, S. M. MYERS & E. STERN. 1965. Urinary excretion of estrone, estradiol, and estriol by patients with lung cancer and emphysema. Amer. Rev. Resp. Dis. **92:** 417–427.
42. BECK, J. C., A. J. BLAIR, M. M. GRIFFITHS, M. W. ROSENFELD & E. E. MCGARRY. 1966. In search of hormonal factors as an aid in predicting the outcome of breast carcinoma. Canad. Cancer Conf. **6:** 3–35.
43. BULBROOK, R. D. 1966. Hormonal factors in the etiology and treatment of breast cancer. Canad. Cancer Conf. **6:** 36–49.
44. JULL, J. W. 1966. Hormonal mechanism in carcinogenesis. Canad. Cancer Conf. **6:** 109–123.
45. CAMIEL, M. L., D. L. BENNINGHOFF & L. L. ALEXANDER. 1967. Gynecomastia associated with lung cancer. Dis. Chest **52:** 445–450.
46. DAUGHTRY, D. C., J. G. CHESNEY, H. C. SPEAR, T. O. GENTSCH & P. B. LARSEN. 1967. Unexplained systemic manifestations of malignant lung tumors. Dis. Chest **52:** 632–639.
47. FISHER, R. A. 1936. The use of multiple measurements in taxonomic problems. Ann. Eugen. **7:** 179–188.
48. STERN, E., C. E. HOPKINS, J. M. WEINER & J. MARMORSTON. 1964. Hormone excretion patterns in breast and prostate cancer are abnormal. Science **145:** 716–719.
49. MARMORSTON, J., J. M. WEINER, C. E. HOPKINS & E. STERN. 1966. Abnormalities in urinary hormone patterns in lung cancer and emphysema. Cancer **19:** 985–995.
50. WEINER, J. M., J. MARMORSTON, E. STERN & C. E. HOPKINS. 1966. Urinary hormone metabolites in cancer and benign hyperplasia of the prostate: A multivariate statistical analysis. Ann. N. Y. Acad. Sci. **125:** 974–983.
51. MARMORSTON, J. 1966. Urinary hormone metabolite levels in patients with cancer of the breast, prostate and lung. Ann. N. Y. Acad. Sci. **125:** 959–973.
52. BRANTIGAN, O. C. 1967. Complacency in carcinoma of the lung. Dis. Chest **52:** 173–185.
53. BOLOOKI, H. & S. MINKOWITZ. 1967. Evaluation of primary carcinoma of the lung and survival rate after curative resection in a large city hospital. Dis. Chest **52:** 680–682.
54. BENNINGHOFF, D. L. & L. L. ALEXANDER. 1968. Treatment of lung carcinoma—radiation versus radiation combined with 5-fluorouracil. New York J. Med. **68:** 532–534.
55. WATSON, W. L. & D. SCHOTTENFELD. 1968. Survival in cancer of the bronchus and lung, 1949–1962—Comparison of men and women patients. Dis. Chest **53:** 65–72.
56. WEINER, J. M. & O. J. DUNN. 1966. Elimination of variates in linear discrimination problems. Biometrics **22:** 268–275.
57. BULBROOK, R. D. & J. L. HAYWARD. 1967. Abnormal urinary steroid excretion and subsequent breast cancer. Lancet **1:** 519–522.
58. TOMKINS, G. M. 1968. Biological regulation by steroid hormones. Canad. Cancer Conf. **7:** 163–174.
59. BUSH, I. E. 1963. Meth. Biochem. Anal. **11:** 149–209.
60. ROBERTS, J. B., I. E. BUSH & N. B. GIBREE. 1968. Urinary steroid analysis: A comprehensive procedure. Anal. Biochem. In press.

DISCUSSION OF THE PAPER

DR. KATZ: Because of my own interests, this was a particularly stimulating presentation. I do, however, want to ask one question: In the work of others who have been interested in a discriminant ratio, such as Bulbrook's group in England and Moore's group at Peter Bent Brigham, they have tended to shy away from inclusion of estrogens, apparently because of the relative variability of estrogens on a day-to-day basis during the monthly menstrual cycle, as well as on a year-to-year basis, because of involutional processes involving the ovaries. Yet, you have included this, and I was wondering if you might comment on your group's feelings about this whole issue.

DR. WEINER: There are two problems, I think, in dealing with estrogens, as the steroid chemists in the audience can discuss much better than I. First, there are problems in determining estrogens and, specifically, the determination of estrone, estradiol, and estriol. These procedures have been discussed (Marmorston *et al.* 1965. Urinary Excretion of estrone, estradiol, and estriol by patients with breast cancer and benign breast disease. Amer. J. Obstet. Gynec. **92:** 460).

Second, we attempted to control for some of the variation within the menstrual cycle by collecting our samples at the tenth or twentieth day of the cycle. These times were selected to obtain a more representative concentration of estrogen. Once the methods of collection and chemical analysis are determined, the question of information potential must be considered. As you know, Bulbrook found from an early study that 17-ketosteroids and 17-hydroxycorticosteroids appeared to provide more information than did other steroids.

I really do not think that Bulbrook feels even today that estrogens are not important. However, the situation in his laboratory at the time of his initial studies was such that from many points of view he felt that he could not do estrogens. In addition, he obtained such nice results with his current discriminant function that he probably decided not to pursue other measures of endocrine activity.

We were more interested in describing a relatively complete urinary steroid pattern in different disease states.

DR. THOMAS L. DAO (*Roswell Park Memorial Institute, Buffalo, N.Y.*): Dr. Weiner, I'm indeed very interested in your work. We have been doing similar studies for years, but have not come near the conclusion you have presented.

The first comment I should like to make is that perhaps, in your small series, judging from your survival data, most of your patients have relatively advanced disease. I wonder whether comparing this type of patient with the normal is entirely justified. Now, we all know that there are many pitfalls in determining steroids, especially the urinary steroid hormones.

I do have one question to ask you. It strikes me quite strongly that in one of your slides it showed that the measurements in normal man by estriol and the andosterone showed a negative discriminant. Would you comment: Where do you find estriol as the source of estrogen in this patient?

DR. WEINER: Let me get to your first point first.

Suffice to say that we intensively sought cases of early cancer. I agree with your feelings that we were not totally successful in doing so, having looked at the survival data about five to eight years later. However, our clinicians, that is, the cancer specialists at our hospital, made an intensive effort to find early cancer.

As you know, the sources of estrogen in males are the adrenals and the testes. The lowered concentration of estriol in the normal and the elevated concentration in cancer is one of the interesting findings associated with our work. The mechanism leading to decreased androsterone and increased estriol is unknown at this time.

NEUROENDOCRINE FACTORS IN EXPERIMENTAL CARCINOGENESIS*

Elizabeth Stern, Max R. Mickey, and Roger A. Gorski

School of Public Health and School of Medicine
University of California
Los Angeles, Calif.

About 150 years ago, Rigoni Stern, working in Italy, reported a disparity in mortality rates for uterine and breast cancer according to marital status. This difference is evident at the present time and suggests that the interplay of psychological and physiological factors that are determinants of marital status may also be related to the localization of cancer in target organs such as the breast and cervix. The same author stated that, among married women, cancer of the uterus is more common in sensitive, frustrated women.[1] In a more recent epidemiological study of cancer of the cervix, Stern and co-workers[2] found an association between a behavioral pattern–expressed in married women as early age at marriage and multiple marital events–and a hormonal factor, in patients with cancer of the uterine cervix.

Leads derived from our studies on human populations have given direction to the experimental work on the association of hormonal factors and tumorigenesis. The emphasis is largely on the hormonal facet, which we suppose, is intermediate in relation to psychological and physiological aspects of cancer. Our experiments have been concerned, in principle, with relating tumor response to endocrine state.

The relevance of endocrine environment to the development of tumors in endocrine and target organs has been established by many investigators. Pertinent examples will be given and followed by observations from our experimental work suggesting that the nervous system may be implicated in setting up and maintaining the hormonal imbalance.

In studies on the relationship of hormonal imbalance to tumorigenesis, we used a chemical carcinogen to accelerate tumor induction and observed endocrine effects associated with the administration of carcinogen.

One modification of hormonal state utilized in our experiments was that of androgen-sterility. The constant estrus feature of the hormonal state provides a convenient baseline for observing effects of treatment. A short-term effect of exogenous carcinogen was interruption of the constant vaginal estrus, a response that may be mediated by the hypothalamus. This response was found to be related to the later development of tumors, and by implication, suggests that the neural effect of the carcinogen is a significant factor in tumorigenesis.

Finally, we shall present some preliminary observations with carcinogen implants in the hypothalamus.

Tumors of endocrine and target organs have been produced by a disturbance in the internal hormonal environment brought about by surgical manipulation of endocrine organs. For example, Muhlbock and Boot induced mammary carcinoma by means of pituitary isografts in mice free of the milk factor and confirmed their hypothesis that excessive hormonal stimulation will lead to mammary-gland carcinogenesis.[3] Johnson and Witschii, using a parabiotic system, induced

* Supported in part by a research grant from NIH-CHHD.

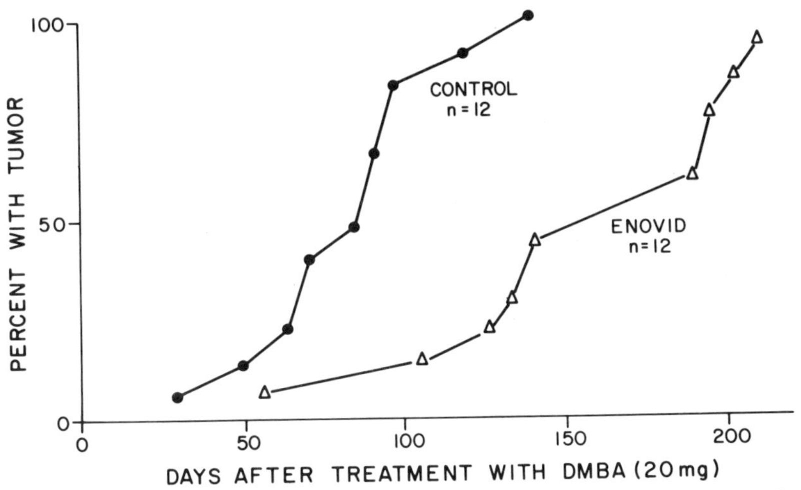

FIGURE 1. Delay in appearance of mammary cancer in rats given Enovid E cyclically.

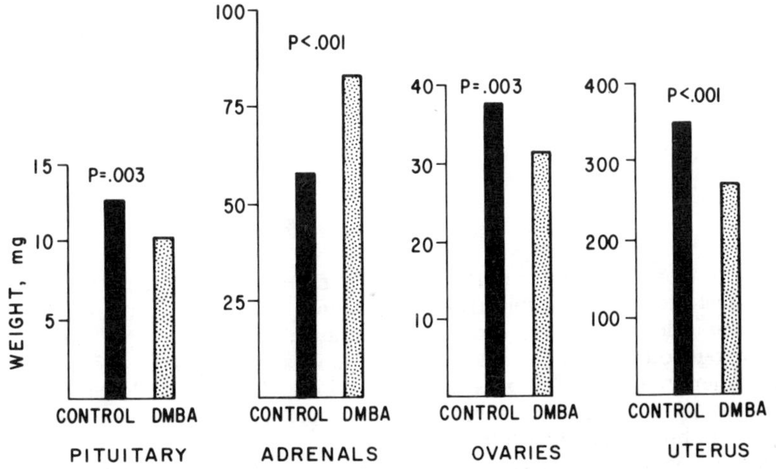

FIGURE 2. Short-term effects of DMBA in androgen-sterile rats necropsied three days after treatment (20 mg DMBA at age 50 days). Sample size: control, n = 21; DMBA, n = 22.

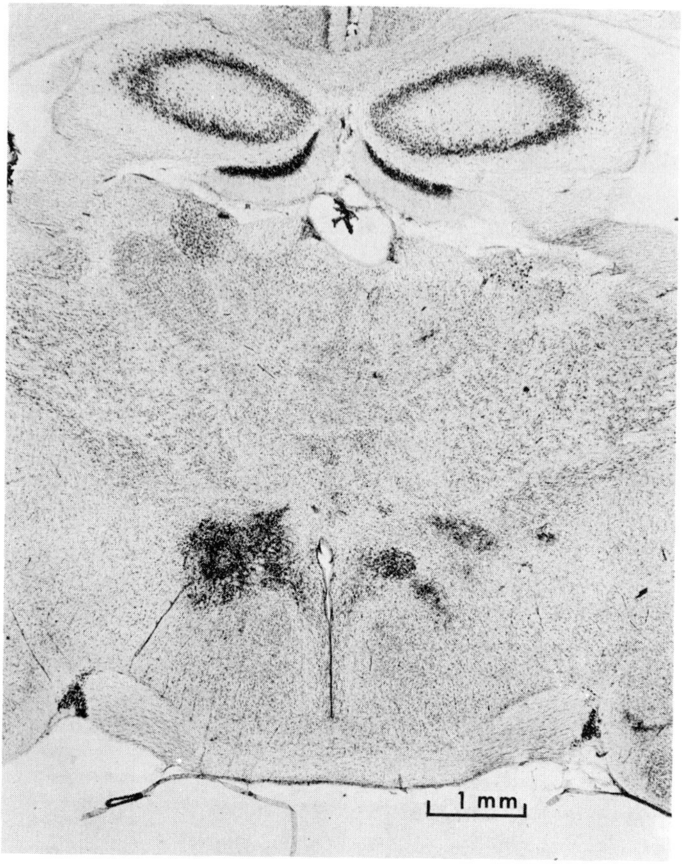

FIGURE 3. Hypothalamus. DMBA implants in the region of the VMN. No. 61 (7) cycling rat; thionine stain. (Mag. × 13.)

ovarian granulosa cell tumors in the nonovulating reactor under constant stimulation by "castrate" gonadotropin from the pituitary of its parabiont and attributed the tumor development to the gonadotropin imbalance.[4]

That exogenous hormones are carcinogenic was first demonstrated by Lacassagne,[5] when mammary tumors developed in male mice following estrogen administration. Uterine tumors have been induced in rabbits by estrogen treatment[6] and in mice treated with testosterone.[7]

About 40 years ago, it was discovered that chemical compounds produced skin tumors at the site of application.[8] When Shay and co-workers administered the chemical carcinogen 3-methylcholanthrene to Wistar rats intragastrically, they were disappointed when stomach cancer failed to develop. However, there was a high incidence of mammary tumors after 6–15 months of treatment.[9] The carcinogen apparently was effective in inducing tumors at a site distant from its point of introduction.

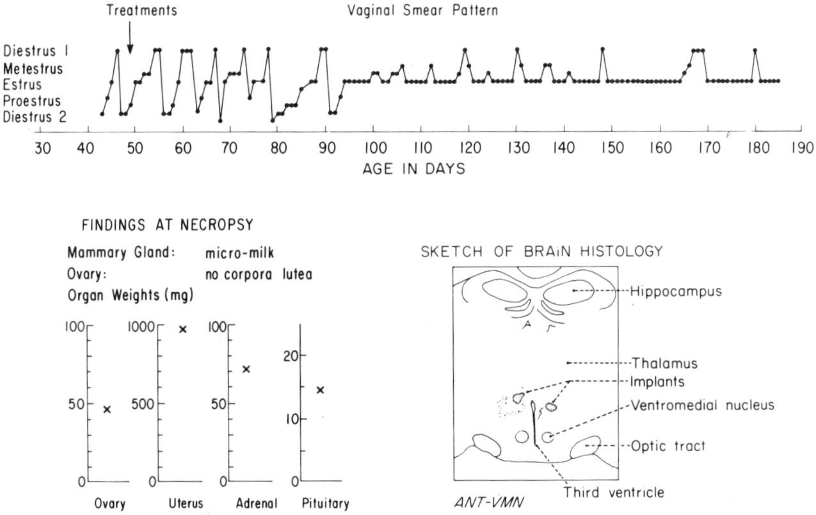

FIGURE 4. Composite: cycling rat, same as in FIGURE 3. In the vaginal-smear record, normal cycling is replaced, after age 95 days, by persistent estrus with occasional episodes of diestrus. Endocrine and target-organ data include milk secretion and an absence of corpora lutea. Brain drawing localizes DMBA implants in VMN in relation to regional structures. Rats also received DMBA intragastrically.

The necessity for long-term administration of chemical carcinogens in the induction of mammary tumors was modified when Huggins demonstrated that a single dose of the carcinogen 7,12-dimethylbenz(α)anthracene (DMBA), given at an optimal age to normally cycling Sprague-Dawley rats invariably resulted in the development of mammary-gland tumors within 60 days, and that there was a dose-response relationship.[10] The use of this model simplified study of the effect of hormones on tumor development. Experiments referred to in the following have used this experimental model for the induction of tumors by chemical carcinogens.

Huggins administered hormones for 30 days, beginning 15 days after the carcinogen administration, and reported profound effects on the latent period of mammary tumors.[11] Progesterone accelerated mammary-tumor development, estrogen retarded the tumors, and a combination of progesterone and estrogen delayed the onset of tumors and reduced their incidence. Hormonal administration during the induction period of the tumors had a marked influence on the course of their development.

That the hormonal environment at the time of carcinogen treatment is related to tumor development is illustrated by the following experiment. McCarthy pretreated normally cycling rats with the progestin-estrogen antifertility compound Enovid® for ten days, and then gave the carcinogen.[12] He found there was an increased incidence of mammary-gland tumors in animals treated with 0.25 mg Enovid daily and no effect on incidence at the 1 mg level. The effectiveness of a comparatively low dose of Enovid is an indication that tumor outcome is sensitive to subtle changes in hormonal environment.

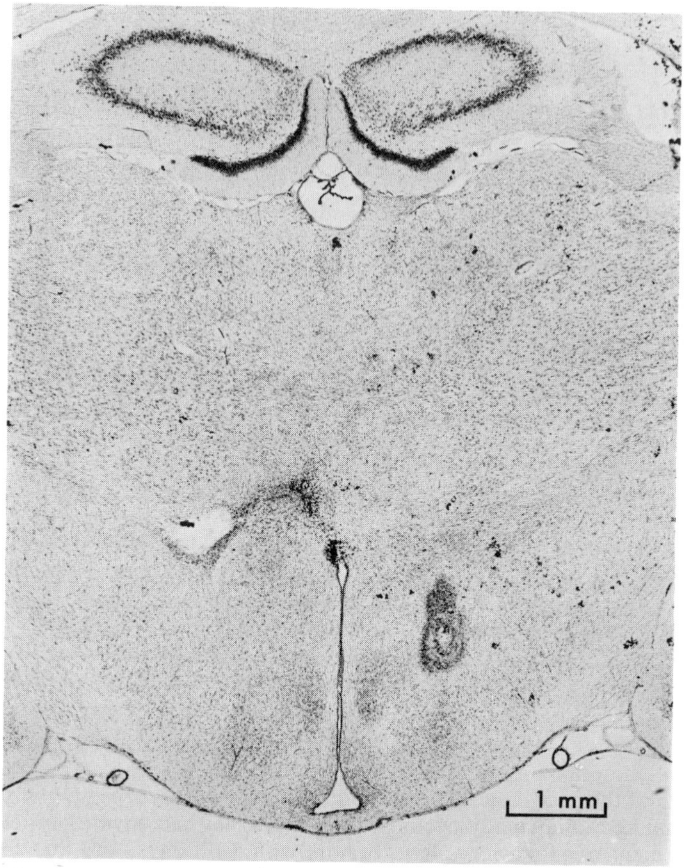

FIGURE 5. Hypothalamus. DMBA implants in the region of the VMN. No. 70 (9) androgen-sterilized rat; thionine stain. (Mag. × 13.)

Effect of a Cyclic Regimen of an Antifertility Compound on Induced Mammary Gland Tumors

We found that long-term experimental administration of Enovid E* retards the development of induced mammary-gland tumors in rats. We used a cyclic regimen of Enovid administration simulating the treatment schedule in women, beginning soon after puberty at approximately 45 days of age, and continuing for the duration of the experiment. Animals were necropsied at 100, 200, and 365 days of age. The carcinogen was given ten days after the Enovid treatment was begun. The effect on latency of induced mammary tumors was somewhat similar to that of Huggins[11] when he used the progesterone-estradiol-17β combination, except that all of our animals eventually developed tumors (FIGURE 1).

In our experiment, the delay in onset of induced mammary-gland tumors may

* Norethinodrel (17α-ethynyl-17-hydroxy-5(10)-estren-3-one) 2.5 parts:Mestranol (ethynyl-estradiol 3-methyl ether) 0.1 parts. Enovid E was generously supplied by G. D. Searle & Co.

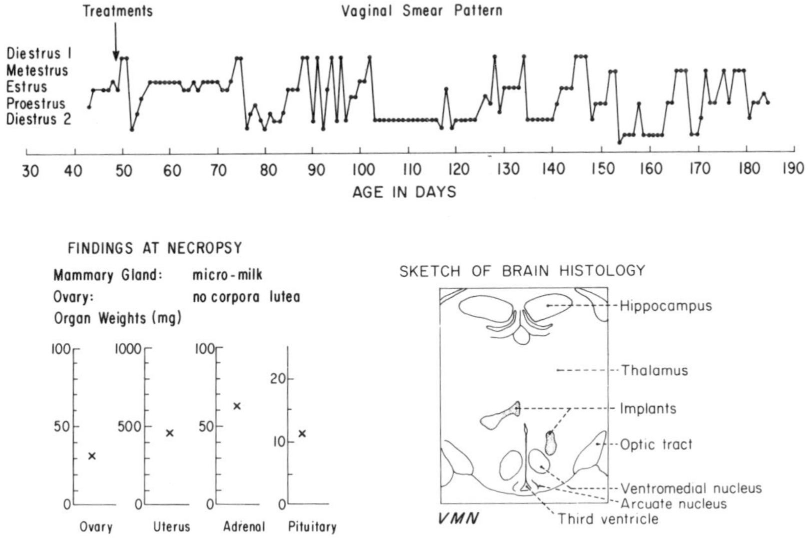

FIGURE 6. Composite: Androgen-sterilized rat, same as in FIGURE 5. In the vaginal-smear record, note the vaginal diestrus response the day after DMBA treatment, the return to constant estrus, and intermitten cycling after age 70 days. There is milk secretion, and an absence of corpora lutea. Brain drawing localizes DMBA implants in VMN in relation to regional structures. Rat also received DMBA intragastrically.

be related to the finding that Enovid-treated animals necropsied at age 100 days showed significant changes in endocrine and target organs. The delayed development of induced mammary-gland tumors, conversely, may be related to the finding that by age 200 days, those changes were no longer evident.

For example, the significant differences between Enovid and non-Enovid treated rats in ovary, uterus, and preputial gland weights at the age—100-days necropsy were not observed in comparable groups necropsied at age 200 days.[13]

The difference in hormonal environment of the Enovid-treated rats 45 days after the carcinogen administration, at a time when induced tumors are developing in non-Enovid animals, may be related to their latency in developing tumors.

Effect of Androgen-Sterility on Induced Tumors

The effect on induced tumors of altering the hormonal environment at a much earlier stage in the animal's development is illustrated by a series of experiments using androgen-sterile rats, in which a persistent, defined, endocrine alteration was possible without complicated surgical intervention. Female S.D. rats, prepared according to the method of Barraclough and Gorski,[14,15] are given a single dose of testosterone postnatally, before hypothalamic maturation is completed, and are sterile as adults.

The hormonal imbalance is characterized by tonic release of gonadotropic hormone, but the rhythmic surge of ovulating hormone is abolished and the animal fails to ovulate. In the ovaries, graafian follicles develop and grow, but corpora lutea are absent. There is constant vaginal estrus.[15] The mammary glands show patchy lobuloalveolar differentiation and milk secretion, changes suggestive of modification of hypothalamic factors normally inhibiting prolactin release by the pituitary.[16]

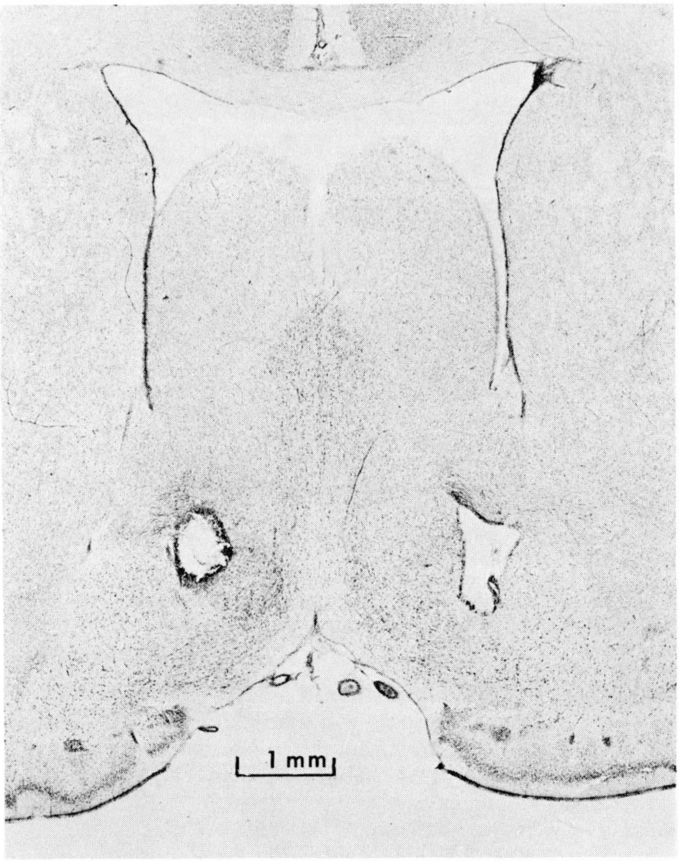

FIGURE 7. Hypothalamus. Localization of DMBA implant sites in the region of the preoptic area. No. 48 (3) androgen-sterilized rat; thionine stain. (Mag. × 13.)

We found a significant drop in the incidence of carcinogen-induced mammary-gland tumors in androgen-sterile rats. The hormonal disturbance provides an internal environment in which the induction of mammary carcinoma is inhibited while the development of ovarian granulosa cell tumors is favored.[17]

A hormonal state comparable to that of the androgen-sterile rat is obtained by administration of steroid antifertility compounds. As in androgen-sterility, the antifertility effect is due to suppression of ovulation by means of a primary action on the hypothalamus.[14,18] In both cases there is inhibition of carcinogen-induced mammary tumors.

In the Enovid experiment, animals were observed over a period of one year and the inhibition is manifest as increased latency, while in the case of the androgen-sterile experiment, terminated at age 150 days, inhibition is indicated by decreased incidence.

Endocrine Effects of Chemical Carcinogen

Endocrine effects are also associated with the administration of carcinogen. Some short-term effects are of special interest.[17] FIGURE 2 shows a decrease in

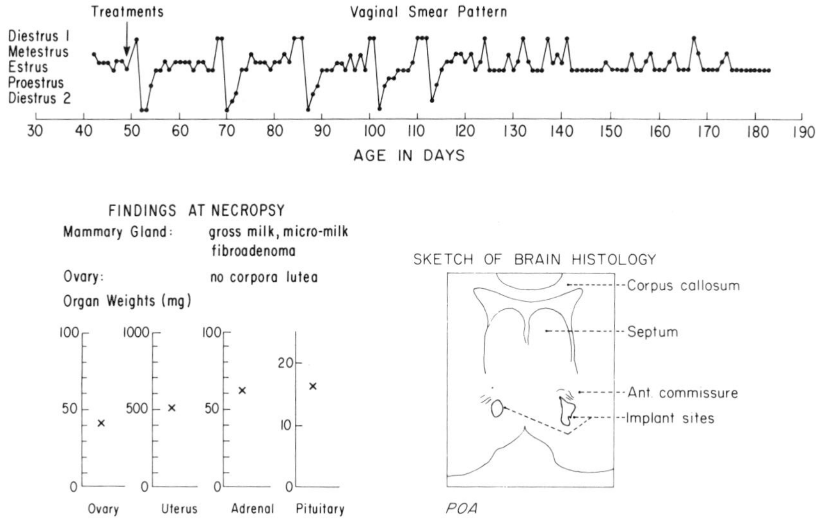

FIGURE 8. Composite: Androgen-sterilized rat, same as in FIGURE 7. DMBA in POA, solvent intragastrically. In the vaginal-smear record, note the vaginal diestrus response two days after DMBA treatment, the return to constant estrus, and the sporadic cycling after age 70 days. There is milk secretion and an absence of corpora lutea. Brain drawing localizes DMBA implant sites to the region of the POA in relation to the anterior commissure.

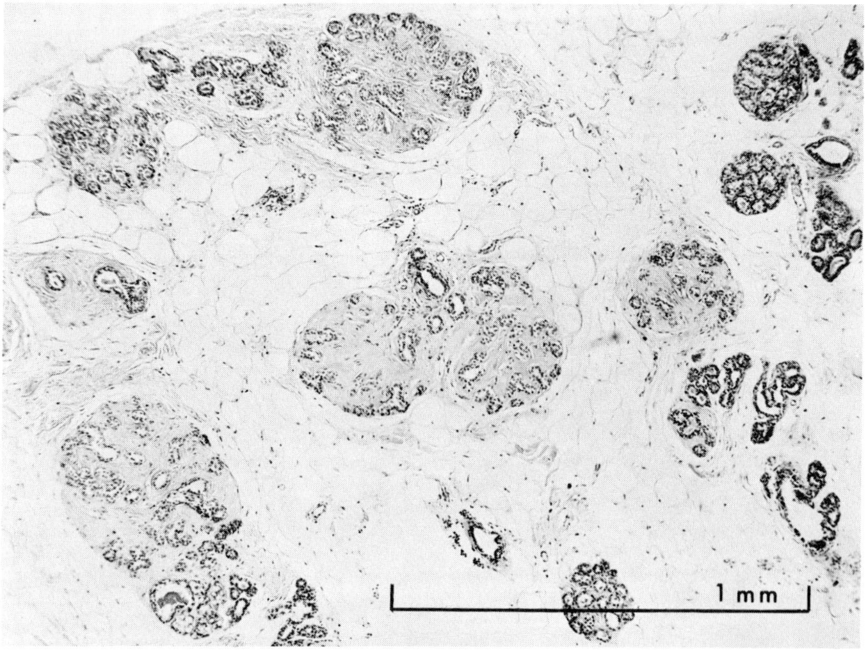

FIGURE 9. Androgen-sterilized rat, same as in FIGURES 7 and 8. Mammary gland. Developing mammary gland tumor of the fibroadenoma type. H. & E. stain. (Mag. × 13.)

pituitary, ovary, and uterus weights in androgen-sterile animals three days after DMBA. Similar effects are found in normally cycling animals. The increase in adrenal weight is attributed to hemorrhagic necrosis of the adrenal cortex, which is the result of a local action of DMBA on the adrenal.[19] It seems likely that the changes in pituitary, ovary, and uterine weights may not be isolated events, but may be interrelated and indicative of a rapid alteration in endocrine state that is additional to whatever direct effect the carcinogen may have on the cells of mammary glands.

Endocrine effects of carcinogen are more readily detected in the androgen-sterile rat because of the essentially tonic hormonal state. Further, endocrine changes that involve a vaginal response can be monitored by daily vaginal smears.

In androgen-sterile animals, a response to the carcinogen was observed in vaginal smears within 48 hours.[16] There is an arrest of keratinization, and neutrophiles appear, in sharp contrast to the constant estrus pattern characteristically present in these animals.

Most of the animals that later developed tumors had a diestrus response. Most of the rats that remained free of tumors did not have the response. The association

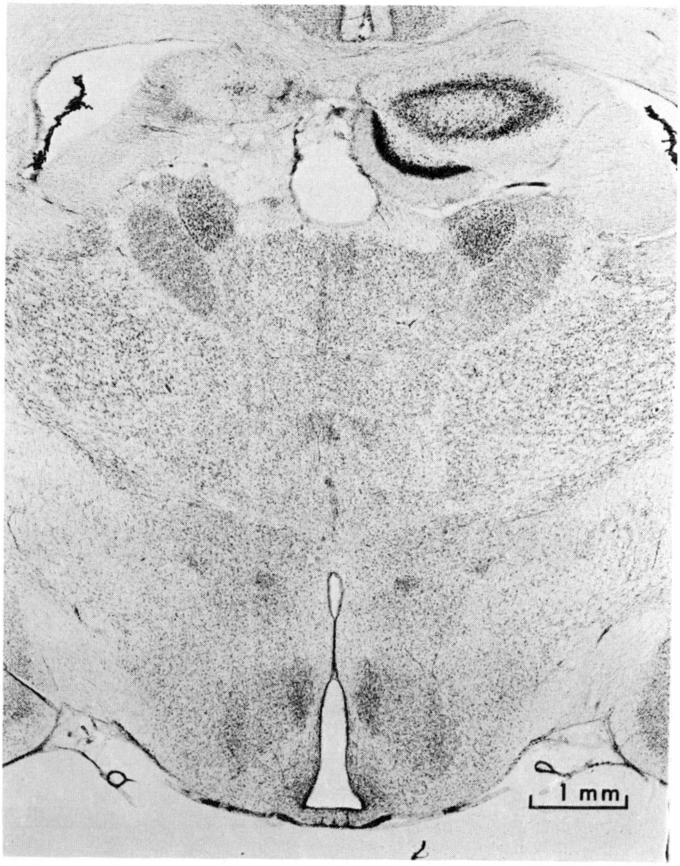

FIGURE 10. Hypothalamus. Sham procedure to VMN. There is no evidence of residual brain damage. No. 82 (4) androgen-sterilized rat; thionine stain. (Mag. × 13.)

does not merely represent a response to the carcinogen, but is related to tumor outcome.[20] Thus, an immediate endocrine effect of the carcinogen–interruption of the constant vaginal estrus–correlated with the later development of tumors.

The correlation is an indication that the tumor fate of the rat may be pretty much settled by the state of the animal at the time of treatment with DMBA and shortly thereafter. This would be consistent, for example, with McCarthy's results, that tumor incidence was increased following pretreatment with small amounts of Enovid.

Perhaps of greater importance to us has been the view that all of the observed endocrine effects could possibly be accounted for by supposing that a predominant effect of the DMBA was a central nervous system reaction, involving the hypothalamic-pituitary axis.

The vaginal response to DMBA resembles the vaginal response to progesterone in persistent estrus rats[21] and in androgen-sterile rats.[22] Barraclough has proposed that the progesterone lowers thresholds of excitability within the hypothalamus of sterile rats.[23] By analogy, the carcinogen, DMBA, may affect the hypothalamus. If this were the case, there would be important implications for the psychophysiological point of view of tumorigenesis.

In order to test this idea, we have implanted the carcinogen in the brain. Some preliminary observations are of interest.

Effect of Intrahypothalamic Carcinogen

The carcinogen DMBA was implanted in crystalline form bilaterally in the hypothalamus in the anterior preoptic area (POA) or in the region of the ventromedial nucleus (VMN). The technique of implantation consisted of extrusion of the crystalline DMBA from a 21-gauge needle, which was then removed. The amount of DMBA implanted, 1.5 mg on each side, was considered to be the maximum quantity that could be placed. The areas were chosen because of their importance in gonadotropin regulation.

We used two main experimental groups, normally cycling and androgen-sterilized rats. Animals in each group received bilateral brain implants or were subjected to bilateral sham procedures, and either supplemental intragastric DMBA at the minimal effective dose level of 1 mg in sesame oil or the vehicle only were given. For each animal, brain and intragastric procedures were carried out on the same day at approximately 50 days of age. A small number of normally cycling rats and of androgen-sterilized rats were given no brain manipulation, but ingested the 1-mg threshold dose of DMBA. The experiment was terminated when the animals were six months old.

For each animal, we prepared a composite showing the lifetime record of daily vaginal smears, necropsy findings on organ weights, presence or absence of corpora lutea in the ovaries, degree of mammary-gland differentiation, and a drawing of the brain histology that identified the sites of DMBA implantation. Photomicrographs were also prepared from the histologic sections of the brain to indicate the topography and the relative amount of space occupied by the implants.

Endocrine effects of the brain manipulation were noted in both cycling and androgen-sterilized animals. There was no apparent difference in endocrine effect whether the site of the implant was POA or VMN.

In four of ten cycling animals an effect of the carcinogen was to induce sterility. Approximately one month after brain implantation or sham surgery, vaginal cycling was replaced by a pattern of persistent vaginal estrus. At necropsy, at age six months, there was a decrease in ovary weight and absence of corpora lutea,

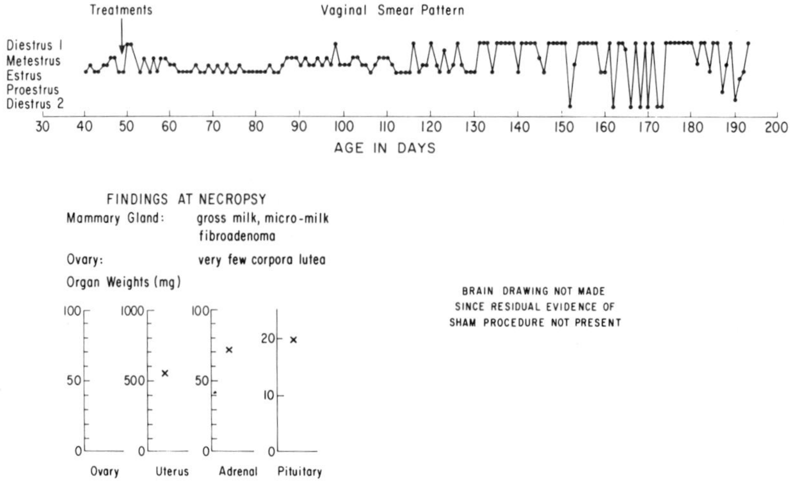

FIGURE 11. Composite: Androgen-sterilized rat, same as in FIGURE 10. In the vaginal-smear record, note the vaginal diestrus response the day after sham brain surgery—intragastric DMBA, the return to persistent estrus, and periodic diestrus episodes after age 100 days. There is milk secretion, and a few corpora lutea are present in the ovary. Brain drawing was omitted, since there was no histologic evidence of the sham procedure.

but antrum-containing follicles were present and interstitial tissue was prominent. In previous experiments, intragastric DMBA alone did not induce sterility.

An example of the effect of brain manipulation in a cycling animal is given in FIGURES 3 and 4. The DMBA implants are shown in the microphotograph (FIGURE 3). In the composite of the same animal (FIGURE 4), the vaginal-smear record shows that cycling was replaced at about age 95 days by persistent estrus with occasional episodes of diestrus. The drawing of the relevant brain section localizes the implants in the region of the ventromedial nucleus. Endocrine and target-organ effects are shown at the lower left.

In 13 of 18 androgen-sterilized animals, the carcinogen induced vaginal cycling. An immediate effect was interruption of the constant estrus pattern—a response similar to that reported in an earlier experiment when 20 mg DMBA was given intragastrically.[20] There were ensuing episodes of diestrus and intermittent cycles. At necropsy at age six months, while in most animals with induced vaginal cycles ovarian histology was consistent with that of the androgenized rat, some ovaries showed one or more recent corpora lutea that might be related to a prenecropsy episode of vaginal cycling.

An example of the effect of brain carcinogen in an androgen-sterilized animal is shown in FIGURES 5 and 6. In the photomicrograph (FIGURE 5), the DMBA implants are noted in the region of the VMN. In the composite (FIGURE 6), the animal is in estrus both before and on the day of the implant, and there is a diestrus response the following day. After the cycle is completed there is a return to constant estrus, which is later interspersed with episodes of diestrus and a pattern of irregular vaginal cycles. The drawing of the brain shows the implant sites in the region of the VMN.

It is of interest to note that two of the four cycling animals with induced sterility and five of the 13 sterile animals with induced cycling were subjected to the sham brain procedure, but given intragastric DMBA.

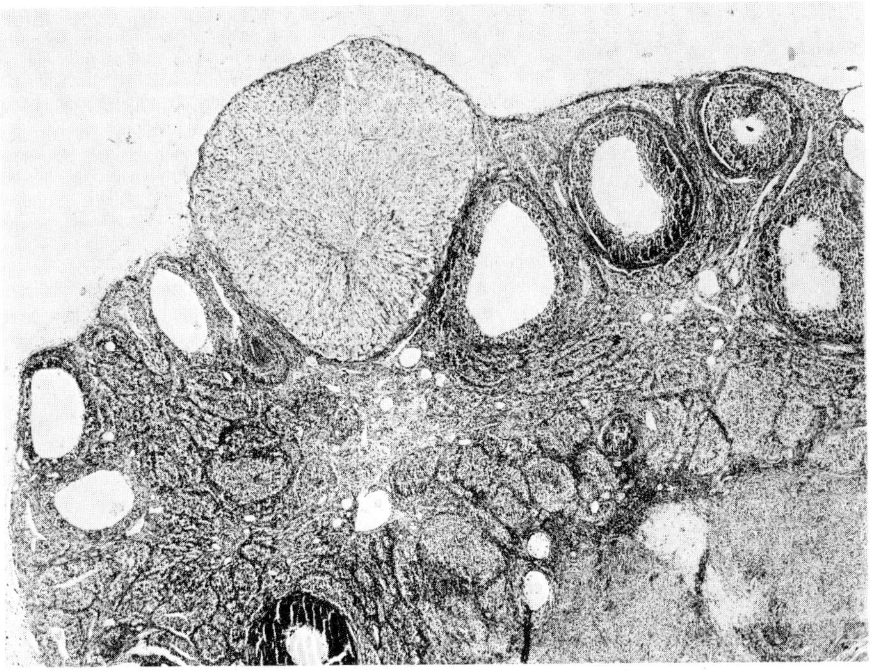

FIGURE 12. Androgen-sterilized rat, same as in FIGURES 10 & 11. Ovary. The corpus luteum can be related to the prenecropsy vaginal cycle charted in FIGURE 11. H. & E. stain. (Mag. × 30.)

Endocrine effects of the sham brain procedure and the intragastric threshold dose of DMBA are comparable to those in animals that received the brain implants of DMBA. This is surprising, in view of the fact that it is well known that the sham procedure does not result in altered endocrine status in cycling animals nor in the constant estrus status of sterile animals. There may be an interrelationship between the intragastric DMBA and the sham procedure. One possible explanation is that the systemic carcinogen might localize in the sham-operated areas of the hypothalamus. The passage of the needle through the brain during the sham surgery may facilitate the transfer of DMBA across the blood-brain barrier.[24] The effects are not observed in animals in which the threshold dose of intragastric carcinogen was given but in which there was no brain procedure.

Although there was a low incidence of mammary-gland tumors in this study, the possible significance of the effect of carcinogen on the brain warrants presentation of individual cases in this preliminary report.

Mammary tumors developed in five carcinogen-treated, brain-manipulated animals. These were found in four of the 18 androgen-sterilized animals and in one of 10 cycling animals. The tumors were small, and were detected only on microscopic examination of mammary glands removed at necropsy.

One tumor-bearing animal (FIGURES 7–9) had received only the brain DMBA. The photomicrograph (FIGURE 7) shows the restricted localization of the bilaterally symmetrical implant sites in the region of the preoptic area into which the DMBA had been implanted four months earlier.

The drawing of the hypothalamus in FIGURE 8 identifies neighboring structures.

The vaginal smear pattern of this androgen-sterilized rat shows the diestrus response and intermittent episodes of vaginal cycling. The small mammary-gland tumor is shown in FIGURE 9.

Although implantation of carcinogen occasionally produced physical lesions of the brain, such lesions were not correlated with the effects of DMBA. For example, FIGURE 7 represents an effective implant of carcinogen with no evidence of a lesion. In addition, animals subjected to sham surgery, in which no lesions were produced (FIGURE 10), displayed changes in endocrine function.

Another tumor-bearing animal (FIGURES 10–13) had been given the sham operation in the region of the VMN and the threshold dose of intragastric carcinogen. The intact brain of this animal is shown in the photomicrograph (FIGURE 10). The composite (FIGURE 11) shows the diestrus response and subsequent cycling in the androgen-sterilized animal. The photomicrograph of the ovary (FIGURE 12) shows a corpus luteum that may be related to the episode of prenecropsy cycling. The mammary-gland tumor is shown in FIGURE 13. It is possible that the threshold dose of intragastric DMBA was facilitated in some manner by the sham surgery in the brain. In androgenized animals without brain manipulation, there was no response to this threshold intragastric DMBA.

Our preliminary observations are consistent with an endocrine effect of carcinogen when implanted in the brain. These effects are related to reproductive physiology. Systemic carcinogen, in addition to direct effects on target tissues, by traversing the blood-brain barrier, may have effects that are mediated by the

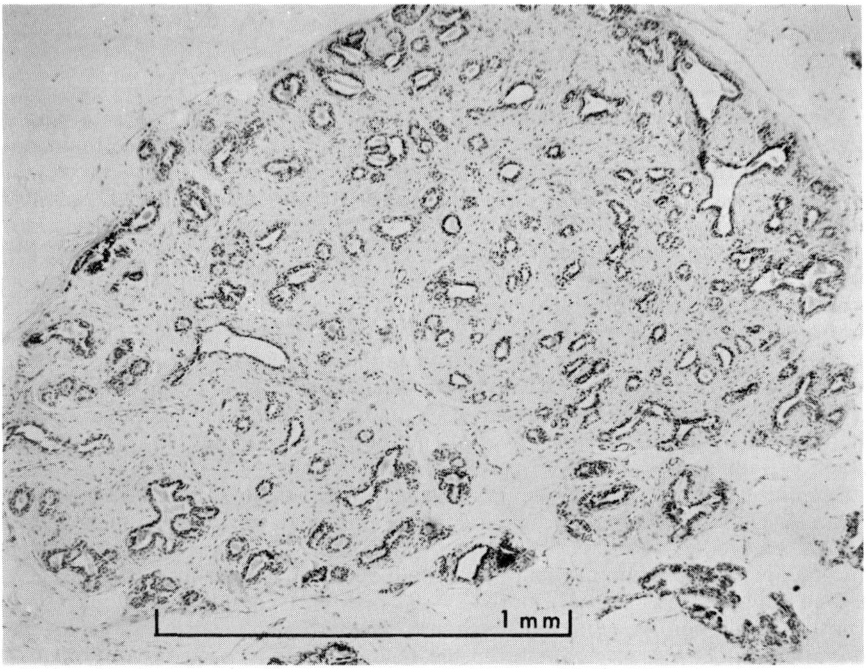

FIGURE 13. Androgen-sterilized rat, same as in FIGURES 10–12. Fibroadenoma, mammary gland. H. & E. stain. (Mag. × 55.)

hypothalamus. Our preliminary observations on the relation between neuroendocrine processes and the induction of tumors are encouraging, and we have taken this opportunity to present individual examples because of their possible significance.

References

1. STERN, R. 1844. Nota sulle richerche de dottor Tanchou intonno la frequenza de cancro. Ann. Univ. Med. Chir. (Milan) **110:** 484–503.
2. STERN, E., P. LACHENBRUCH & W. J. DIXON. 1967. Cancer of the uterine cervix. II: A biometric approach to etiology. Cancer **20:** 190–201.
3. MUHLBOCK, O. & L. M. BOOT. 1959. Induction of mammary cancer in mice without the mammary tumor agent by isografts of hypophyses. Cancer Research **19:** 402–412.
4. JOHNSON, D. C. & E. WITSCHI. 1961. Endocrinology of ovarian tumor formation in parabiotic rats. Cancer Res. **21:** 783.
5. LACASSAGNE, A. 1932. Apparition de cancers de la mamelle chez le souris male, soumise a des injections de folliculine. C. R. Acad. Sci. (Paris) **195:** 630–632.
6. MEISSNER, W. A., S. C. SOMMERS & G. SHERMAN. 1957. Endometrial hyperplasia, endometrial carcinoma, and endometriosis produced experimentally by estrogen. Cancer **10:** 500–509.
7. VAN NIE, R., E. L. BENEDETTI & O. MUHLBOCK. 1961. A carcinogenic action of testosterone provoking uterine tumors in mice. Nature **4809:** 1303.
8. COOK, J. W., I. HIEGER, E. KENNAWAY & W. V. MAYNEORD. 1932. The production of cancer by pure hydrocarbons. Proc. Roy. Soc. (London) Series B. **III:** 455–496.
9. SHAY, H., E. A. AEGERTER, M. GRUENSTEIN & S. KOMAROV. 1949. Development of adenocarcinoma of the breast in the Wistar rat following the gastric instillation of methylcholanthrene. J. Nat. Cancer Inst. **10:** 255–266.
10. HUGGINS, CHARLES, L. C. GRAND & F. P. BRILLANTES. 1961. Mammary cancer induced by a single feeding of polynuclear hydrocarbons, and its suppression. Nature **189:** 204–207.
11. HUGGINS, CHARLES, R. C. MOON & S. MORII. 1962. Extinction of experimental mammary cancer. I. Estradiol-17β and progesterone. Proc. Nat. Acad. Sci. (USA) **48:** 379–386.
12. MCCARTHY, JACK. 1965. Influence of two contraceptives on induction of mammary cancer in rats. Amer. J. Surg. **110:** 720–723.
13. STERN, E. & M. R. MICKEY. 1969. The effect of a cyclic steroid contraceptive regimen on induced mammary gland tumors in rats. Brit. J. Cancer **23:** 391.
14. BARRACLOUGH, C. A. 1961. Production of anovulatory sterile rats by single injections of testosterone propionate. Endocrinology **68:** 62.
15. BARRACLOUGH, C. A. & R. A. GORSKI. 1961. Evidence that the hypothalamus is responsible for androgen induced sterility in the female rat. Endocrinology **68:** 68.
16. STERN, E., M. R. MICKEY & L. OSVALDO. 1965. Lactogenesis in the androgen sterile rat: augmentation following 7,12-dimethylbenz(α)anthracene. Nature **206:** 369–371.
17. STERN, E., M. R. MICKEY & L. OSVALDO. 1967. Tumorigenesis in the androgen sterile rat: reciprocal incidence of carcinogen induced mammary gland and ovarian tumors. First International Symposium on Biorhythms in Clinical and Experimental Endocrinology (Italy). Rass. Neurol. Veg. **21:** 1–2.
18. MINAGUCHI, H. & J. MEITES. 1967. Effects of norethynodrel-mestranol combination (Enovid) on hypothalamic and pituitary hormones in rats. Endocrinology **81:** 826.
19. HUGGINS, CHARLES & S. MORII. 1961. Selective adrenal necrosis and apoplexy induced by 7-12-dimethylbenz(α)anthracene. J. Exp. Med. **114:** 741–760.
20. STERN, E. & M. R. MICKEY. 1967. Neural mechanism in induction of dioestrus and tumour in the androgen sterile rat. Nature **216:** 185–187.
21. EVERETT, J. W. 1940. The restoration of ovulatory cycles and corpus luteum formation in persistent estrus rats by progesterone. Endocrinology **27:** 681.
22. GORSKI, R. A. & C. A. BARRACLOUGH. 1963. Effects of low dosages of androgen on the differentiation of hypothalamic regulatory control of ovulation in the rat. Endocrinology **73:** 210.
23. BARRACLOUGH, C. A. 1966. Second International Congress on Hormonal Steroids (Milan) abstract. Excerpta Medica **111:** 85.
24. DANIEL, P. M., O. E. PRATT & M. PRICHARD. 1967. Metabolism of labelled carcinogenic hydrocarbons in rats. Nature **215:** 1142–1146.

DISCUSSION OF THE PAPER

DR. BENNETTE: I do not feel competent to comment on this excellent paper, but I just want to make an observation with which Dr. Stern may not be familiar, because I think it has not yet been published.

In Edinburgh, Dr. Hamilton has been doing some very interesting work on pinealectomy and on the exposure of rats to continuous light and the administration of melatonine, and finds substantial numbers of mammary tumors arising in various combinations of these treatments. I wondered whether there were any observations of your work that implicated pineal pathways in the induction of mammary tumors.

DR. STERN: I do not know much about pineal physiology, but if there are any specialists in that field in the audience, they might correct me. I am under the impression that there is a relationship between the activity of the pineal gland and the reproductive function of the hypothalamus.

DR. DAO: The question I really want to ask you is related to your mentioning that these hydrocarbons commonly do concentrate in these areas. Have you actually determined the concentration of the hydrocarbon that you administered systematically?

DR. STERN: Determined it how?

DR. DAO: The concentration of the hydrocarbon in these areas.

DR. STERN: In the brain?

DR. DAO: Yes.

DR. STERN: No, we have not made any such determination yet. We intend to do this.

DR. DAO: Another question that I would like to ask you is: Did you notice any lactation in these animals? I mean extensive lactation in the lesioned rats.

DR. STERN: We did not lesion these rats, and this is a complicated question, because our androgen-sterile rats develop lactation without any brain treatment. We have a slight indication that what happens in androgen-sterile rats, with the type of brain manipulation which we have done, is that lactation is inhibited. In the cycling animal, we do not have clear-cut indications yet as to what is happening with respect to lactation.

DR. DAO: I should like to point out that these, perhaps, are different mechanisms involved, because if you do put lesions in the hypothalamus, you produce enormous lactation in the mammary gland of these rats.

DR. STERN: This is very true, and a lesion not only produces lactation because you are isolating the pituitary, but it produces ovarian atrophy, which we did not find in any of our animals.

PSYCHOENDOCRINE CONSIDERATIONS IN CANCER OF THE BREAST

Jack Katz, Thomas Gallagher, Leon Hellman, Edward Sachar, and Herbert Weiner

Montefiore Hospital and Medical Center
and Albert Einstein College of Medicine
Bronx, N. Y.

Introduction

On the basis of empirical steroid analysis, Bulbrook[1] and his coworkers in England have found that women with cancer of the breast fall into two groups: In one, the ratio of corticoid to androgenic steroids is relatively high, and the prognosis of the illness and the response to treatment are poor; in the other, the ratio between these steroids is lower, and the prognosis and response to treatment are better. The underlying basis for this differential prognosis remains unclear, although Bulbrook speculates that implicit in this ratio characteristic of the poor-prognosis group may be some decreased efficiency in immunologic functioning or increased vulnerability to estrogens.

It is not known why differences in this ratio occur. Genic, constitutional, and possibly perinatal factors have been postulated to account for them, and starvation or a rise in body temperature can transiently alter the ratio. Breast neoplasms themselves have not, we might add, been found to account for the elevation of the corticosteroids by virtue of any adrenocorticotropic hormone (ACTH) secretion.

However, in view of the now well-established fact that psychological events can influence corticosteroid levels, it seems legitimate to ask whether they cannot significantly affect this ratio, either acutely or in a more enduring manner.

With this question in mind, we have been studying a group of women with breast tumors by making assessments of their psychological state and then investigating possible correlations with production rates of hydrocortisone and excretion of the principle hydrocortisone and androgen metabolites and the ratio between these hormones.

Methods

Thirty-two women, 33 to 79 years of age and from lower and middle class backgrounds, were hospitalized in the Clinical Research Center of the Montefiore Hospital and Medical Center. Each woman had what was considered to be a potentially operable lesion. The patients were aware that they would be staying on the ward for approximately five to 10 days for complete diagnostic and endocrine evaluations before being transferred to a surgical ward for biopsy of the tumor. All medication, except chloral hydrate for sleep, was withheld during this period.

After at least three or four days in the Research Center, each patient received an intravenous infusion of ^{14}C-labeled hydrocortisone, and three-day pooled urines were then collected. By means of radioactivity dilution technique, daily hydrocortisone *production* rate could then be calculated from the two metabolites in the urine uniquely derived from hydrocortisone, namely, tetrahydrocortisone and tetrahydrocortisol. The daily *excretions* of the principal hydrocortisone metabolites (tetrahydrocortisone, tetrahydrocortisol, and allotetrahydrocortisol) and the principal androgen metabolites (etiocholanolone and androsterone) were also determined by means of rigorous isolation and purification techniques. The data were then calculated in terms of milligrams per gram creatinine excreted.

Psychiatric interview generally took place one-half to six hours after the infusion of the radioactive tracer. Nineteen of the 32 interviews were tape recorded and assessed by three other raters to check interrater reliability. Two patients were eliminated from the study because they were found to have disseminated metastases, and consequently the possible influence of such conceivable variables as pain, central nervous system involvement, or adrenal or pituitary metastases on corticosteroids could not be ruled out. During the study, the clinical diagnosis and all hormonal data were withheld from the raters.

The assessment of the interviews was modeled after the criteria described by Wolff and coworkers[2] in 1964 and validated by Poe, Rose, and Mason[3] in 1967. These criteria, as adapted in FIGURE 1, consisted of three psychological dimensions that presumably reflected defensive failing under threat. These were (1) affective distress, such as anxiety or despair, (2) disruption of autonomous ego and psychophysiological functions, such as impaired concentration or insomnia, and (3) impairment of defensive reserve, as reflected, for instance, in sudden subject agitation when confronted in interview with possible impending loss. The critera permitted them to predict urinary 17-OHCS levels in parents of dying leukemic children with dramatic accuracy.

We attempted, however, to further refine these criteria. Thus, we devised seven point scoring scales to allow global ratings of each patient for each of the defensive adequacy criteria. The affective scale was made bipolar to include pleasant as well as unpleasant affects. The rater's global assessments were to take

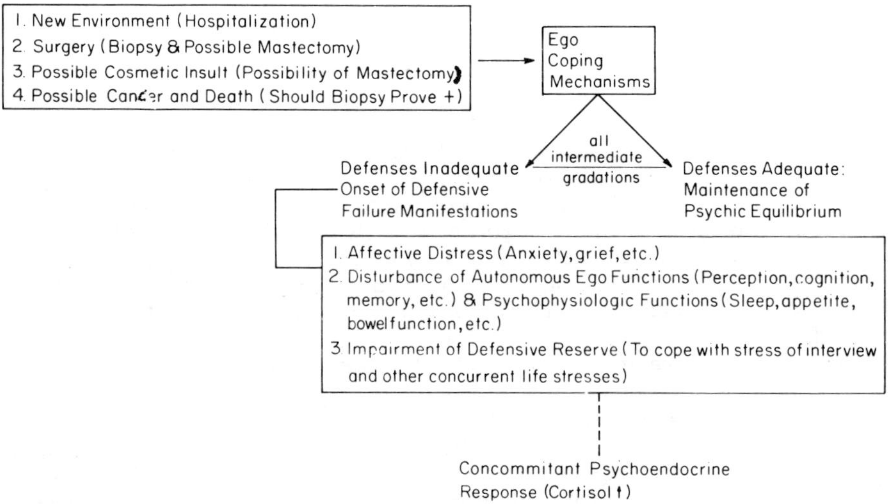

FIGURE 1. Threats faced by breast tumor patients preoperatively.

into consideration the number and intensity of the prebiopsy affects, pleasant as well as unpleasant, the extent and variety of functions disrupted, and the severity of defensive breakdown elicited by confrontations during the interview–all of these being viewed wherever possible in the framework of the patient's overall personality style. The individual category scores were then summed to give a total score. The higher this value, the greater the presumed defensive failing.

Furthermore, each rater was asked to specify which pleasant and/or unpleasant affects were noted and which functions disrupted and whether these were explicit or inferred. The raters were also asked to specify the defenses primarily employed in the acute situation and the apparent premorbid personality style. Finally, wherever discernible, each rater was to indicate which stress seemed most threatening to the patient: hospitalization, various ward procedures, biopsy and surgery, loss of the breast, cancer and death, or even the interview itself.

Results and Discussion

The following summarizes our findings:

1. Of 30 women in our series, 22 were found to have malignant lesions and eight, benign lesions.

2. Hydrocortisone production rates (FIGURE 2) were in the normal range of 9.0 to 24.5, and the total excretion rates of the principal metabolites of hydrocortisone ranged from 2.2 to 7.0. It will be seen from this illustration that many of the values cluster about the low middle part of the distribution; in fact, mean values for production and excretion were slightly less than mean values for a normal population in our laboratory.

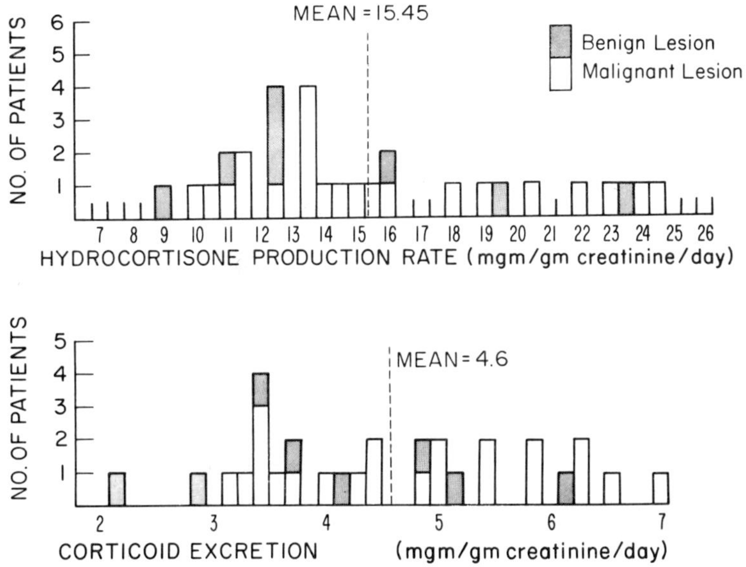

FIGURE 2. Distribution (above) of preoperative hydrocortisone production rates to the nearest .5 mg and distribution (below) and preoperative corticoid excretion.

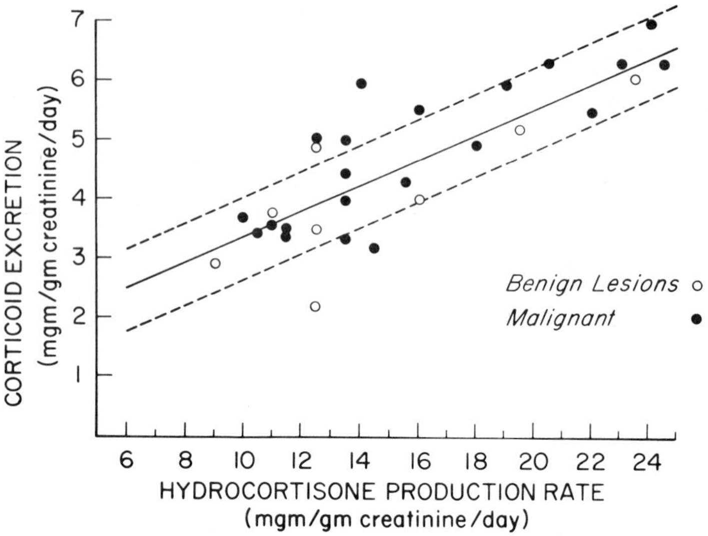

FIGURE 3. Preoperative hydrocortisone production rate versus corticoid excretion $r_{PM} = .821, p < .001$).

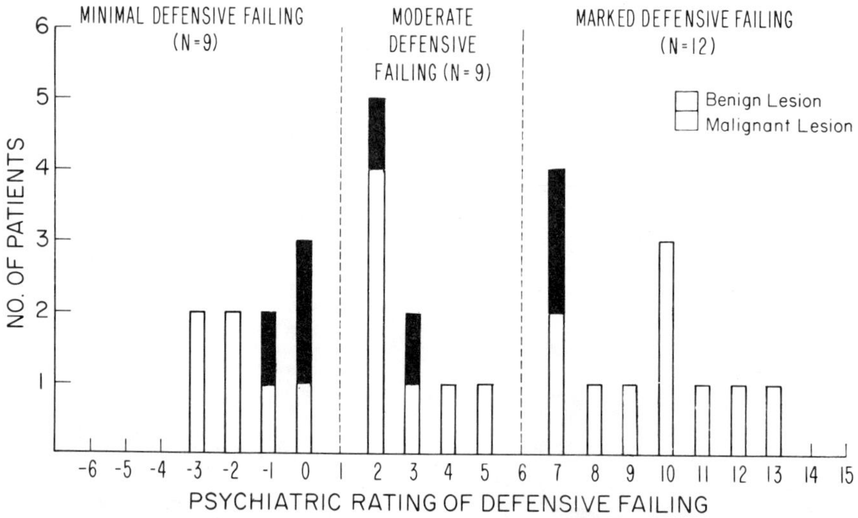

FIGURE 4. Distribution of preoperative scores for defensive failing based on sum of ratings of pleasant affect ($0 \rightarrow -6$), unpleasant affect ($0 \rightarrow +6$), functional disruption ($0 \rightarrow +6$), and impairment of defensive reserve ($0 \rightarrow +6$).

3. As seen in FIGURE 3, production rates of hydrocortisone and excretion of its principal metabolites correlated quite well, although not perfectly.

4. Total androgen metabolite excretion ranged from 0.9 to 8.0 mg per g creatinine, with an unremarkable distribution and mean value.

5. We come now to the psychological variables. Interrater reliability among the three raters and the interviewer on the 19 taped interviews was .83 (Kendall Coefficient of Concordance), which is highly significant ($p < .001$). The raters and interviewer did not differ significantly on their evaluations, and thus this report will deal with the interview assessments of the interviewer himself on all 30 patients.

6. The total defensive effectiveness score showed a distribution that was again characterized by a cluster around the lower middle part of the distribution, as shown in FIGURE 4. As a lower score presumably reflects more effective defensive coping, we take this distribution and those of the hydrocortisone production rates and metabolite excretion to indicate that many women actually do surprisingly well under this particular threat. We can only conclude, as have others, that it is not a stress situation per se that evokes psychic distress and adrenal corticosteroid response, but rather that these are dependent upon how the stress is perceived, interpreted, and defended against.

7. On the basis of her total defensive effectiveness score, each subject was placed in a well-defended, moderately failing, or severely failing group. As FIGURE 5 shows, the mean *production* rate values were 11.9, 14.9 and 18.6 respectively, the differences being significant at less than the .01 level by analysis of variance. As this illustration also shows, differences between the *excretion*

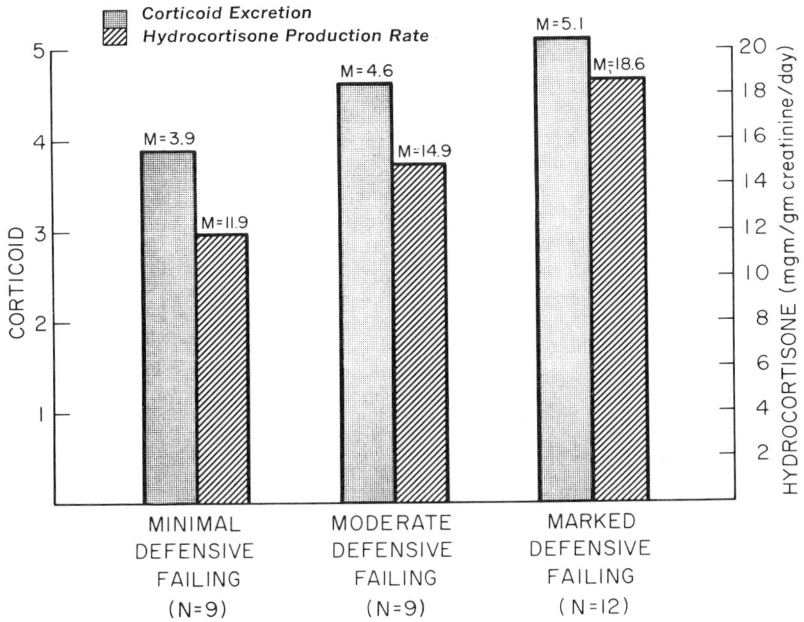

FIGURE 5. Mean preoperative hydrocortisone production rates and corticoid excretion for patients grouped on basis of rated adequacy of defensive functioning.

levels of the principal metabolites were less striking and less statistically significant ($p < .05$).

8. The respective total defense scores were also matched against the production rates, and, as FIGURE 6 shows, the product-moment correlation coefficient was .56, which is significant at less than the .01 level. A similar plotting against cortisol metabolite excretion revealed a correlation of .42, which again is significant only at the .05 level. In summary, then, the psychological ratings of defensive effectiveness were very highly correlated with hydrocortisone production rates, although somewhat less with metabolite excretion.

9. None of the individual criteria, that is, affect, function disruption, or reserve impairment, when taken alone, could predict hydrocortisone production at the same level of significance as the assessment utilizing all three dimensions together. Affect, however, came the closest.

10. No correlation of any kind could be found between our psychological variables and androgen excretion.

11. No striking differences could be defined in either the psychological or the hormonal characteristics between women with benign and those with malignant tumors.

12. With regard to the critical corticosteroid-to-androgen ratio itself, we found that of the eight women predicted and also found to be high cortisol producers, six revealed relatively elevated ratios; of the nine women predicted and found to be low cortisol producers, only one had a relatively elevated ratio, and this was by virute of extremely low androgens, which obviously also affect the final figure.

Our findings suggest that not only should the Bulbrook[1] discriminant ratio be calculated when a woman is in a state of relative emotional equilibrium, but if the Bulbrook formulation is indeed correct, it is conceivable that women whose defensive coping mechanisms are markedly limited may possess a poor prognosis

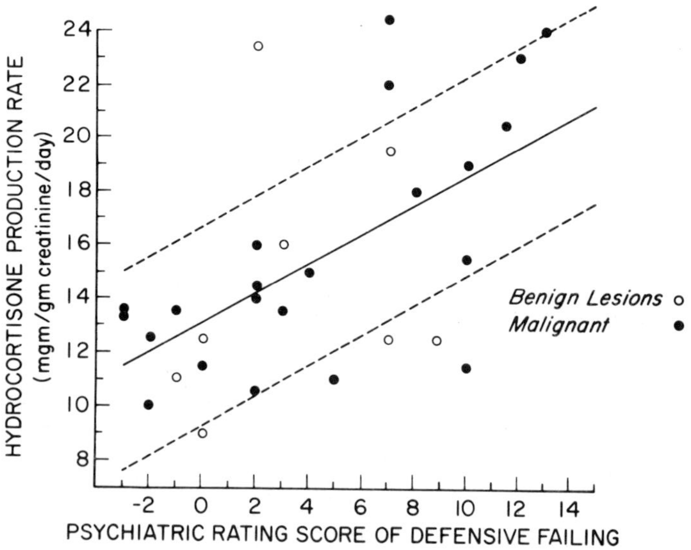

FIGURE 6. Preoperative defensive failing score versus hydrocortisone production rate ($r_{PM} = .566$, $p < .01$).

in this disease by virtue of frequent hydrocortisone elevations. It might also be speculated that breast cancer exacerbations during periods of emotional crisis may be mediated via this psychoendocrine pathway.

13. We would like to emphasize, however, that despite the significant correlations obtained in this cross-sectional report, we do not know how reliable and valid they are until longitudinal assessments of these patients are completed. For example, some production rates may show relatively small changes with time, despite large psychological fluctuations, because of constitutional influences, or psychological state and corticoid levels may both dramatically vary from their preoperative values as adaptation to the illness changes with time.

14. A close look at the psychological characteristics revealed no simple correlation between a single specific affect and hydrocortisone production. Those with elevated rates frequently were apprehensive, worried, or fearful, as well as dejected, discouraged, or despairing, while those with low rates generally reacted with hope, faith in God or fate, and pride in their ability to handle such situations. With regard to defenses, we observed that stoicism, fatalism, and/or prayer were frequently the basic maneuvers that allowed the expression of these pleasant affects. We might note also that effective denial of the lesion's potential significance was frequently inferred and indeed generally did correlate with low production rates, but ironically it was often precisely these women who tended to be the slowest to seek medical attention after their breast lesions were discovered.

15. At least several sources for those occasional discrepancies that did exist between prediction and production are likely. The psychological criteria themselves require further refinement: On the one hand, there is probably some overlap between the assessment categories; on the other, we found, as did the Wolff[2] group, that we frequently had difficulty in evaluating present symptomatology in the light of overall style and ego structure. For instance, two women who were strongly expected to be high cortisol producers were found to have two of the lowest rates; both were chronically masochistic, hysterical women whose wallowing in their misery apparently led to incorrectly inflated scores. We were also aware of the limitations of a single interview as a source of reliable data about a subject. Finally, individual differences in adrenal responsiveness to ACTH were also not taken into consideration.

Summary and Conclusions

In conclusion, we have found that psychological covariants of hydrocortisone production rates do exist in women with breast tumors. The potential consequent influence of this finding on the prognostic Bulbrook[1] corticosteroid-androgen ratio appears to raise significant questions about the possible effects of psychological variables on the course of cancer of the breast.

References

1. Bulbrook, R. D. 1965. Hormone assays in human breast cancer. Vits. and Hormones **23:** 329.
2. Wolff, C. T., S. B. Friedman, M. A. Hofer & J. W. Mason. 1964. Relationship between psychological defenses and mean urinary 17-hydroxycorticosteroid excretion rates. Parts I and II. Psychosom. Med. **26:** 576.
3. Poe, R. O., R. M. Rose & J. W. Mason. 1967. Multiple determinants of 17-hydroxycorticosteroid excretion in recruits during basic training. (abst.) Psychosom. Med. **29:** 542.

DISCUSSION OF THE PAPER

DR. EMERSON DAY (*Strang Clinic and Preventive Medicine Institute, New York, N.Y.*): I should like to ask Dr. Katz one question: whether or not he has looked at the hormonal levels and the defensive levels in terms of concurrent social stresses in these people.

The other comment is related to a clinical experience. I have, unfortunately, had the current experience of seeing a patient, who initially had her mastectomy three years ago at a time when she had to make a move from her home. Three years later, after she had moved to a new place–she again was going to have to move–she developed massive metastases, following which she had an oophorectomy and adrenalectomy and took 15 or 20 mg of cortisone a day for another three years. Again, three years later, she had to make a move, during which time I assume that her adrenal cortical levels and her hormonal cycling were approximately the same, and she again developed an exacerbation of her malignancy.

Now, I think that if we looked at this woman at this point and saw certain kinds of changes in her tumor, and certain kinds of changes in her hormonal levels, we might have associated them as being the cause of the exacerbation of her tumor. But I do not think this is so. I think, as you have pointed out, that there is probably something else going on.

DR. KATZ: I might just comment that during the period that these people were seen in the hospital, most of the women who showed significant affective disturbance were preoccupied primarily with the impending biopsy and possible mastectomy, rather than other concurrent life problems. However, two things might be added to this. First of all, of the 30 women, at least 12 had experienced a significant object loss during the preceding year or year-and-a-half. Second, we have also, as I indicated, had a chance to follow many of these women subsequent to the preoperative studies, and there is no doubt that environmental influences can have a significant effect on the corticosteroid levels. How this influences the patient's coping, psychologically and physiologically, with her neoplasm and her corticosteroid to androgen ratio, is still not completely definable. We are finding it a very complicated task, indeed, to tease out which factors are relevant in our follow-up studies.

INDUCED CARCINOGENESIS UNDER VARIOUS INFLUENCES ON THE HYPOTHALAMUS

R. E. Kavetsky, N. M. Turkevich, R. N. Akimova, I. K. Khayetsky and Y. D. Matveichuck

Laboratory of Tumor Endocrinology
Kiev Research Institute for Experimental and Clinical Oncology
Ministry of Health of the Ukrainian SSR
Kiev, USSR

Investigations of recent years have shown that the hypothalamic area of the brain is the center in which the influences of the environment are effected and the endocrine functions of the organism are coordinated.[1,9,14] It is also a well-known fact that disturbance of the endocrine regulation plays an important part in the development of hormone-dependent tumors.[4,5,7] It is quite evident that to understand the mechanisms of the effect of the nervous system on carcinogenesis, it is necessary to ascertain the role of the hypothalamus in this process.

The question of the role of the hypothalamus in carcinogenesis was advanced and discussed at the eighth anticancer congress in Moscow in 1963. In his report, A. Lacassagne said that the time had come when we must establish the endocrine disturbances accelerating or inhibiting the development of tumor that may be linked with the disturbance of hypothalamic function.[8]

There are very few indications in the literature of the role of the hypothalamus in tumor development.

Some psychopharmacological substances possessing properties affecting the hypothalamic centers may be used to analyze the role of the hypothalamus.[8] When these drugs are administered, substantial changes occur in endocrine balance, which cannot but affect the emergence and development of hormone-dependent tumors.

In earlier researches we studied the effect on carcinogenesis of various influences on the hypothalamus. We applied reserpine[12] in DMBA-induced carcinogenesis of the mammary glands in rats. Administration of reserpine together with DMBA led to a decrease in the number of diseased animals and a prolongation of the latent period. However, in the case when reserpine was administered after termination of DMBA administration, it was found to have a stimulating effect on tumor development. One of us (I.K. Khayetsky[13]) showed that electrolytic lesions of various zones of the hypothalamus and prolonged illumination of the animals alter the latent period and frequency of DMBA-induced tumors of the mammary glands in rats.

The present experimental study is devoted to induced carcinogenesis of the mammaries in rats upon administration of ipraside and to induced thyroid gland tumors following electrolytic influences on the hypothalamus.

Effect of Ipraside on the Development of DMBA-Induced Tumors of The Mammary Glands

When conducting these researches, we proceeded on the assumption that there is a two-phase character to induced carcinogenesis of the mammaries.[2,3]

Ipraside was administered during introduction of the carcinogen, when interaction of the carcinogen occurs with the mammary gland cells, or some time after introduction of DMBA, i.e., when development of the tumor takes place.

Mature female albino rats weighing 110–120 g were used in the experiment. The carcinogen was injected i.v. in quantities of 2 mg per animal, five times at intervals of one week. The total dose was 10 mg. The latent period of development of the tumor was defined as the time elapsing between the last carcinogen injection and the appearance of a palpable tumor. The tumors were removed for histological examination. During the administration of pharmacological substances, vaginal washings were examined for estimation of the endocrine state of the organism. Ipraside was injected s.c. daily in the course of 30 days. The initial dose was 100 mg/kg during the first five days, then 6 mg/kg until the end of the course. The control animals received s.c. injections of physiological solution. The results of the investigation are presented in TABLE 1.

A study of the effect of ipraside on carcinogenesis is of great interest, since reserpine and ipraside are known to produce opposite effects in the central divisions of the nervous system and in the periphery.[6]

It has been shown that ipraside retards sexual maturity in rats as a consequence of suppression of the gonadotropic function of the pituitary.[10] No data on the effect of ipraside on carcinogenesis of the mammary gland were found in the literature, but in experiments with dithiocarbamoyl—a substance similar to ipraside in its mechanism of action—inhibition of methyl cholanthrene mammary gland carcinogenesis was revealed.[11]

Our data (TABLE 1) also indicate that ipraside, when administered together with the carcinogen, suppresses tumor formation and prolongs the latent period of the tumor's appearance. On the other hand, ipraside did not substantially affect the development of tumors.

Effect of Lesions of the Anterior Hypothalamus on the Development of Tumors of the Thyroid Gland Induced by 8-Methylthiouracil

Experiments were conducted on male golden hamsters weighing 90–115 g. A stereotaxic device was used to produce bilateral electrocoagulations of symmetrical areas of the anterior hypothalamus in intact hamsters and in hamsters with tumors of the thyroid gland developing after prolonged ingestion of 6-methylthiouracil (MTU). The nature of the development of these tumors was evaluated by comparing their histological structure at the time of lesion of the hypothalamus (or sham operation) and at the end of the experiment.

The investigations showed that lesions of the hypothalamus involving the paraventricular (PV) and ventromedial (VM) nuclei and the walls of the third ventricle led to a decrease in J-131 accumulation by the thyroid gland in most of the animals attended by a certain decrease in the protein-bound iodine of the serum.

TABLE 1
EFFECT OF IPRASIDE ON THE APPEARANCE AND GROWTH OF DMBA-INDUCED TUMORS OF THE MAMMARIES

	Number of Animals at End of Experiment	Number of Animals with Tumors of the Mammaries	Average Number of Tumors of the Mammaries per Rat	Latent Period of Appearance of Tumors (in Days)
DMBA	26	11 (42%)	2.7	76.0
DMBA + ipraside simultaneously with carcinogen	24	7 (29%)	1.3	103.0
DMBA + ipraside after carcinogen	13	6 (46%)	1.3	72.0

A histological study of the thyroid gland showed signs of its hypofunctional state in many of these animals.

Lesion of the above-mentioned hypothalamus structures in animals receiving 6-MTU for a long time (6–15 months) led to an acute decrease (by 47–50%) in the capacity of the thyroid gland to absorb J-131 and to a decrease in thyroid weight by 32–50%, as compared to the sham-operated animals that received strumogen.

A slight destruction of the marginal region of the PV hypothalamus nuclei (preserving their anterior divisions) with simultaneous lesion of the VM nuclei did not arrest the symptoms of hyperstimulation of the thyroid gland with pituitary thyroid-stimulating hormone (TSH) under the effect of 6-MTU.

In the case of total adenomatosis of the thyroid gland, three months after lesion of the PV and partial destruction of the dorsomedial nuclei a reduction is found in the signs of thyroid stimulation by pituitary TSH. Morphological investigations indicated various stages of the regression of adenomatosis and, in some areas, signs of "normalization" of the gland structure.

In the case of glandular and cystopapillary forms of thyroid gland cancer, proliferation of connective tissue may be observed in the thyroid gland three months after lesion of the above-mentioned nuclei of the anterior hypothalamus. This proliferation leads in rare cases to fibrosis of the gland, reduction of the number of follicles, and a fall in their activity.

The investigations indicate that destruction of the above-mentioned nuclei of the anterior hypothalamus in golden hamsters leads in most cases to a fall in the functional activity of the thyroid gland, to depression of the thyrogenic reaction, and with tumorous processes in the gland, to proliferation of connective tissue.

On the basis of the facts obtained it may be inferred that lesion of the anterior hypothalamus leads to a decrease in thyroid gland stimulation by TSH and to attenuation of the signs of malignancy of tumors of the gland induced by 6-MTU.

Thus our investigations offer evidence of the fact that by acting on the hypothalamus it is possible to alter the course of hormone-dependent carcinogenesis. There are grounds for inferring that the influence of the hypothalamus on carcinogenesis is through the endocrine function of the organism.

References

1. Alyoshin, B. V., N. S. Demidenko, S. V. Zhukov & L. A. Us. 1966. *In* Physiology and Pathophysiology of the Hypothalamus. : 131–134. Nauka. Moscow, USSR.
2. Briziarelli, G. 1966. Z. Krebsforsch. **68**(3): 217–223.
3. Dao, T. L. 1964. Progr. Exp. Tumor Res. **5**: 157–216.
4. Desaive, P., W. Smets, P. Dar, H. Taynon & M. Van Rymenant. 1958. Hormones et Cancers. Bruselles, Belgium.
5. Kavetsky, R. E. 1962. Tumour and the Organism. Kiev, USSR.
6. Kraneberg, G. *et al.* 1960. Arch. Exp. Pathol. Pharmakol., **239**: 29. After Lacassagne, A. & L. C. Hurst. 1966. R. Acad. Sci. **263**: 701–703.
7. Lazarev, N. I. 1963. Theoretical Foundations of the Prevention and Treatment of Dyshormonal Tumours. Moscow, USSR.
8. Lacassagne, A. 1963. Trudy VIII Mezhdunarodnovo Protivorakovovo Kongressa. **3**: 342–345. Moscow, USSR.
9. Sentagotai, Y., B. Flerko, B. Mes & B. Halasz. 1965. Hypothalamic Regulation of the Anterior Hypophysis. Budapest, Hungary.
10. Setnikar, J., W. Murmann & M. J. Magistretti. 1960. Endocrinology **67**(4): 511–520.
11. Shay, H., M. Gruenstein & M. B. Shimkin. 1964. Cancer Res. **24**(6): 998–1001.
12. Turkevich, N. M., L. K. Kunitsa & Y. D. Matveichuk, Vop. Eksp. Onkol. **1**: 94–102.
13. Khayetsky, I. K. 1965. The influence of hypothalamo-pituitary disturbances produced by continuous light on development of induced mammary tumours in rats. Vop. Exp. Oncol. **1**: 87–94.
14. Jules, M. & I. Hollo. 1967. Diagnosis and Pathophysical Foundations of Neuroendocrine Disease. : 309–346. Budapest, Hungary.

SOME ELECTROPHYSIOLOGICAL PECULIARITIES OF THE NERVOUS SYSTEM IN MALIGNANT GROWTH

K. P. Balitsky, A. P. Kapshuk and V. F. Tsapenko

Laboratory of Pathogenesis of Tumours, Kiev Research Institute for Experimental and Clinical Oncology of the Ministry of Health, Ukrainian SSR
Kiev, USSR

The origin of any pathological process, including tumorous processes, is intimately linked with the reactivity of the organism, which is determined to a great extent by the functional state of the nervous system (Kavetsky *et al.*, 1958; Balitsky, 1952; Kavetsky *et al.*, 1966). The changes in the functional state of the higher divisions of the central nervous system under the effect of the tumorous process have been elucidated to a far lesser extent (Turkevich, 1955; Latmanizova, 1956). At the same time, the nervous system, being the basic mechanism of communication of the organism with its environment, the starting lever of its compensatory and defensive reactions, cannot but be injured by the effect of the malignant process.

The aim of this research was the study of the dynamics of the alterations of the bioelectric activity of the cerebral cortex in tumors and the afferent impulsation of some peripheral nerves, innervating the area of development of the tumorous process.

The bioelectric activity of the cerebral cortex was recorded on a 15-channel Alvar electroencephalograph (Kapshuk & Tsapenko, 1965; Tsapenko, 1967). The investigations were conducted on 68 rabbits of the chinchilla breed, each weighing 1.8–2.5 kilograms. Transplantation of the Brown-Pearce carcinoma was carried out by means of intratesticular (group I), subcutaneous (s.c.) (group II), and intramuscular (i.m.) (group III) injection of 1 ml of a 20%-suspension of tumor cells.

The results of the investigations show that in rabbits with intratesticularly inoculated Brown-Pearce carcinoma, characterized by progressive development, an increase in the amplitude and frequency of the basic EEQ rhythm occurs on the second to the third day after inoculation. The amplitude then attains a value of 92.5 ± 4.0 μv, and the frequency of the basic rhythm 8.1 ± 0.6 osc/second. The increase in amplitude and frequency reaches a maximum on the 10th–12th day after inoculation. The amplitude increases to 145.0 ± 8.2 μv, and the frequency to 10.8 ± 0.9 osc/second. At this time, tumors appear in the testicles in the form of pea-shaped nodules with cords; the testicles are strained. After the 10th–12th day, the amplitude and frequency of the basic rhythm begins to decrease, and by the 20th–22nd day do not exceed 66.2 ± 4.2 μv and 9.2 ± 0.7 osc/sec respectively. After the 20th–22nd day, shortly before the death of the animals from numerous metastases, the amplitude and frequency of the biopotentials begin to fall below the initial level, decreasing sharply during the last days of life of the animals. The amplitude in those days does not exceed 20–30 μv, with slow oscillations predominating. (FIGURE 1).

In rabbits with s.c. inoculated Brown-Pearce carcinoma, the changes in the bioelectrical activity of the cerebral cortex occurs on the seventh to the eighth day after inoculation. By this time the tumors can be palpated under the skin in the experimental animals. A further increase in the amplitude and frequency of the basic rhythm of the EEG occurs before the 18th–21st day after inoculation. The amplitude increases to 118.8 ± 3.7 μv, while the frequency of the basic rhythm reaches a value of 7.6 ± 0.5 osc/second. By this time the s.c. inoculated tumors

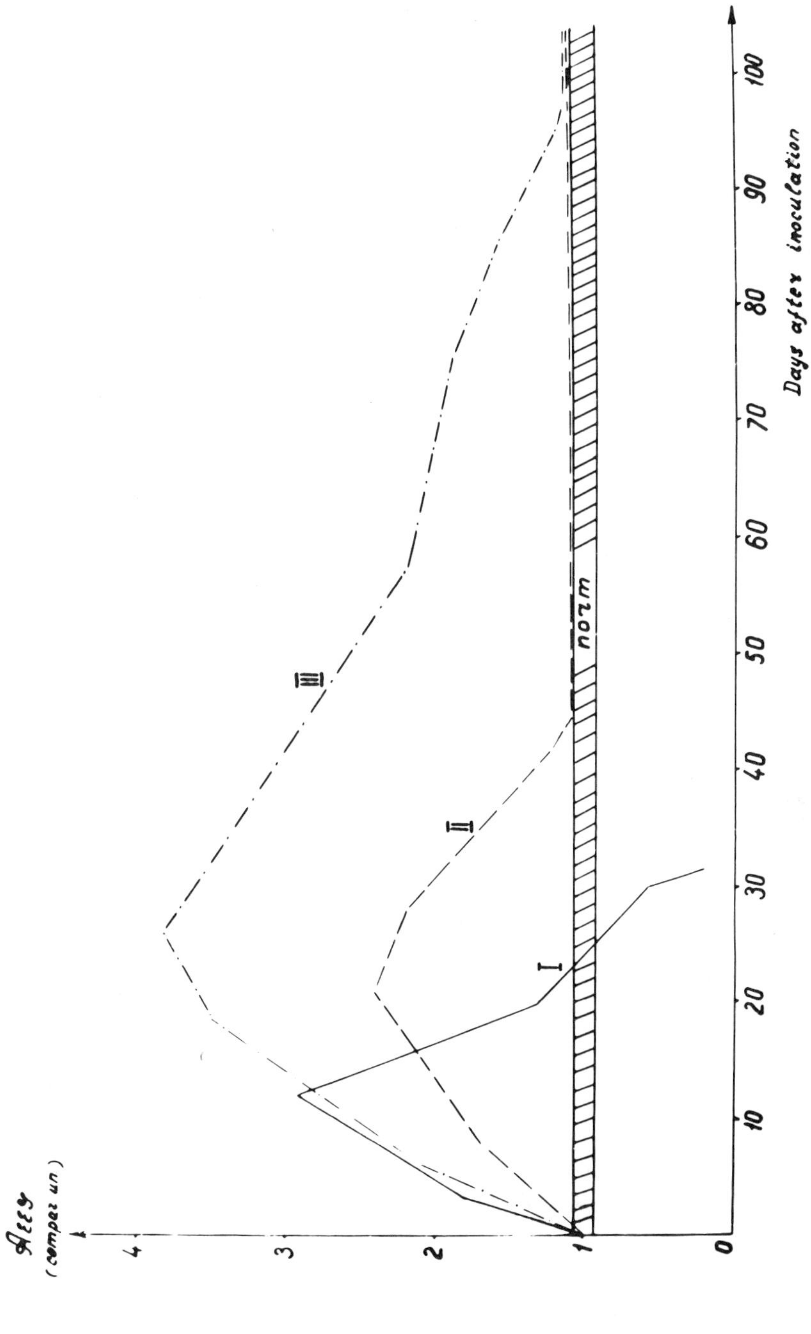

FIGURE 1. Changes in the amplitude of the basic rhythm of the EEG in rabbits with intratesticular (I), subcutaneous (II), and intramuscular (III) inoculation of Brown-Pearce tumor.

increase in diameter to 27.5 ± 1.3 mm, on the average, and then begin to diminish. From the 18th–21st to the 28th-30th day, the bioelectrical activity, decreasing slightly, remains at an elevated level. After the 28th–30th day, when the s.c. inoculated tumors have been considerably reduced, there is a fall in the bioelectrical activity of the cerebral cortex, which returns to the normal level on the 42nd–45th day after inoculation, when the s.c. inoculated tumors are resolved (FIGURE 1).

In animals with i.m. inoculated Brown-Pearce carcinoma, the change in the bioelectrical activity of the cerebral cortex occurs beginning with the sixth to eighth day after inoculation to the twelfth to fourteenth day; the amplitude increases to 140.3 ± 2.7 μv, and the frequency of the basic rhythm to 11.1 ± 0.9 osc/second. The i.m. inoculated tumors during this period reach a weight of 19.3 ± 4.2 g, on the average, during this period, and continue increasing. On the days following the inoculation, the principal indices of the EEG increase, and on the 26th–30th day the amplitude attains a value of 196.2 ± 11.6 μv, while the frequency of the basic rhythm is 16.4 ± 1.5 osc/second. During this period the i.m. inoculated tumors weigh an average of 72.2 ± 4.0 grams. During the period when the tumors begin to resolve – from the 26th–30th day to the 57th–65th day – the amplitude and frequency of the biopotentials begin to fall. After the 57th–65th day a further drop in the bioelectrical activity occurs, and on the 85th–90th day after inoculation, the amplitude does not exceed 80.0 ± 7.0 μv, while the frequency of the basic rhythm is 7.8 ± 0.4 osc/second. The return to normal of the bioelectrical activity of the cerebral cortex in rabbits with i.m. inoculated Brown-Pearce carcinoma occurs on the 95th–102nd day after inoculation; i.e., at the moment of complete resolution of the i.m. inoculated tumors (FIGURE 1).

Investigation of the afferent impulsation in the peripheral nerves during development of the tumorous process yields data for objectively judging the change in the information flow along the corresponding nerves from the area of tumor development to the central nervous system.

We investigated the afferent impulsation of nervus tibialis and nervus paeroneus of rabbits during the development and resolution of Brown-Pearce carcinoma inoculated into the shank muscles, and of nervus splanchnicus major during irreversible carcinoma inoculated intravenously. The biopotentials were recorded on a UPB I-0I Biofizpribor electrophysiological device.

The investigations were conducted under conditions of a chronic experiment, for which we designed a special electrode device (Kapshuk, 1966) implanted in the corresponding nerves, making it possible to lead off and record the biopotentials during a period of more than three months (FIGURE 2). The afferent impulsation was separated out of the general stream by blocking the conductance of the nerve by means of local cooling proximally to the implanted electrodes (Nozdrachev, 1966), for which purpose a special cooling system was provided in the electrode setup. The experiments were carried out on 60 chinchilla rabbits weighing 2–2.5 kg each.

It was found that in healthy animals the afferent impulsation of nervus tibialis is characterized by impulses having a frequency that, remaining relatively stable in each individual rabbit, falls within a range of 48–81 imp/sec with an amplitude of up to 20 microvolts. The afferent impulsation of nervus paeroneus accordingly falls into a frequency range of 78–130 imp/sec with an amplitude of up to 25 μv, and the impulsation of nervus splanchnicus major into a range of frequency of 24–62 imp/sec with an amplitude of up to 25 microvolts.

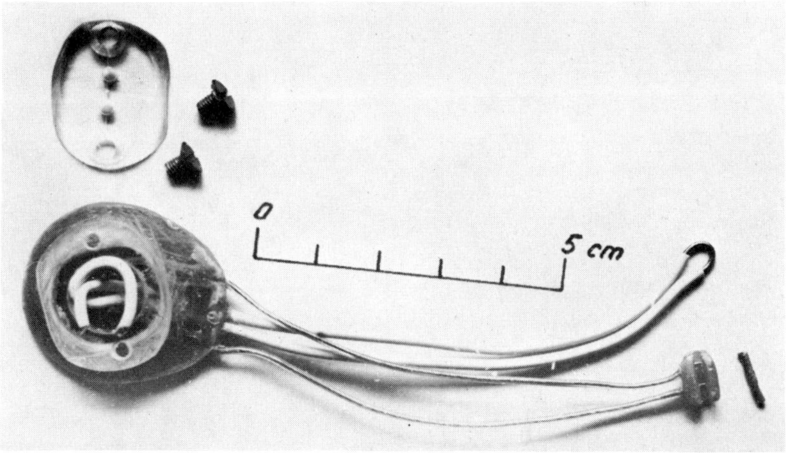

FIGURE 2. Electrode setup for recording action currents of nerves in a chronic experiment.

In the case of inoculation of Brown-Pearce carcinoma into the shank muscles by injection of 1 ml of a 20%-suspension of tumor cells, there is first an active growth of tumor, and then the growth stops and the tumor is gradually resolved spontaneously. The entire cycle of growth and resolution of the tumor lasts from 80–90 days. Investigation of the afferent impulsation in nervus tibialis and nervus paeroneus with such a method of tumor inoculation showed that the frequency of impulsation of the two nerves as the tumor grows is gradually reduced, and by the 30th–40th day after inoculation of the tumor, was at the minimum. The tumors attained their maximum dimensions during that period. Subsequently, as the tumors were resolved, the frequency of the biopotentials in the above-mentioned nerves gradually increased, and by the 80th–90th day after inoculation, differed little from the initial frequency (FIGURE 3).

Another picture is observed in the change in afferent impulsation of nervus splanchnicus major in i.v. inoculation of Brown-Pearce carcinoma by injecting 1 ml of a 20%-suspension of tumor cells in the vein of the ear. In this case, rapid lesion of the organs of the abdominal cavity by the tumor occurred, involving the liver and kidneys particularly. During the first days after i.v. inoculation of the tumor, the frequency of the afferent impulsations of nervus splanchnicus major exceeded the initial level, reaching a maximum on the fifth day. A rapid fall in the frequency of the impulsation then set in, and from the 10th–12th day after inoculation it proved to be below the initial value. By the moment of death of the rabbit, occurring 20–30 days after tumor inoculation, the frequency of the afferent impulsation of nervus splanchnicus major was considerably lower than the initial value (FIGURE 3).

The investigations indicate that the nature and stage of the tumorous process have a substantial effect on the functional state of various divisions of the nervous system. The dynamics of the changes in the electroencephalogram is, to a certain extent, evidence of the nature of the course of the malignant process. The development of the tumor affects the character of the afferent impulsation. A considerable alteration in the nature of the information transmitted along the investigated nerves to the central nervous system indicates the existence of law-governed neuroreflex correlations between the tumor and the organism.

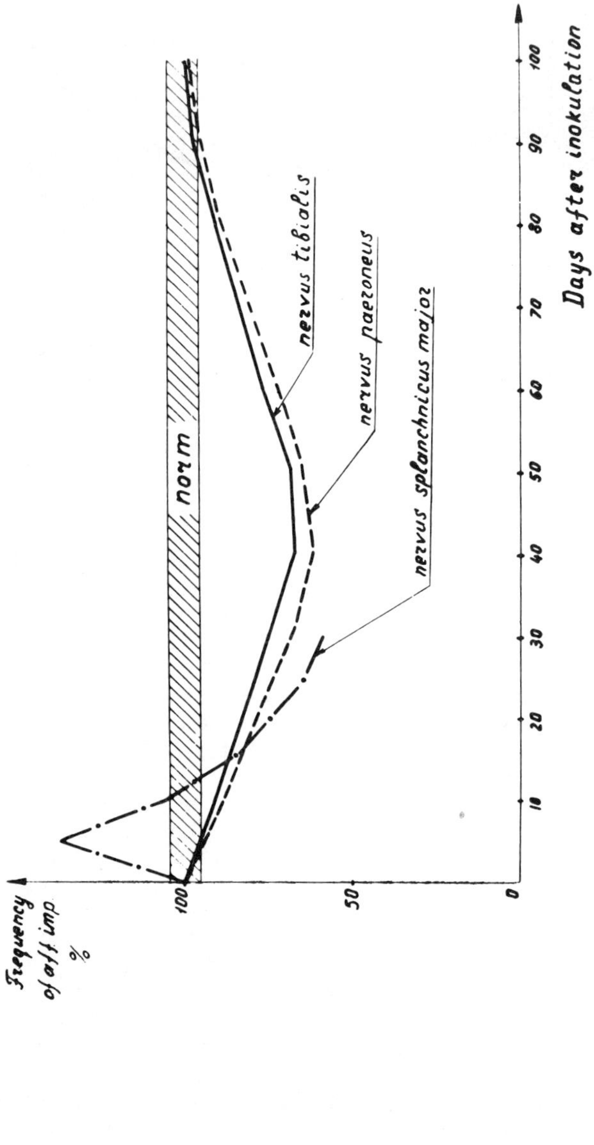

FIGURE 3. Changes in the frequency of the afferent impulsation in nerves during development of Brown-Pearce carcinoma.

References

BALITSKY, K. P. 1952. Some data from the literature on the role of the nervous system in the pathogenesis of malignant neoplasms. Klin. Med. (Moskva) **30**(9): 41–49.

KAPSHUK, A. P. 1966. Electrodes for recording action currents of peripheral nerve conductors in a chronic experiment. Fiziol. Zh. SSSR. **12**(3): 413–414.

KAPSHUK, A. P. & V. F. TSAPENKO. 1965. Method of implanted electrodes for electroencephalographic observations on rabbits. Fiziol. Zh. SSSR **1**(5): 626–627.

KAVETSKY, R. E., K. P. BALITSKY, L. I. KORENEVSKY, G. A. LEVCHIK, B. S. RUCHKOVSKY, S. P. SIZENKO & N. M. TURKEVICH. 1960. The Neoplastic Process and the Nervous System. National Science Foundation. Washington, D. C.

KAVETSKY, R. E., N. M. TURKEVICH & K. P. BALITSKY. 1966. On the psychophysiological mechanism of the organism's resistance to tumor growth. Ann. N. Y. Acad. Sci. **125**(3): 933–945.

LATMANIZOVA, L. V. 1956. Functional peculiarities of the nervous system in cancer. Uchoniye zapiski Leningradskovo gosudarstvennovo pedagogicheskovo instituta. **20**(6).

NOZDRACHEV, A. L. 1966. Electrophysiological characteristics of afferent and efferent impulsation in vegetative nerves in a chronic experiment. Fiziol. Zh. SSSR **50**(1): 46.

TSAPENKO, V. F. 1967. Peculiarity of changes in the electroencephalogram in rabbits with different character of development of Brown-Pearce carcinoma. Dopov. Akad. Nauk. Ukr. RSR 357–360.

TURKEVICH, N. M. 1955. Significance of the typological peculiarities of the nervous system in the emergence and development of cancer of the mammaries in mice. Vop. Onkol. **1**(6): 64–70.

DISCUSSION

PHYSIOLOGIC RESPONSES TO AVOIDABLE AND UNAVOIDABLE PSYCHOLOGIC STRESS IN RELATION TO GENETIC DIFFERENCES*

Samuel A. Corson

Laboratory of Cerebrovisceral Physiology, Division of Behavioral and Nurobiological Sciences, Department of Psychiatry
Ohio State University College of Medicine
Columbus, Ohio

What we have been trying to do in our laboratory during the last few years is to make some small contribution toward the transformation of psychosomatic medicine from an anecdotal phase to some semblance of an exact science.

We have been trying to study physiological and endocrine effects of psychological stress in relation to genetic differences. These experiments were done on dogs.

FIGURE 1 is a drawing of a dog with a chronically implanted urinary-bladder cannula. This cannula has a tightly fitting obturator that can be removed during the experiments so that one can study the effects of psychologic stress on renal function without the complication of urinary-bladder reflexes.

The experimental procedure (FIGURE 2) was as follows: dogs kept on a constant regimen of food and water intake were placed in a pavlovian stand in a sound-shielded, air-conditioned chamber maintained at 20°–22° centigrade. The experiments were started exactly at the same time of day. Before each experiment, the dogs received a water load of 25 ml/kg. In the control room (first pair of bar graphs on the left), this water load led to a diuresis, accompanied by a fall in the urine osmolality, which can be taken as an indication of a decrease in the circulating antidiuretic hormone.

The other five pairs of bar graphs represent experiments performed in the Pavlovian conditioning room, where the animal on previous occasions had been presented with 20 tones reinforced with electrocutaneous stimuli to a foreleg, so that the animal developed a motor defense reflex (leg withdrawal). The excitatory tones (reinforced with shock) were arbitrarily referred to as A tones. In some experiments, excitatory A tones were intermingled at random with inhibitory differentiating tones arbitrarily referred to as B tones. On some experimental days, differentiating B tones alone were presented. On other days, extinction experiments were run wherein 20 A tones were administered without reinforcement. In some experiments, the animal was placed on the pavlovian stand, but no stimuli were given. All the tones were administered during the same time of day for a period of 20 minutes, as indicated on the graphs by broken vertical lines. The details of the method have been published elsewhere.†

Note that under all circumstances the animal in the pavlovian conditioning

* Supported in part by research grants MH 12089 and LM NB 00635 from the NIH, and the NIH General Research grant to the Ohio State University College of Medicine.

† Corson, Samuel A. 1966. Conditioning of water and electrolyte excretion. *In* Endocrines and the Central Nervous System. Res. Publ. Ass. Nerv. Ment. Dis. **43:** 140–199. Williams and Wilkins. Baltimore, Md.

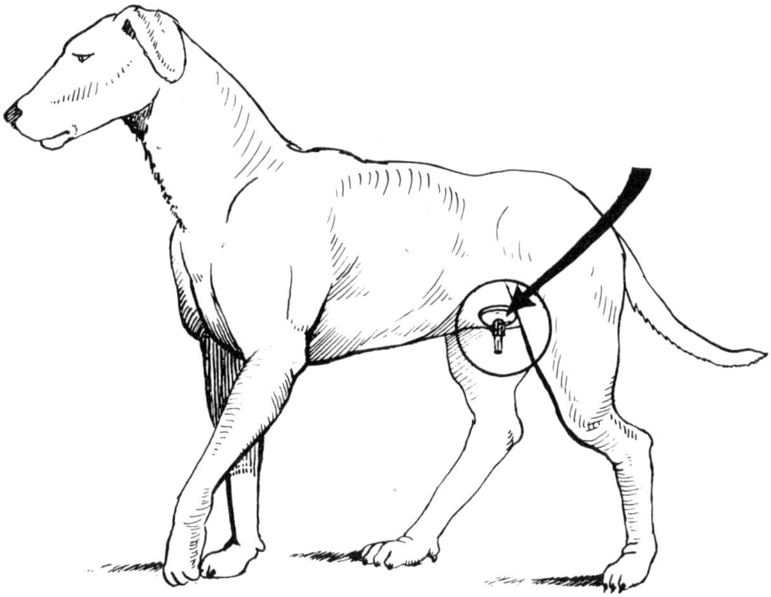

FIGURE 1. Drawing of a dog with a surgically implanted urinary-bladder cannula. Between experiments the dog can use the normal urinary tract. During the experimental sessions, the obturator is removed from the cannula in order to permit continuous collection of urine samples.

chamber showed a consistent antidiuresis, with a high urine osmolality (suggesting the possible participation of antidiuretic hormone) even when no tones whatsoever were given, or when only inhibitory differentiating B tones were presented.

I now want to call your attention to another phenomenon. It is well known that somatic motor defense responses are stimulus-bound. As far as these somatic responses are concerned, the animals learn to differentiate between the excitatory and inhibitory tones rather rapidly. For example, when we conduct an extinction session, the motor defense response is extinguished with ease; in fact, after the animal has been exposed to a number of extinction sessions, then in any given extinction session, after the first or certainly the second nonreinforcement, the motor defense responses disappear. In other words, the animal has learned that if the first tone is not reinforced, then none of the tones will be reinforced.

By contrast, the conditional visceral responses, as exemplified by the renal parameter, persist throughout the entire experiment under all circumstances, as long as the animal is in the pavlovian conditioning room. These conditional visceral responses persist even in experiments involving the presentation of inhibitory tones or 20 unreinforced tones, or even in the absence of any tones at all. In other words, the entire pavlovian chamber becomes converted into a conditional aversive stimulus. We refer to this discrepancy between the conditional somatic (leg withdrawal) and visceral responses as somatovisceral di-

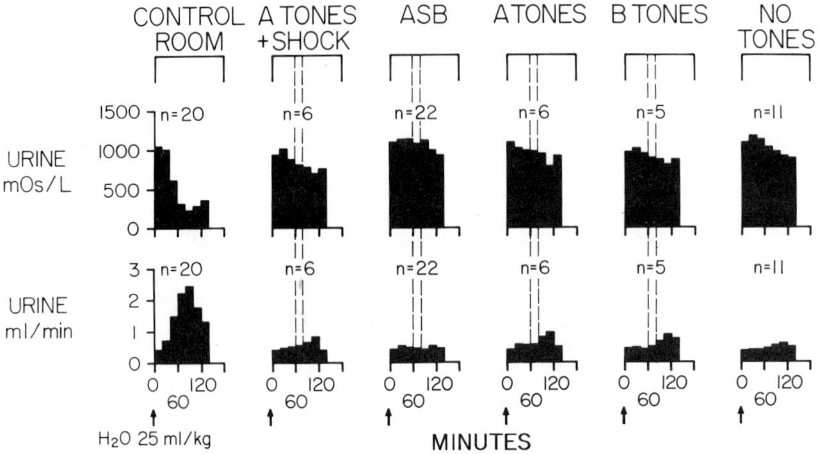

FIGURE 2. Development and stabilization of conditional antidiuretic responses in dog Harry (male, 17 kg), studied for a period of four years. On the ordinates are plotted urine osmolality and rates of urine flow. From left to right are plotted mean values (n = number of experiments in a given design) for experiments conducted in the control room (where the animal was never exposed to reinforced or unreinforced signals), and five groups of experiments conducted in the conditioning room. Water administration (25 ml/kg per os) is indicated by an arrow at time O. Broken vertical lines indicate the 20-minute period during which reinforced (A + shock), unreinforced (A) or inhibitory (B) tones were presented. "A tones + shock" indicates that 20 reinforced tones were administered at one-minute intervals. "ASB" indicates that 10 reinforced tones were interspersed at random with 10 inhibitory B tones. "A tones" signifies extinction sessions during which 20 unreinforced A tones were presented at one-minute intervals. "B tones" signifies the presentation of 20 inhibitory tones. "No tones" signifies that the animal was placed in the conditioning room, but no conditional or unconditional stimuli were presented. "Control Room" represents experiments performed by a different experimenter in a neutral room where the dog was never exposed to aversive stimuli. Note that as far as the renal responses are concerned, the conditioning-room complex acted as a conditional stimulus, the dog exhibiting conditional antidiuretic responses regardless of the experimental design, as long as the animal was in the conditioning room.

chotomy. This phenomenon is a demonstration of the principle of schizokinesis described some years ago by W. H. Gantt.‡

When we bring the animal back to a control room (where the animal was never presented with any reinforced or unreinforced tones), we can again observe the normal diuretic responses comparable to those observed before the dog was given electrocutaneous stimuli.

FIGURE 3 demonstrates the responses of another dog exposed to exactly the same kind of experiment as indicated in FIGURE 2. Notice that this dog exhibited a very mild antidiuresis for only the first three experiments. Moreover, even in these three experiments, the urine osmolality was not markedly different from that observed in the control room. Thereafter, all the renal responses exhibited in the pavlovian conditioning room were essentially indistinguishable from those observed in the control room.

We found that in the case of some animals, even when we did nothing but

‡ Gantt, W. H. 1953. Principles of nervous breakdown–schizokinesis and autokinesis. Ann. N. Y. Acad. Sci. **56** (2): 143–163.

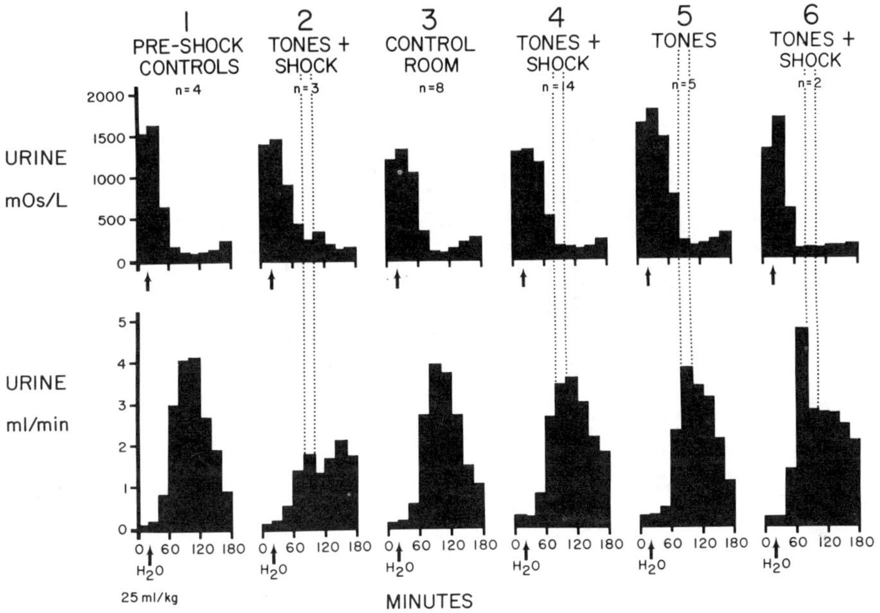

FIGURE 3. Case history of diuretic dog (Mary, female, 20 kg) studied for a period of more then 18 months. After a 14-hour period of food deprivation and a five-hour period of water withdrawal, the dog was placed in a pavlovian stand. Water was administered by stomach tube in the conditioning chamber or the control room, after a 20-minute urine-collection period, at the time indicated by an arrow. Tones reinforced or unreinforced with shock were always administered during the fifth urine-collection period, indicated by vertical dotted lines. In column 1 are represented experiments conducted in the control room before the dog was ever shocked. In column 3 are represented experiments conducted in the same control room (never associated with shock or tones) and interspersed throughout the experimental series. Note that this dog responded with mild antidiuresis for only three experimental sessions (column 2). Moreover, during these three sessions the urine osmolality values were not much higher than those in the control room. After the first three antidiuretic experiments, the renal responses in the conditioning room were essentially similar to those observed in the control room.

place them in a pavlovian chamber and close the door of the chamber, the mere isolation developed in them an antidiuretic response, as can be seen in FIGURE 4. This was an extreme source of frustration for us, because we were trying in this particular case to develop a conditional diuretic response. We were reinforcing tones with water, expecting to elaborate a diuretic response to the tones, comparable to the conditional salivary responses to tones when reinforced with food. But instead, we observed an antidiuresis.

At the first Conference on Psychophysiological Aspects of Cancer, I presented data to suggest that the two types of dogs differ endocrinologically. The renal responses of the diuretic dogs appear to involve primarily adrenergic pathways. If you administer an alpha-adrenergic blocking agent such as phentolamine (Regitine) to a diuretic dog, you find that this dog now shows antidiuretic responses. And if you give the dog enough phentolamine, some sedation will be observed. If a diuretic dog is given a drug like chlorpromazine, which has adrenergic blocking properties, you observe similar effects.

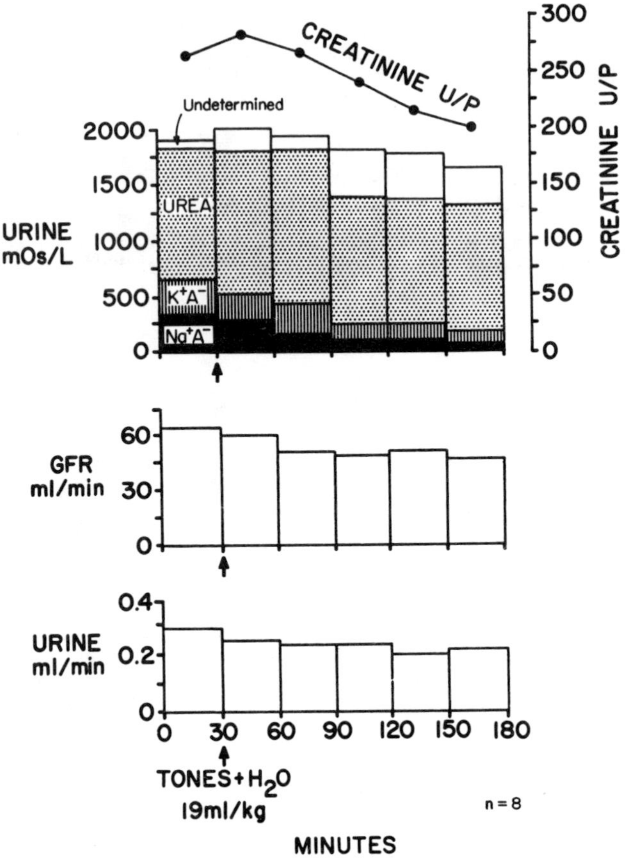

FIGURE 4. Paradoxical antidiuretic responses (mean of eight experiments) to the administration of tones and water in experiments designed to develop conditioned diuretic responses. (Dog Audrey, female, 17 kg.) Time (in minutes) and urine-collection periods are plotted along the abscissae. Along the ordinates are plotted the rate of urine flow, the glomerular filtration rate (GFR, based on endogenous creatinine clearance), and urine osmolality, represented as a diagram of the Gamble type. The Na and K on the Gamble diagram are plotted in terms of the milliosmol values of their salts (Na^+A^- and K^+A^-). The urine/plasma creatinine ratios are plotted as points connected by a straight line. Note that following the administration of tones and water, there was a decrease in the rate of urine flow. The urine osmolality and the creatinine U/P ratios remained high, and even increased, suggesting increased renal tubular water reabsorption in spite of the fact that the dog received a large water load.

What is the significance of the difference in the renal responses of the two types of dogs? What adaptive functions are represented by the psychogenic antidiuresis? Some of the answers to these questions came from a careful study of the responses of other physiological systems of the two types of dogs, after repeated exposure to psychologic stress. It turned out that the antidiuretic dogs also respond to the pavlovian conditioning chamber with persistent hyperpnea, tachycardia, and copious salivation (FIGURE 5). This salivation is not related to con-

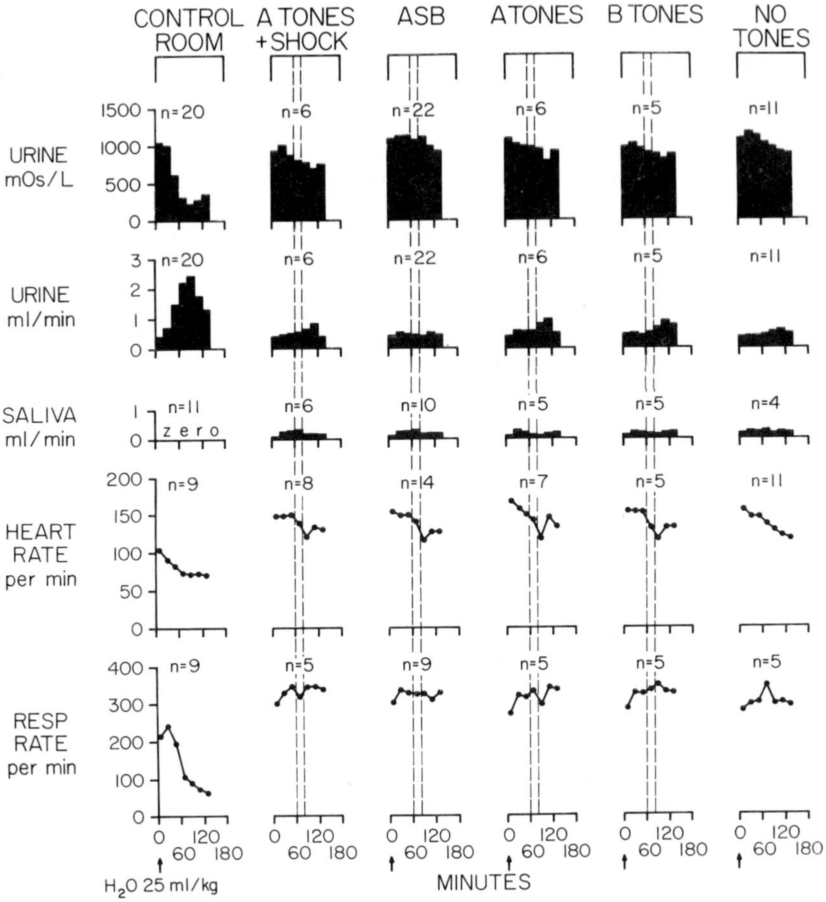

FIGURE 5. Conditional visceral responses to psychologic stress in antidiuretic dog Harry. In the pavlovian conditioning room, this dog exhibited a tetrad of responses: antidiuresis, salivation, tachycardia, and polypnea. Note that in the control room, where the animal was never exposed to reinforced or unreinforced signals, none of these responses occurred.

ditioned alimentary reflexes, since food reinforcement was never used in these particular experiments.

This tetrad of responses to the aversive environment represented by the pavlovian conditioning chamber suggested to us that the antidiuretic dogs behave physiologically in the pavlovian conditioning room as though they were engaged in intense muscular effort. These responses would be comparable to those described by Walter B. Cannon as a "fight or flight" situation.

The primary response of the antidiuretic dogs to psychological stress appears to be a conditional anticipatory increase in heat production characteristic for muscular exertion. The hyperpnea then would serve the purpose of dissipating the heat. The salivation provides the water for evaporative cooling on the buccal surfaces. The antidiuresis serves the function of conserving body water so that it will be available for evaporative cooling.

This is therefore a good example of the transformation of an integrated complex of adaptive responses into a maladaptive pattern, because all of these responses in our dogs represent a Don Quixote type of fighting against windmills. All of these physiological responses in a pavlovian conditioning chamber are not geared to reality. In reality, these dogs should be responding with a diuresis, in view of the fact that these animals are faced with a water excess (since a large quantity of water was administered to the dogs at the beginning of each experiment). Instead of responding physiologically to the real stimulus of a water excess by a diuresis, the dog responds psychologically to a symbol of fighting or running, which the animal is not capable of carrying out under the circumstances. It should be pointed out at this time that pavlovian conditioning experiments involving electrocutaneous reinforcement do not permit the animal to achieve a consummatory adaptive response, in contrast to pavlovian conditioning experiments involving food reinforcement. Thus the antidiuretic dogs under conditions of pavlovian aversive reinforcement can be considered to be in a chronic state of

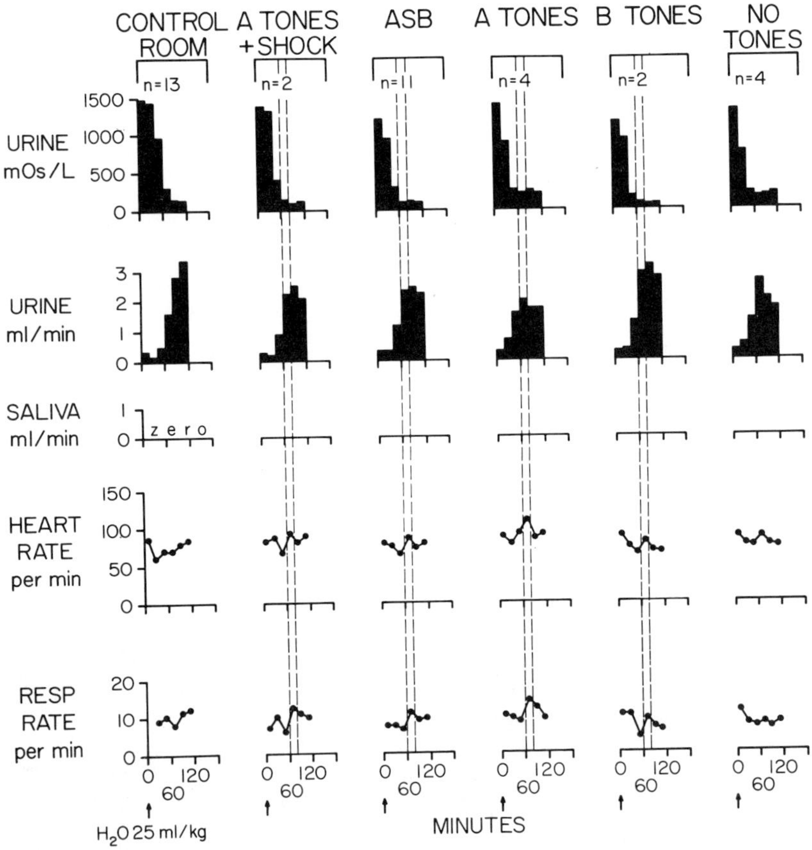

FIGURE 6. Stability of visceral functions in diuretic dog David exposed to psychologic stress. Whether in the pavlovian conditioning room or in the control room, this dog exhibited none of the tetrad of responses seen in FIGURE 5 in an antidiuretic dog.

frustration. They exhibit a discordance between physiologic and behavioral adaptive processes. This discordance may be looked upon as one aspect of the biological foundation of anxiety.

FIGURE 6 shows a complex of physiological responses of a diuretic dog to the pavlovian conditioning chamber. The animal shows no salivation; the heartbeat and respiration remain at about the same level as observed in the control room.

Therefore, we may conclude that psychogenic antidiuresis can be looked upon as a diagnostic sign of the fact that the organism is responding to symbols of stress with a series of physiologic responses signifying attempts at maintaining thermal homeostasis. Preliminary measurements of oxygen consumption in the

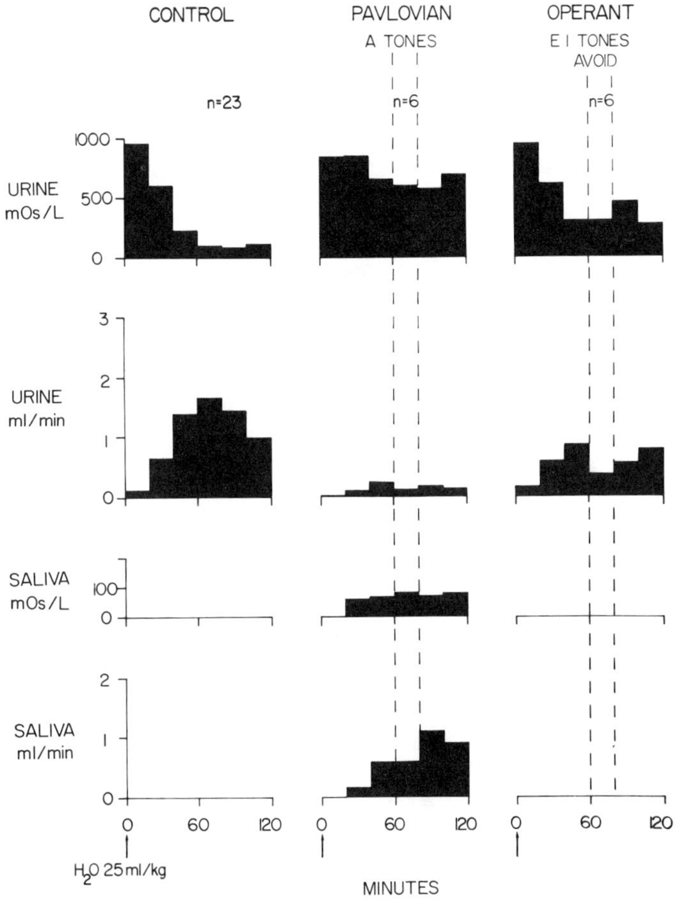

FIGURE 7. Comparative renal and salivary responses in antidiuretic dog Mitzi (female wirehaired fox terrier, 10 kg) in pavlovian and operant conditioning rooms. In the pavlovian room are depicted the mean values of renal and salivary responses in six extinction sessions. In the operant room the mean values of six experiments are depicted after the dog reached a 90–100% level of avoidance. Note the amelioration of the antidiuresis and the decrease in urine osmolality in the room where avoidance experiments were conducted. Note also that in the avoidance experiments the psychogenic salivary responses disappeared.

two types of dogs indicate that the antidiuretic dogs have a consistently higher metabolic rate than the diuretic dogs.

It is interesting to note that most of the wirehaired fox terriers, which have been selectively bred for their fighting propensity, are consistently antidiuretic and exhibit the tetrad of responses described above, whereas most beagles are diuretic and do not exhibit any other components of the tetrad.

FIGURE 7 demonstrates the fact that this psychophysiologic tetrad in the antidiuretic dogs is related primarily to frustration and inability to achieve a consummatory adaptive response. When the antidiuretic dog is studied by another experimenter in another conditioning room, where the animal is permitted to develop an escape and eventually a discriminated avoidance response, then all the components of the psychophysiologic tetrad either disappear or become markedly attenuated.

This observation would fit in well with the general idea proposed in Dr. Bahnson's and in Dr. Kissen's work, that it is the inability to express one's feelings, or to express one's responses, that may be responsible for many psychovisceral disturbances in individuals with certain constitutional predispositions. It must be emphasized that it is probably not appropriate to speak of psychologic stress *per se* as being responsible for psychosomatic disturbances; instead, the question should be phrased: how may different kinds of psychologic stress contribute to the development of different diseases, including carcinogenesis, in individuals with different genetic endowments?

PART V. PSYCHODYNAMIC PROCESS AND CANCER

A FURTHER REPORT ON PERSONALITY AND PSYCHOSOCIAL FACTORS IN LUNG CANCER*

David M. Kissen,† R. I. F. Brown, and Margaret Kissen

The Psychosomatic Research Unit
University Department of Psychological Medicine
Southern General Hospital
Glasgow, Scotland

In the monograph derived from the first conference on the psychophysiological aspects of cancer held under the auspices of this Academy, D. M. Kissen (1966a) presented a clinically derived hypothesis that lung cancer patients have diminished outlets for emotional discharge compared with noncancer patients. Among the empirical evidence supporting this was the finding that lung cancer patients had a lower mean score on the neuroticism scale of the Short Maudsley Personality Inventory than did noncancer patients. This was taken to indicate a lesser ability to discharge emotion (Kissen & Eysenck, 1962; Kissen, 1963; Kissen, 1964) and was independent of smoking habits. Significant differences between the same lung cancer patients and the controls were later found in the reported incidence of certain environmental and social factors such as adverse events in childhood and adulthood (Kissen, 1967).

As in the work reported in the earlier studies, all the findings to be presented in this report are derived from samples of lung cancer patients and control patients drawn from the same hospital wards and suffering from other chest diseases. The samples were selected in the same way, without deliberate bias, and seen under the same conditions, in which the interviewer never knew the diagnosis and more often than not neither did the patient at that time (Kissen, 1966b). The present report covers preliminary results from further samples of more than 550 male patients.

The neuroticism scale of the short form of the Maudsley Personality Inventory is described by Eysenck (1959a) as measuring general emotional lability, emotional overresponsiveness, and liability to breakdown under stress. This scale (N-SMPI) was administered to 539 patients—249 lung cancers and 290 controls. As expected, there was a slight but significant negative correlation between age and neuroticism (TABLE 1), and since the cancer group was slightly older than the control, it was necessary to control statistically for age effects. Therefore a sample of matched pairs was composed, matching each lung cancer and control pair for age to within one year (TABLE 2). The resulting sample yielded a mean N-SMPI for lung cancer patients of 4.57 and for controls of 5.34. A Wilcoxon Matched-Pairs Sign-Rank Test showed this difference to be significant ($p<.01$).

Even using relatively crude statistical methods, reducing the sample by age-matching, these preliminary results are an unequivocal confirming replication of the first work done by D. M. Kissen and H. J. Eysenck using the Short MPI, and more sophisticated statistical methods can only be expected to yield higher

* The Council for Tobacco Research, U.S.A., supported this work for the year July 1 1967–1968 as a special project.

† Dr. David Kissen died on February 23, 1968, prior to this conference.

TABLE 1

NEUROTICISM SCALE OF SHORT MPI: CORRELATION BETWEEN AGE AND N-SMPI

249 Cancers + 290 Controls N = 539
Spearman rho = −0.10 (N-SMPI tends to drop with advancing age) ($p < .025$)
Mean Age Difference between Cancers and Controls
$\bar{x}$ cancers = 57.59 years
$\bar{x}$ controls = 53.29 years
($p < .001$)

TABLE 2

NEUROTICISM SCALE OF SHORT MPI: PAIRS OF LUNG CANCERS AND CONTROLS MATCHED ON AGE

Lung Cancers		Controls
$\bar{x}$ (N-SMPI) = 4.57		$\bar{x}$ (N-SMPI) = 5.34
	Wilcoxon Matched-Pairs Sign-Rank Test ($p < .01$)	
n (cancers) = 206		n (controls) = 206
	Total N = 412	

significances. Once again it has been shown that lung cancer patients are less emotionally reactive as measured on this scale when used in Britain, and this is interpreted as consonant with the germinal clinical impression that, as a group, they are lacking in outlets for emotional discharge. Cultural differences may vitiate the transfer of a scale standardized in one country from that country to another, and it would be interesting to check whether this scale will differentiate between lung cancers and controls equally well in North America, Eastern Europe, and the rest of the world.

The newer Eysenck Personality Inventory (EPI), designed to supercede the MPI, comprises neuroticism and extraversion scales (N-EPI and E-EPI) of 24 items each and a lie scale of nine items. Neuroticism EPI is a refinement of neuroticism SMPI and can be described in the same terms (Eysenck & Eysenck, 1964). Extraversion EPI is described as measuring sociability, tendency to impulsive behavior, stimulus seeking, etc. (Eysenck & Eysenck, 1963a & 1964). The lie scale attached to this inventory is designed to measure desirability response set or the tendency to answer questions according to the favorable light that the answer would throw on the subject. Extensive item analyses and factor analyses have shown this scale to be valid, reliable, and useful in detecting individuals "faking good" (Eysenck & Eysenck, 1964; Eysenck, 1959b; Gibson, 1962). Eysenck recommends that if an individual produces an L score above four or five, the E and "particularly the N" scores should be regarded with considerable scepticism. Tendency to have high L scores may, in itself, be an interesting personality trait (Eysenck & Eysenck, 1963b).

The EPI was administered to 489 patients—221 with lung cancer and 268 controls. Previous studies have shown significant negative correlations between N-EPI and age, but on this sample the correlation was not significant and it was not necessary to control statistically for age (TABLE 3). Without controlling for social desirability set, that is, including all subjects whatever their lie score, the lung cancer group had a mean of 8.10 on the N-EPI and the controls had one of 9.34 (TABLE 4). This difference was highly significant (Mann-Whitney

TABLE 3
NEUROTICISM SCALE OF THE EPI

Cancers		Controls
$\bar{x} = 57.95$ years		$\bar{x} = 53.29$ years
	Approx. 4 years difference ($p < .001$)	
	Correlation between N EPI and Age	
	Spearman rho = −0.061	
	Not significant ($p > .20$)	
n (cancers) = 221		n (controls) = 268
	Total N = 489	

TABLE 4
NEUROTICISM SCALE OF THE EPI
UNCORRECTED FOR SOCIAL DESIRABILITY

Cancers	(N = 489)	Controls
$\bar{x} = 8.10$		$\bar{x} = 9.34$
	Mann-Whitney U: $p < .003$	
	Corrected for Social Desirability	
Cancers	(N = 289)	Controls
$\bar{x} = 8.68$		$\bar{x} = 11.23$
	Mann-Whitney U: $p < .0003$	

U Test; $p<.003$). When social desirability is controlled for, that is, when only individuals with lie scores of four or under are considered, the lung cancer mean is 8.68 and the control 11.23. This difference is also very highly significant (Mann-Whitney U Test: $p>.0003$).

Previous work relating the N and L scales of the Maudsley family of tests has shown that people who appear less neurotic also appear to lie more (Gibson, 1962), and we did find a small negative correlation between neuroticism and lying. The change in EPI scores when social desirability set is controlled for is mainly confined to the control sample, and it appears that correcting for social desirability yields significantly higher N scores in the controls ($p<.0005$), but not in the cancers ($p>.20$). There is also a lower and less significant correlation between high neuroticism and lying in the cancer sample (TABLE 5). than there is in the combined sample of controls and cancers. This peculiarity of the cancer patients, that their neuroticism scores are less affected by the tendency to show themselves in a favorable light, may point to a personality trait in itself. One possibility is that the denial characteristic of the cancer patient is too deep to be affected by a mere wish to show oneself in a favorable light. Another is that the cancer patients as a group are relatively depressed, in which state they may be more likely to give an unvarnished account of themselves.

On this particular sample, there was again no need to control for age effects on the scores for extraversion. (TABLE 6). Mean extraversion scores, uncontrolled for social desirability set, for the lung cancer group are 11.32 and for the controls 11.41. The difference is not significant (Mann-Whitney U Test: $p>.40$). Even when corrected for social desirability set, the difference between cancers and controls is not significant (Mann-Whitney U Test: $p>.45$).

TABLE 5
LIE SCALE OF THE EPI:
CORRELATIONS BETWEEN NEUROTICISM (N-EPI) AND LYING (L-EPI)

	Whole Sample (Cancers + Controls)	
	Spearman's rho: $-.270$ ($p < .0001$)	
	Cancer Patients Only	
	Spearman's rho: $-.199$ ($p < .01$)	
	Difference between Cancers and Controls	
Cancer $\bar{x} = 4.56$		Control $\bar{x} = 4.56$
	Mann-Whitney U: $p > .50$	

TABLE 6
EXTRAVERSION SCALE OF THE EPI:
CORRELATION BETWEEN E-EPI AND AGE

Cancers		Controls
	Spearman rho = .0598 ($p > .20$)	
	Uncorrected for Social Desirability	
Cancers	(N = 456)	Controls
$\bar{x} = 11.32$		$\bar{x} = 11.41$
	Mann-Whitney U: $p > .40$	
	Corrected for Social Desirability	
Cancers	(N = 289)	Controls
$\bar{x} = 11.61$		$\bar{x} = 11.70$
	Mann-Whitney U: $p > .45$	

Eysenck (1965) has suggested that both smoking and lung cancer may be a a product of a common cause in a personality factor of extraversion. He has shown that cigarette smokers, if not pipe smokers, are extraverted (Eysenck, 1964; Eysenck, 1963), and in support of his suggestion that the extraverted person is more likely to develop lung cancer, he cites a joint paper with D. M. Kissen. In this, lung cancer patients between 55 and 64 years were found to be more extraverted than controls ($p<.05$), and this was even more marked provided only patients with a history of psychosomatic disorder were considered in this age group (TABLE 7). On the present sample considering patients with a history of psychosomatic disorder alone from the age group 55–64, the mean score for the lung cancer group does not differ significantly from the controls (Mann-Whitney U Test: $p>.13$). Although these findings could hardly be said to support Eysenck's argument, we cannot rule it out of court yet either. If, as seems likely, however, relatively low extraversion as compared to that of other cigarette smokers is a feature of the lung cancer patient, this factor can aid in identifying the cancer-prone (Kissen, 1965b).

Rudimentary figures on smoking habits have been extracted on our sample that show broadly the same trends as previously reported by D. M. Kissen (1963) (TABLE 8), but more detailed and sophisticated analyses have yet to be carried out.

TABLE 7

EXTRAVERSION SCALE OF THE EPI:
PSYCHOSOMATIC PATIENTS AGED 55–64

Cancers	(N = 143)	Controls
$\bar{x} = 11.58$		$\bar{x} = 10.84$
	Mann-Whitney U Test: $p < .13$	

TABLE 8

SMOKING HABITS

Current + Ex-Smokers	Cancers	Controls
Pipe smokers	17.06	15.93
Cigarette smokers (all)	94.05	93.22
Cigarettes (1–14)	27.78	34.24
Cigarettes (15–24)	42.46	37.63
Cigarettes (25+)	24.21	21.70
All figures percent	N = 252	N = 295

Psychosocial variables such as the patient's recollection of various adversities and disturbing situations in adulthood and childhood have also been recorded on the same large samples of cancer patients and controls. To control for possible age effects, only the 55–64 age group was examined. There is no significant difference in numbers of lung cancer patients compared to controls reporting any one or more adversities in adult life ($x^2 = .2 : p > .50$). Similarly, there is no significant difference between cancers and controls in numbers reporting various deprivations and adversities before age 15, such as death of father or death of mother (TABLE 9). Interviews were much more structured and shorter than they were in D. M. Kissen's earlier studies (1967).

Potentially important differences *were* found in the way in which reports of adult adversities emerged in the course of the interview with the patient. During the course of the interview, many adverse events and situations in the adult life of the patient were touched on or casually elicited in enquiries as to the medical history of the patient's relatives and his relationships with his workmates and boss, to give only two examples. These reported events or situations were recorded under the heading Incidental Reports. At the end of each interview, the patient was asked the general question, "At some time, recently or long ago, you probably experienced some event or state of affairs that you found particularly disturbing, upsetting, or worrying?" The interviewer then paused for an answer. Any disturbances reported at this point were recorded under the heading Immediate Reports. If there was no reply, the interviewer proceeded: "Did this have anything to do with your work, your boss, or your colleagues at work? Money worries? Your married life?" and so on. Any events reported at this point were recorded under the heading Prompted Reports. It was thus possible for both cancer patients and controls to report adverse situations in adult life as Incidental Reports, Immediate Reports, and Prompted Reports.

There is no difference between cancer patients and controls in the way in which they tend to report events other than deaths (TABLE 10).

Regarding reports of deaths, there was no difference in the numbers of cancer

TABLE 9
REPORTED CHILDHOOD ADVERSITIES:*
INCIDENCE IN CANCERS AND CONTROLS

	x^2	
Death of father	1.06	$p > .30$
Death of mother	1.84	$p < .20$
Death of sibling	0.27	$p > .50$
Father away	0.05	$p > .50$
Mother away	0.85	$p > .30$
n cancer = 194	n controls = 217	N = 411

* All adversities pre-15 years of age.

TABLE 10
EMERGENCE OF REPORTS OF ADULT ADVERSITIES: PATIENTS REPORTING
ANY ONE OR MORE DISTURBANCES OTHER THAN DEATHS

	x^2 Cancers versus Controls	
	x^2	p
Immediate reports	0.00	$< .50$
Prompted reports	0.84	$< .50$
Incidental reports	0.33	$< .50$
	n = 66 cancers, 56 controls	
	Total N = 122	

patients and controls reporting at least one death immediately or when prompted. (TABLE 11). But more lung cancer patients report at least one death incidentally $x^2 = .82 : p < .01$), in spite of the fact that no more cancer patients report at least one death overall (Immediate plus Prompted plus Incidental reports) than do the controls. We infer that the cancer group, in contrast to the controls, report deaths incidentally rather than associate them with a question about disturbing or worrying events. Whether this is because they are less heavily invested emotionally in people or because they tend to deny disturbing emotions is not clear, but an inability to consciously accept and express disturbing emotion fits in with the hypothesis of D. M. Kissen that lung cancer patients as a group are less able to discharge emotion.

A new 11-item scale, here called Awareness of Autonomic Activity (AAA), was constructed by amending original work by Mandler, Mandler, and Uviller (1958). The following is a specimen item (TABLE 12): "When you are feeling worried, anxious, or frightened, how often are you aware of the beating of your heart or palpitations?" Scores for each item are awarded on a five-point self-rating scale, and scores for items are summed to produce an AAA score for each individual. Other items cover, besides heart rate and gastrointestinal disturbances, respiration, muscle tension, etc. The scale is, of course, unvalidated in its present form, and no figures are available for reliability.

This scale was administered to 120 lung cancer subjects and 167 controls, making 287 in all. A Spearman Rho showed that AAA correlated negatively but significantly with age, and since the cancer sample was again older than the control, an Analysis of Covariance was completed, finding for differences between lung cancers and controls over and above age effects. This shows (TABLE 13) a difference between cancers and controls at $p < .05$ when all liars are included

TABLE 11

EMERGENCE OF REPORTS OF ADULT ADVERSITIES: PATIENTS REPORTING ANY ONE OR MORE DEATHS

	x^2 Cancers versus Controls	
	x^2	p
Immediate reports	0.82	$< .50$
Prompted reports	1.32	$< .30$
Incidental reports	6.60	$< .01$
	n = 66 cancers, 56 controls Total N = 122	

TABLE 12

AWARENESS OF AUTONOMIC ACTIVITY SCALE: SPECIMEN ITEMS

1. When you are feeling worried, anxious or frightened, HOW OFTEN ARE YOU AWARE OF THE BEATING OF YOUR HEART OR PALPITATIONS?

	seldom	sometimes	often	
NEVER				ALWAYS

2. When you are feeling worried, anxious or frightened, HOW OFTEN DO YOU GET THE FEELING THAT YOUR STOMACH IS RISING OR FALLING AS YOU MIGHT EXPERIENCE IN A LIFT OR A FEELING LIKE "BUTTERFLIES IN THE STOMACH"?

TABLE 13

AWARENESS OF AUTONOMIC ACTIVITY: ANALYSIS OF COVARIANCE

Sample Uncontrolled for Social Desirability ($L \rightarrow \infty$) N = 286
Lung cancers score lower than controls F = 3.283 (df = 2 and 283): $p < .05$
Sample Controlled for Social Desirability ($L \rightarrow 4$) N = 110
Lung cancers score lower than controls F = 7.131 (df = 2 and 106): $p < .005$

and at $p<.005$ when the high liars are excluded. Including all liars, the cancer mean is 10.56 and the control is 12.37, and excluding high liars, the cancer mean is 11.84 and the control is 14.98.

It would be premature at date of writing to go into the complex interaction effects of age, diagnosis, and presence or absence of a history of psychosomatic illness. Some of these effects have been worked out on age-matched samples, but a complex multivariate analysis of variance with disproportionality is planned as soon as computer programs become available. Until then, it would be fascinating but unwise to theorize, because the available information is incomplete.

Nevertheless, at this stage it is in order to discuss the theoretical significance of the finding of significantly lower awareness of autonomic activity in lung cancer patients as compared to controls. On this sample, scores for both lung cancers and controls correlate highly with scores on N-MPI and with scores on N-SMPI after the effects of age have been partialled out. This strongly suggests that per-

TABLE 14
AWARENESS OF AUTONOMIC ACTIVITY:
CORRELATIONS WITH N-SMP, N-EPI AND E-EPI

AAA and N-EPI (Spearman's rho)	rs = 0.59 $p < .001$
AAA and E-EPI (Spearman's rho)	rs = −0.032 $p > .50$
AAA and N-SMP (Kendall's tau partialling out age) T = 0.334	$p > .00003$

haps the most important component of what we have been measuring all along in our studies as lower neuroticism in lung cancer patients is a lack of awareness of autonomic activity.

Mandler and others using the original APQ scale from which the AAA was derived have shown that people who experience less autonomic activity actually *have* less, although those who experience little are aware of even less than they have and those who report much exaggerate what they have (Mandler *et al.*, 1958; Mandler and Kremen, 1958; Mandler *et al.*, 1961). Quite apart from work with this particular kind of scale, the literature of psychophysiology contains many reports of work linking scales of manifest anxiety, neuroticism, and related phenomena to actual autonomic activity (Duffy, 1962). It seems probable, then, that lung cancer patients actually have less autonomic activity.

To be more specific yet, inspection of the items of the AAA scale suggests that high scorers probably experience much activity of the sympathetic or adrenergic division of the autonomic nervous system, and conversely, the lung cancer patients with lower scores may experience reduced activity of the sympathetic nervous system. In terms of modern psychophysiological arousal theory, the lung cancer patients may have low arousal (Duffy, 1962) and low emotional lability, or in Wenger's older conception of autonomic balance, they may be parasympathetically dominant (Wenger, 1941 & 1942; Wenger & Ellington, 1943). In any case, one hardly needs to point out how findings at the psychological level lead to work at the psychophysiological level and beyond that have implications in the biochemical field of hormone secretions.

Finally, on the one hand it is possible that the low neuroticism and lack of awareness of autonomic activity associated with lung cancer patients represents the actual presence of *less* autonomic, or more specifically, sympathetic, activity. On the other hand it may be that a psychological mechanism similar to denial or repression such as reported by Bahnson and Bahnson (1966) is at work here, and cancer patients may actually have greater or equal sympathetic activity while at the same time contriving to deny it to themselves or at least remaining unaware of it. Work on two levels simultaneously (on the psychological level of denial and repression and on the psychophysiological level of concurrent autonomic activity) is being undertaken in an attempt to throw light on the relative importance of these two possibilities.

Summary

To summarize:

1. The original work of D. M. Kissen showing lower neuroticism in lung cancer patients as measured with the Short MPI has been replicated and confirmed.

2. Additional confirmation comes from use of a newer neuroticism scale also showing significantly lower neuroticism in lung cancer patients.

3. The tendency of lung cancer patients' answers on a neuroticism scale to be less affected by social desirability response set than those of controls is commented upon.

4. Failure to find significant differences between lung cancer patients and controls on an extraversion scale is discussed in relation to Eysenck's work and is noted as another possible way of distinguishing potential sufferers from lung cancer from the mass of cigarette smokers.

5. Differences between lung cancers and controls in the way in which psychosocial data emerge at interview are reported in connection with the patient's reporting of deaths, and these differences are related to Kissen's hypothesis of lack of outlet for emotional discharge.

6. Differences between lung cancer patients and controls in awareness of autonomic activity are reported and discussed in relation to the twin possibilities: (a) that cancer patients actually *have* less autonomic or sympathetic activity and (b) that they have as much autonomic activity as controls, but tend to repress or deny awareness of it.

Acknowledgments

We acknowledge with gratitude the contributions made to this investigation by Miss Dorothy D. Hayes, Cert. Soc. Stud., Cert. Inst. Almon., and Miss Edith M. Taylor, Cert. Soc. Stud., Cert. Inst. Almon., who collected much of the psychosocial data, by Mr. R. A. Elton, B. A., and Mr. P. A. K. Covey-Crump, B.A., Department of Statistics, University of Glasgow, who vetted the statistics, and by Miss Olive F. Pogue, B.Sc., who collected some of the psychological data and together with Miss Elizabeth H. Girvan performed most of the calculations.

References

BAHNSON, C. B. & M. B. BAHNSON. 1966. Role of the ego defences: Denial and repression in the etiology of malignant neoplasm. Ann. N. Y. Acad. Sci. **125:** 827–845.

DUFFY, E. 1962. Activation and Behaviour. John Wiley & Sons, Inc. New York, N. Y.

EYSENCK, H. J. 1959a. Das Maudsley Personality Inventory bestimmer der neurotischen tendency und extraversion. Z. Exp. Angew. Psychol. **6:** 167–190.

EYSENCK, H. J. 1959b. Manual of the Maudsley Personality Inventory. University of London Press. London, England.

EYSENCK, H. J. 1963. Smoking, personality and psychosomatic disorders. J. Psychosom. Res. **7:** 107–130.

EYSENCK, H. J. 1964. Personality and cigarette smoking. Life Sci. **3:** 777–792.

EYSENCK, H. J. 1965. Smoking Health and Personality. Wiedenfeld and Nicholson. London, England.

EYSENCK, H. J. & S. B. G. EYSENCK. 1963a. The validity of questionnaires and rating assessments of extraversion and neuroticism and their factorial validity. Brit. J. Psychol. **54:** 51–62.

EYSENCK, H. J. & S. B. G. EYSENCK. 1964. Manual of the Eysenck Personality Inventory. University of London Press. London, England.

EYSENCK, S. B. G. & H. J. EYSENCK. 1963b. An experimental investigation of desirability response set in a personality questionnaire. Life Sci. **5:** 343–355.

GIBSON, H. B. 1962. The lie scale of the Maudsley Personality Inventory. Acta Psychol. **20:** 18–23.

KISSEN, D. M. 1963. Personality characteristics in males conducive to lung cancer. Brit. J. Med. Psychol. **36:** 27–36.

KISSEN, D. M. 1964. Relationship between lung cancer, cigarette smoking, inhalation and personality. Brit. J. Med. Psychol. **37:** 203–216.

KISSEN, D. M. 1965. The possible contribution of the psychosomatic approach to the prevention of lung cancer. The Medical Officer (No. 2996) **CXIV** (26): 343–345.

KISSEN, D. M. 1966a. The significance of personality in lung cancer in men. Ann. N. Y. Acad. Sci. **125**(3): 820–826.

KISSEN, D. M. 1966b. Psychosomatic histories in the relatives of male hospital chest unit patients with special reference to lung cancer. Int. J. Soc. Psychiat. **12**: 199–208.

KISSEN, D. M. 1967. Psychosocial factors, personality and lung cancer in men aged 55–64. Brit. J. Med. Psychol. **40**: 29–43.

KISSEN, D. M. & H. J. EYSENCK. 1962. Personality in male lung cancer patients. J. Psychosom. Res. **6**: 123–127.

MANDLER, G. & I. KREMEN. 1958. Autonomic feedback: A correlational study. J. Personality **26**: 388–399 & **28**: 545.

MANDLER, G., J. M. MANDLER, L. KREMEN & R. D. SHOLITON. 1961. The response to threat: relations among verbal and physiological indices. Psychol. Monogr. **75**(9): (Whole No. 513).

MANDLER, G., J. M. MANDLER & E. T. VILLER. 1958. Automic feedback: The perception of autonomic activity. J. Abnorm. & Soc. Psychol. **56**: 367–373.

WENGER, M. A. 1941. The measurement of individual differences in autonomic balance. Psychosom. Med. **3**: 427–434.

WENGER, M. A. 1942. The stability of measurement of autonomic balance. Psychosom. Med. **4**: 94–95.

WENGER, M. A. & M. ELLINGTON. 1943. The measurement of autonomic balance in children. Method and normative data. Psychosom. Med. **5**: 241–253.

DISCUSSION OF THE PAPER

DR. LEONARD M. LIEGNER (*St. Luke's Hospital Center, New York, N.Y.*): I realize that society is changing, and that we are seeing a change in attitudes. How does this study explain or concern itself with the rising incidence of cancer of the lung? I remember that in the 1940's, in medical school, it was a rare occasion to see a cancer of the lung at autopsy. Now, it is a most common disease. Could you explain this, please?

MR. BROWN: I doubt that I could relate the rising incidence of cancer of the lung to data from this study. However, I wonder whether possibly, and this is merely heresay, it may be related to the rising consumption of cigarettes in the older generation today. I am sorry that I cannot answer any more definitely than that.

UNIDENTIFIED SPEAKER: There are a few points I should like to comment on, and about which I would like some clarification from you. The limited experience I have indicated that the postlobectomy lung cancer patient actually lies, in the sense that, for a long time, he minimizes the number of cigarettes that he smokes. This is one area in which, as with other drug addicts, it is very difficult to arrive at the truth. It is not at all easy to get accurate cigarette-smoking histories from these people, which certainly is in contrast to what one generally says.

The other point is that I think it is misleading to use the word "neuroticism," because (at any rate, as many of us see it) these patients, even prior to any cancer or lesion, seem to have certain kinds of character neuroses and certain kinds of characterological anomalies. They are not suffering from psychoneuroses; this word, I think, tends to be misleading. Similarly, there is some semantic confusion around Eysenck's views about extraversion, which certainly do not coincide with those of Jung, who invented the term.

I also think that there are some other difficulties with these questionnaires, as you have given them, because they do not tap what one gets in psychiatric interviews with these people. One finds that what is important is the total life cycle and how these people may have changed during it. They may have had, at one time, perhaps superficial relationships with large numbers of people, and may have been socially active in a superficial sense, but they are poor in relating deeply to people, and later on, as they get discouraged (which, I think, precedes the onset of the cancer), their relationships with other people, and the affective communication with other people, is very bad. So it seems as though the test describes more of a cross section, rather than what is going on in the total history of a person.

MR. BROWN: I will start with the question about smoking and the accuracy of the patient's reports. We have not tested this accuracy, as I suppose we might. It is possible to do so by having the patients observed on the wards, and so on. I should imagine that possibly the social desirability of responses may influence reports of smoking. To pass on to your comments about Eysenck's scales, let me say this: Eysenck's idea of neuroticism and his ideas of extraversion are, I must agree, peculiar to Eysenck. We have been trying to break down the concept of neuroticism, using, for instance, the AAA scale, which I was talking about, and we think that we have succeeded in doing this to some extent. We found a component of it, which at least has a more meaningful face validity. The important point is that it does not matter what the neuroticism actually turns out to be in the long run. The differences between the cancers and controls are there, and keep turning up. Our next step now is to find out in more detail what this means.

EGO DEFENSES IN CANCER PATIENTS

Marjorie Brooks Bahnson*

Eastern Pennsylvania Psychiatric Institute
Philadelphia, Pa.

and

Claus Bahne Bahnson*

Eastern Pennsylvania Psychiatric Institute, Institute of Pennsylvania Hospital, Philadelphia, Pa., and University of Connecticut, Storrs, Conn.

Theoretical Introduction

A theory of complementarity between physiological and psychological regression has been proposed previously by us (Bahnson & Bahnson, 1964a & 1966). From this general psychosomatic theory, we have predicted that cancer patients make extensive use of repressive and denying ego defenses in order to cope with a number of psychological conflicts related to loss and depression, aggression, hostility and dominance, and libidinal as well as narcissistic creative urges. Within the framework of this theory of complementarity between different ego defensive modalities and psychosomatic manifestations of repression, the ego defenses repression and projection are conceptualized as extreme, opposing, and mutually exclusive coping mechanisms. Ego adaptive rather than ego defensive coping patterns are represented somewhere near a midpoint between the operation of repression and projection.

The type of repression specified herein is secondary repression in contrast to primary repression, which, according to psychoanalytic theory, antecedes the projecting and displacing defenses that are engaged when the primarily repressed impulse returns and is discharged in action or ideation. Secondary repression refers to a continual defense process that successfully prevents the conflictual impulse from ever discharging in ideational or behavioral form. Thus, according to our conceptual framework, a person who utilizes repression blocks any behavioral or cognitive outlet of the disturbing impulse; rather, he must cope with the drive, not psychologically, but somatically, through internal discharge mechanisms.

In this more specific definition of repression, the most extreme examples of both defenses, secondary repression and projection, are thought to operate substitutively, or temporally exclusive of each other. Most persons utilize both defenses to varying degrees, but each person at particular points in time probably could be described by his tendency to utilize one defense more readily than the other. If, for the moment, one disregards ego adaptive mechanisms and considers only ego defensive solutions, one may conclude that absence of projection indicates the operation of repression, whereas absence of repression indicates the operation of projection. This conceptualization is central to our theory of complementarity and provides a necessary foundation for the hypothesis evaluated herein; i.e., that cancer patients make use of projective defenses to a lesser extent than do normal subjects.

As has been demonstrated so aptly by the Midtown Manhattan Study (Srole *et al.*, 1961; Langner & Michael, 1963), most "normal" subjects definitely make

* Formerly at Jefferson Medical College, Department of Psychiatry, Philadelphia, Pa.

use of neurotic defenses. Such occurrences, which obviously must be interpreted in cultural and social psychological terms, shall not be elaborated upon here, but the fact that neuroticism is widespread in our culture allows us to expect that a normal random sample of the population will include subjects exhibiting projective defenses in addition to others with adaptive and nondefensive coping patterns. Theoretically, then, the expectation that cancer patients should show less projection on tests and procedures designed to measure this dimension than a matched population sample is basically sound.

Hypotheses

In order to permit its testing by the particular methodology used in this study, the hypothesis that cancer patients utilize less projection (and by implication, more repression) than do normal control subjects can be operationally expressed in the following way. Cancer patients will be less prone than normal subjects to assign to neutral environmental events disturbing, distressing, or threatening emotional states such as anxiety, depression, hostility, guilt, or socially undesirable attitudes. To express the same tendency reciprocally, cancer patients, compared to normal subjects, are prone to assign more positive emotional attitudes to the environment, such as feelings of security, happiness, friendliness, and self-acceptance, as well as more socially desirable attitudes, because the lack of projection of undesirable qualities defended against predisposes these subjects to perceive the environment as nonthreatening, benign, and socially desirable. Since the methodology used in this study makes use of self-referent and environment-referent (projected) check lists comprised of negative and positive polarities of adjectives, and of affirmation and denial of these adjectives as appropriately descriptive, these hypotheses can be expressed in different parallel ways. One way of expressing proneness to assign to the environment disturbing emotions is to affirm more unpleasant and threatening adjectives that refer to the environment than such adjectives that refer to oneself. Another way of expressing the same is to deny more positive and desirable adjectives that refer to the environment than such adjectives that refer to oneself. Similarly, assignment of positive emotional states to the environment can be expressed either by affirming more pleasant and desirable, or by denying more disturbing and undesirable, adjectives that refer to the environment than those that refer to oneself.

A secondary hypothesis has been specified on the following basis. Several studies, including our own, have suggested that cancer patients have special problems with the resolution of depression and despair after loss of important cathected objects or circumstances. Since, according to psychoanalytic theory, the most intense ego defenses (in this case in the form of repression) are mobilized when the threatening emotion or impulse is most alarming, we expect that cancer patients, in comparison with normal controls, will repress more (project less) on this dimension than on other emotional and interpersonal dimensions not considered to be as problematic for these patients. The specific additional hypothesis is: Cancer patients and normal control subjects will be most discrepant on the dimension of depression, a feeling state that cancer patients will be especially unlikely to project onto a neutral environmental event.

Subjects

Thirty white males, ages 34 to 64 (mean of 53.9), comprised the cancer subjects, all currently in treatment at the time of testing. The majority was contacted through a general hospital outpatient clinic (Jefferson Medical College Hospital), others from the inpatient services of three general hospitals (Jefferson

Medical College Hospital, Philadelphia, Lawrence, and Memorial Hospitals, New London, and Backus Hospital, Norwich, Conn.).† Sites of cancer for these subjects were as follows: Nine lung, six colon, two bladder, two rectum, two neck, two lymphoma, and one each of bronchus, parotid, ileum, kidney, prostate, generalized abdominal, and abdominal mesentery. None of these patients had been informed of his diagnosis, nor would any consciously acknowledge his illness to be malignant. This was ascertained during a clinical interview in which each patient talked about his illness and life situation.

Sixty-four randomly selected white males from southeast Connecticut, ages 35 to 65 (mean of 52.2), served as the normal subjects. These men, well and normally functioning, had been drawn by a street-sampling technique from the total Standard Metropolitan Statistical Area population as controls in a larger ongoing study on sociopsychological aspects of coronary heart disease.

Procedure

Data from two adjective checklists were collected from the subjects according to the following procedure. The subject first checked a 50-word alphabetized list of adjectives, the Bahnson Adjective Check List (BACL), according to his present mood state, having been instructed to check the words differentially to describe his feeling state: "Definitely applies," "Probably so, or somewhat applies," "Probably does not apply" (or "Don't know"), or "Definitely does not apply."

The subject then listened to a neutral stimulus (regular temporal and unstructured clicks of white noise), during which he checked another 50-word alphabetized list of "projective" adjectives, the Bahnson Projective Check List (BPCL), applicable to qualities in the environment (e.g. dark, barren, clean, pretty), marking each word again in one of four ways, according to how this auditory stimulus sounded to him.

The two lists of adjectives describe mood and emotion in terms of five bipolar dimensions: Anxiety (anxiety +, secureness −), Hedonic Level (depression +, elation −), Hostility (hostility +, friendliness −), Guilt (guilt +, self-acceptance −), and Social Interaction (dominance +, submission −) (TABLE 1). Note that the + sign has been given to the pole carrying adjectives that generally reflect psychopathology.

The four checking categories on each adjective checklist were reduced to two scoring categories by combining the number of adjectives checked as either "Definitely applies" or "Probably so, or somewhat applies" into one scoring category, *Affirmation*, and combining the number of adjectives checked as either "Probably does not apply" or "Definitely does not apply" into the other scoring category, *Denial.* In the very few instances where particular adjectives were not checked at all, the score was determined by prorating.

Then the following steps were made to obtain what is termed "Projection Score," a single score for each of the five dimensions:

1. The ratios of projected checklist affirmation to self-referent checklist affirmation; that is, BPCL ÷ BACL for Affirmation, (BPCL/BACL Affirm), and projected checklist Denial to self-referent checklist Denial, (BPCL/BACL Deny), were computed for each of the two poles of the five dimensions.

† The cancer patients and normal subjects residing in Connecticut were drawn from a larger group of the subjects studied in the research project Socio-Psychological Factors in Myocardial Infarction, supported by grant HE 07522 from the National Heart Institute and conducted by W. I. Wardwell and C. B. Bahnson.

TABLE 1
ADJECTIVES COMPRISING THE BAHNSON CHECK LISTS

Bahnson Adjective Check List (BACL)		Bahnson Projective Check List (BPCL)	
Anxiety		Anxiety	
Anxiety +	Secureness −	Anxiety +	Secureness −
afraid	calm	breathless	content
anxious	comfortable	disturbed	peaceful
frightened	relaxed	nervous	trustful
jittery	safe	uneasy	restful
scared	secure	upset	at ease
Hedonic Level		Hedonic Level	
Depression +	Elation −	Depression +	Elation −
blue	cheerful	barren	light
gloomy	elated	dark	playful
hopeless	glad	dead	sparkling
sad	happy	desolate	gay
unhappy	pleased	heavy	joyful
Hostility		Hostility	
Hostility +	Friendliness −	Hostility +	Friendliness −
aggressive	affectionate	rude	gentle
angry	friendly	sharp	mild
bitter	good-natured	stinging	smooth
hateful	kindly	war-like	soothing
irritable	warm-hearted	savage	soft
Guilt		Guilt	
Guilt +	Self-Acceptance −	Guilt +	Self-Acceptance −
ashamed	decent	foul	clean
guilt	honest	rotten	pretty
no good	proud of myself	ugly	pure
sinful	self-confident	evil	noble
unworthy	upright	dirty	confident
Social Interaction		Social Interaction	
Dominance +	Submission −	Dominance +	Submission −
bossy	dependent	commanding	delicate
dominating	helpless	firm	hesitating
forceful	submissive	powerful	frail
independent	timid	stern	vague
strong	weak	penetrating	yielding

2. The ratio for the BPCL/BACL Affirm −pole was subtracted from the ratio for the BPCL/BACL Affirm +pole, and the ratio for the BPCL/BACL Deny +pole was subtracted from the ratio for the BPCL/BACL Deny −pole.

3. These two ratio differences for Affirmation and Denial were then added algebraically.‡

‡ Since the two poles of a dimension utilize adjectives opposite in quality (e.g. beautiful −, ugly +, according to the terminology of this paper) and since the operation of denial may logically be considered the negation of affirmation, in order to obtain a single score incorporating both bipolarity *and* mode of response, two operations must follow: (a) Affirmation +pole must be equated with Denial −pole and (b) Affirmation −pole must be equated with Denial +pole. Since denial checking on the +pole is logically the affirmation of −pole qualities and vice versa, for the affirmation mode of response the −pole was subtracted from the +pole, whereas for the denial mode of response the +pole was subtracted from the −pole. An alternative operation to obtain the same score is to add Affirmation +pole to Denial −pole and add Affirmation −pole to Denial +pole, and then summate these totals.

This single score indicated for a particular dimension the extent to which a subject projected emotional qualities onto the neutral stimulus (as measured by the BPCL), compared with his attributing these qualities to himself (as measured by the BACL). The Projection Score is either positive or negative, corresponding to the polarity of the dimension.

Results

The mean difference in projection scores between the normal control and cancer groups for each dimension of emotion and for the five dimensions totaled were compared by means of the t-test (Edwards, 1960; Hays, 1963). These results are presented in TABLE 2.

All mean differences occurred in the predicted direction. The cancer group scored below the normal control group in the projection of anxiety, depression, hostility, guilt, and dominance. The probability of obtaining these mean differences on the basis of chance ranges from beyond the .005 point for the dimension of depression, to somewhat less than .12 for the dimension of dominance. As predicted, the greatest mean difference between cancer and control subjects was obtained for depression. Although the mean difference between the two groups on dominance is not statistically significant, the significance of the mean difference for the five dimensions totaled is less than .001.

Mean total denial and affirmation on either pole of the dimensions were compared between the two groups. These results are presented in TABLE 3, where the summation of projection scores by mode of response (i.e., denial or affirmation) for either +pole or −pole of the dimensions totaled are evaluated by means of t-tests of the mean differences found between the normal control group

TABLE 2

COMPARISON OF MEAN PROJECTION SCORES FOR EACH DIMENSION OF EMOTION FOR NORMAL CONTROL AND CANCER GROUPS

Dimensions of Emotion	Normal Control Group: Mean & S.D.	Cancer Group: Mean & S.D.	Mean Difference	t*	p†
Anxiety	1.245 3.291	−0.691 4.112	1.936	2.451	<.01
Hedonic level	3.799 2.776	1.724 3.311	2.075	3.173	<.005
Hostility	2.296 3.245	0.667 3.321	1.629	2.252	<.02
Guilt	2.056 2.047	1.099 2.409	0.957	1.995	<.025
Social interaction	0.753 2.498	0.053 2.609	0.700	1.250	<.12
Total	10.148 8.439	2.853 10.709	7.295	3.578	<.001
Age	52.2	53.9			
Number	64	30			

* All F ratios testing for homogeneity of variance were not significant at the .05 level.

† The probability values have been determined for a one-tailed test of significance for 92 degrees of freedom.

TABLE 3

COMPARISON OF MEAN TOTAL PROJECTION SCORES FOR MODE OF RESPONSE ON EACH POLE OF THE DIMENSIONS FOR THE NORMAL CONTROL AND CANCER GROUPS

Mode of Response for Each Pole	Normal Control Group: Mean & S.D.	Cancer Group: Mean & S.D.	Mean Difference	t*	p†
$\Sigma \frac{BPL}{ACL}$	14.901	10.069	4.832	4.478	$< .001$
Deny, − poles	4.694	5.260			
$\Sigma \frac{BPL}{ACL}$	2.826	3.972	1.146	2.741	$< .005$
Affirm, − poles	1.713	2.231			
$\Sigma \frac{BPL}{ACL}$	6.721	7.405	.684	0.860	$< .20$
Deny, + poles	3.521	3.748			
$\Sigma \frac{BPL}{ACL}$	4.605	3.355	1.250	1.522	$= .08$
Affirm, + poles	3.586	3.971			

* All F ratios testing for homogeneity of variance were not significant at the .05 level.

† The probability values have been determined for a one-tailed test of significance for 92 degrees of freedom.

and the cancer group. These mean differences again occurred according to prediction. The normal subjects obtained higher total projection scores from denying −pole adjectives (i.e., adjectives with a pleasant or socially desirable connotation) than did the cancer subjects ($p < .001$), while the cancer subjects obtained higher total projection scores from affirming −pole adjectives than did the normal subjects ($p < .005$). These two statements are, of course, reciprocal, according to our statement of the hypothesis tested. The mean differences in denying and affirming +pole adjectives do not attain statistical significance, although the trend of the differences are consistent both with prediction and with the direction of the differences for the −poles. On the +poles, the cancer group projected through denial more adjectives ($p < .20$), and conversely, through affirmation, fewer adjectives ($p = .08$), than did the normal control group.

This analysis indicates that the cancer subjects definitely described the "environment" by affirming −pole adjectives (here such qualities as clean, gentle, peaceful, pure, trustful, etc.), in contrast to the control subjects, who strongly tended to affirm the opposite qualities in their description of the environment. Or stated in another way, cancer subjects tended through denial of +pole adjectives (here such qualities as dirty, frail, nervous, rude, ugly, etc.) to describe the environment as good and desirable, while normal subjects quite definitely projected through denial of emotionally positive, pleasant, and desirable qualities in describing the environment.

Comparable adjective checklist data on two additional groups of subjects, which could serve, in addition to the normal street sample, as controls for the cancer group, became available shortly after the above results were formally presented. Their description and comparison with the cancer group provide both an expanded base of control subjects for reference and an interesting, theoretically relevant distribution of projection scores, since the utilization of denial and repression is expected, according to our general theory of complementarity of somatic and psychologic illness, to be less pronounced in other somatic groups than in cancer, but generally greater than in well, normal subjects.

Thirty-three white males, ages 36 to 63 (mean age of 50.9 years), hospitalized following a first myocardial infarction (coronary group), and 26 white males, ages 38 to 64 (mean age of 50.4 years), hospitalized for various serious illnesses and accidents (mixed sick group), were given the two adjective checklists as described above.§ Data collection on these subjects was carried out during the same time period that all subjects were studied. The mixed sick group comprised cases of the following: Six pyloric or duodenal ulcer, including one with cirrhosis and esophageal varices, two acute appendix with abdominal abscesses, three herniated lumbar discs, two third-degree burns, five hyperplastic prostate, and one each of serious fractures, emphysema, acute bronchial asthma, nephrectomy, uretheral lithotomy, cirrhosis of liver, viral hepatitis, and idiopathic thrombocytopenic purpura bleeding.

Analyses of mean differences between the coronary and mixed sick groups showed no differences statistically significant at a probability level less than .20. Therefore, the two groups were combined. The means and standard deviations of projection scores on the five dimensions of emotion and their total for the two groups, combined and singly, are presented in TABLE 4, which includes the data for the normal control and cancer groups for easy comparison.

TABLE 4
MEANS AND STANDARD DEVIATIONS OF PROJECTION SCORES FOR EACH DIMENSION OF EMOTION FOR THE SUBJECT GROUPS

Dimension of emotion	Normal Group Mean & S.D.	Mixed Sick and Coronary Group Combined Mean & S.D.	Cancer Group Mean & S.D.	Mixed Sick Group Mean & S.D.	Coronary Group Mean & S.D.
Anxiety	1.245	0.903	−0.691	1.110	0.740
	3.291	4.079	4.112	4.200	4.039
Hedonic level	3.799	2.915	1.724	3.452	2.492
	2.776	3.323	3.311	3.698	2.985
Hostility	2.296	2.063	0.667	1.442	2.552
	3.245	3.269	3.321	3.536	3.006
Guilt	2.056	1.179	1.099	1.328	1.061
	2.047	2.719	2.409	3.190	2.326
Social interaction	0.753	1.127	0.053	0.644	1.508
	2.498	3.012	2.609	2.965	3.039
Total	10.148	8.187	2.852	7.976	8.354
	8.439	11.344	10.709	12.845	10.213
Mean age	52.2	50.7	53.9	50.4	50.9
Number	64	59	30	26	33

§ These subjects also are drawn from the Southeastern Connecticut Heart Study.

Results from mean difference evaluation of projective scores between the cancer group and coronary and mixed sick groups, combined and singly, are found in TABLE 5. Normal- and cancer-group comparisons have again been included for reference.

In summarizing the results from TABLE 5, the following points stand out. 1. The cancer group obtained lower mean projection scores than any of the control groups on each of the five dimensions and total, with the single exception of the coronary/cancer comparison on Guilt, for which the mean of the coronary group was just slightly lower than the cancer group. 2. In comparing the mean differences among the various control/cancer groups, the largest differences are between the normal and cancer groups for three of the dimensions: Anxiety, Hedonic Level, Guilt, and total projection score, while the largest mean differences are obtained between the coronary and cancer groups for the two dimen-

TABLE 5
COMPARISON OF MEAN PROJECTION SCORES FOR EACH DIMENSION OF EMOTION FOR CANCER AND COMPARISON GROUPS*

Dimensions of Emotion	Groups Compared	Mean Difference	t	p	Interpretation
Anxiety	normal/cancer	1.936	2.451	<.01	N > Ca
	coronary-sick/cancer	1.594	1.691	<.05	Cor-S > Ca
	coronary/cancer	1.431	1.392	<.08	Cor > Ca
	sick/cancer	1.801	1.618	<.06	S > Ca
Hedonic Level	normal/cancer	2.075	3.173	<.005	N > Ca
	coronary-sick/cancer	1.191	1.561	<.07	Cor-S > Ca
	coronary/cancer	0.768	0.968	<.18	Cor > Ca
	sick/cancer	1.728	1.845	<.04	S > Ca
Hostility	normal/cancer	1.629	2.252	<.02	N > Ca
	coronary-sick/cancer	1.396	1.848	<.04	Cor-S > Ca
	coronary/cancer	1.885	2.364	<.01	Cor > Ca
	sick/cancer	0.775	0.847	<.21	S > Ca
Guilt	normal/cancer	0.957	1.995	<.025	N >Ca
	coronary-sick/cancer	0.079	0.132	<.45	Cor-S ∼ Ca
	coronary/cancer	−0.038	0.058	>.50	Cor ∼ Ca
	sick/cancer	0.229	0.306	<.40	S ∼ Ca
Social Interaction	normal/cancer	0.700	1.250	<.12	N > Ca
	coronary-sick/cancer	1.074	1.620	<.06	Cor-S > Ca
	coronary/cancer	1.455	2.029	<.025	Cor > Ca
	sick/cancer	0.591	0.793	<.22	S > Ca
Total	normal/cancer	7.295	3.578	<.001	N > Ca
	coronary-sick/cancer	5.334	2.084	<.025	Cor-S > Ca
	coronary/cancer	5.501	2.087	<.025	Cor > Ca
	sick/cancer	5.123	1.628	<.06	S > Ca

* The normal/cancer comparisons have been included again in this table for ease of reference. Degrees of Freedom for computation of t are: normal/cancer = 92, coronary-sick/cancer = 87, coronary/cancer = 61, mixed sick/cancer = 54. The mean differences between the coronary and mixed sick groups for all dimensions were not statistically significant. F ratio computation indicated no significant departure from homogeneity of variance for any of the groups compared. Probability values have been determined for one-tailed tests of significance, with the single exception of the coronary/cancer comparison on the dimension of Guilt > in the interpretation column is to be read "higher projection score than." ∼ is to be read "neither higher nor lower projection score than."

sions: Hostility and Social Interaction. 3. Both coronary and mixed sick groups, singly or combined, showed projection scores significantly higher than the cancer group ($p < .05$), with the exception of Guilt. Such results would support the contention that the cancer subjects on this measurement most likely comprise a group distinct from the other two somatic groups.

Discussion

Previous research into psychosomatic aspects of neoplastic disease has resulted in two main trends for data interpretation. One group of workers has pointed toward loss, separation, depression, and despair as important antecedents to the manifest development of cancer (Greene, 1966; Greene *et al.*, 1956; LeShan, 1966; LeShan & Worthington, 1956a, 1956b; LeShan & Reznikoff, 1960; Meerloo, 1954; Kowal, 1955; Schmale, 1958; and Schmale & Iker, 1964, 1966); whereas another group, probably influenced by ego psychology, has commented on the characteristic inhibition, blandness, and denial in cancer patients (Kissen & Eysenck, 1962; Kissen, 1963, 1964, 1965, 1966a, 1966b, 1966c; Kissen & Rao, 1968; Blumberg *et al.*, 1954; Renneker, unpublished observations;† Bahnson & Bahnson, 1964a, 1964b, 1965a, 1965b, 1966). Although we have been impressed by depressive aspects in cancer patients, we have emphasized that repressive ego defenses are the most outstanding and characteristic features. The results obtained from our most recent study lend firm support for this latter hypothesis.

These results are significant for several reasons. First, they show for the cancer group a consistently decreased level of projection of unpleasant emotions on all the dimensions measured, statistically significant for all but one dimension. These differences between the two groups occurred in the predicted direction. Second, these results cannot be considered an artifact of checking style utilized on the two check lists, since the score used was a ratio, derived from dividing each projective checking category score by each self-reported category score. Individuals, of course, differ in their frames of reference, checking style, and test-taking attitudes, and the advantage of a ratio score derived from the checking of adjectives on two lists as compared with a simple frequency or difference score between the two lists, is that these individual differences are controlled for, thus permitting the evaluation of content of checking.

Also of special interest is the finding that the greatest discrepancies between the projection scores of normal control subjects and cancer patients were on the dimensions: Hedonic Level and Anxiety, followed by Hostility, Guilt, and Social Interaction, in that order. Since depression and anxiety are emotions that might be considered consequences of, rather than antecedents to, a subliminal knowledge in the subjects of the disease process, and since the projection score is computed on the basis of a ratio between projected and self-reported emotion, the question arose whether the low projection score simply might result from a higher degree of manifest depression and anxiety as reflected on the self-reporting check list. This was explored in the data, which clearly showed that the two groups hardly differed in the mean scores of self-reported distressing emotion (+poles on Hedonic Level and Anxiety dimensions). Therefore, the differences between the cancer and normal control groups reflect differences in projective checking, rather than differences in self-descriptive checking. This finding corroborates the interpretation that cancer patients project to a lesser extent (i.e., repress more) than do normal subjects.

† In a paper presented at the First Conference on Psychophysiological Aspects of Cancer, April, 1965, held by the New York Academy of Sciences, but not included in the subsequent, published monograph based on the conference.

That the difference in projection score between cancer and control subjects is least impressive on the Social Interaction dimension may derive from the particular ambiguity presented by the relative social desirability values implicit in its two opposite poles. Whereas friendliness decidedly is more desirable than hostility, or secureness more desirable than anxiety, submissiveness may be only slightly, if at all, more desirable than dominance for mature American males. The differences in means, although slight, however, are in the predicted direction, and do contribute to the overall difference in the total projection score, which is significant at a high level of probability.

The prediction that the lack of projection of distressing or conflictual emotions and attitudes to the environment in cancer patients would result in a more benign perception of this environment was also clearly borne out in the results. As indicated in TABLE 3, the cancer group showed significantly higher projection scores than normal control subjects when these were computed in terms of affirmation of pleasant, socially desirable, and nonthreatening emotions; whereas conversely, the normal control subjects obtained significantly higher projection scores in the case of denial of pleasant and desirable emotions. These results indicate that the cancer subjects we studied, when compared with the normal controls, extended to deny unpleasantness in the world around them, describing it instead, as a benign place in which "all is for the best." The absence of release of undesirable affect resulting in this Pollyanna outlook, is one of the strongest indicators of repression we found at work in these patients. Consistent with this result, although not significant, is the finding that cancer patients also have lower projection scores in terms of assigning unpleasant and threatening emotions to the "environment," and, correspondingly, higher scores of denial of such undesirable emotion.

This analysis indicates that cancer patients have lower projection scores not because they are unable to respond to the environment, but because they do not describe it in terms of negative or threatening emotions to the extent that normal subjects do. To us, the gratifying finding is that the double-barreled expectation of divergent projection by the two groups, which might have tended to obscure or negate each other (since the projection score for each dimension of emotion is derived from a composite of responses to plus and minus poles), were both clearly supported by the results. This particular pattern of results, supporting rather intricate and mutually obscuring predictions, could only have been obtained by chance at a very low level of probability.

The addition of two somatically ill comparison groups has confronted the question regarding the use of a street sample of well subjects, although matched for age, sex, and SES, as an adequate, valid, or meaningful control for a group of subjects whole illnesses are life-threatening, irrespective of these subjects denying, being unaware of, or acknowledging their conditions. The coronary and seriously ill patients, matched by age, sex, and SES with the cancer patients, were selected to duplicate these conditions. The differences in projection scores between the normal and cancer groups do hold up when the comparison group comprises patients seriously ill with diseases other than cancer. This finding indicates that the cancer patients' utilization of less projection cannot result merely from their being sick and/or hospitalized with a life-threatening illness, but must reflect other than circumstantial reactions to the illness. These results support our basic hypothesis about cancer patients and cast doubt on the frequently expressed belief that illness and life-threat are the main variables to facilitate the use of repression; on the contrary, for the dimensions Hostility and Social Interaction, the coronary group was more discrepant from the cancer group than was the normal group. Thus, on the basis of the levels of statistical significance obtained between the various mean differences (TABLE 5), the group of cancer patients in this study can be differentiated from groups of patients hospitalized with coronary heart disease and other serious diseases, illnesses, and accidents.

Whether the magnitude of the differences in ego defenses found in this study can be applied in a predictive diagnostic fashion at the present time is not the point for evaluation here. The fact that the distributions of projection scores overlap for the different groups studied here indicates that predicting "health" or "disease" for a given individual on the basis of this measure of ego defense is exceedingly tenuous for the simple reason that defensive ego characteristics very probably account for only a small proportion of the variance between cancer and noncancer groups. The answer to a future predictive approach must lie in a multifactorial discriminant analysis type of procedure by which improved assessments of ego functions comprise one of several interrelated predictive parameters. Certainly, the procedures used here to evaluate projection (and thereby to infer repression) must be refined and other complementary methods to assess ego functions must be developed. Further, methods need to be invented by which to determine the particular conditions that affect, and in which manner they affect, ego functioning. However, the first steps have been taken. Specific hypotheses were operationally stated, experimentally evaluated, and held to be basically tenable. From these results and the interpretation we have given them, we have concluded that the particular predictions made on the basis of the theoretical framework developed previously have been supported. We are proceeding with further research to verify these results and to amplify them with regard to age and types of cancer.

References

BAHNSON, C. B. & M. B. BAHNSON. 1964a. Cancer as an alternative to psychosis: A theoretical model of somatic and psychological regression. *In* Psychosomatic Aspects of Neoplastic Disease. D. M. Kisesen & L. L. LeShan, Eds. : 184–202. Pitman. London, England.

BAHNSON, C. B. & M. B. BAHNSON. 1964b. Denial and repression of primitive impulses and of disturbing emotions in patients with malignant neoplasms. *In* Psychosomatic Aspects of Neoplastic Disease. D. M. Kissen & L. L. LeShan, Eds. : 42–62. Pitman. London, England.

BAHNSON, C. B. 1965a. Psychodynamics of cancer. Presented at Fourth International Conference on Psychosomatic Aspects of Neoplastic Disease. Turin, Italy. (Paper available in mimeograph form.)

BAHNSON, C. B. & M. B. BAHNSON. 1965b. Ego defensive functioning in cancer patients: The utilization of denial and projected mood and emotion. Presented at Fourth International Conference on Psychosomatic Aspects of Neoplastic Disease. Turin, Italy. (Paper available in mimeograph form.)

BAHNSON, C. B. & M. B. BAHNSON. 1966. Role of the ego defenses: Denial and repression in the etiology of malignant neoplasm. Ann. N. Y. Acad. Sci. **125**(3): 827–845.

BLUMBERG, E. M., P. M. WEST & F. W. ELLIS. 1954. A possible relationship between psychosomatic factors and human cancer. Psychosom. Med. **16**: 277–286.

EDWARDS, A. L. 1960. Experimental Design in Psychological Research. Holt, Rinehart, and Winston. New York, N. Y.

GREENE, W., L. E. YOUNG & S. N. SWISHER. 1956. Psychological factors and reticuloendothelial disease. II. Observations on a group of women with lymphomas and leukemias. Psychosom. Med. **18**: 284–303.

GREENE, W. A. 1966. The psychosocial setting of the development of leukemia and lymphoma. Ann. N. Y. Acad. Sci. **125**(3): 794–801.

HAYS, W. L. 1963. Statistics for Psychologists. Holt, Rinehart and Winston. New York, N. Y.

KISSEN, D. M. & H. J. EYSENCK. 1962. Personality in male lung cancer patients. J. Psychosom. Res. **6**: 123.

KISSEN, D. M. 1963. Personality characteristics in males conducive to lung cancer. Brit. J. Med. Psychol. **36:** 27–36.

KISSEN, D. M. 1964. Lung cancer, inhalation, and personality. *In* Psychosomatic Aspects of Neoplastic Disease. D. M. Kissen & L. L. LeShan, Eds. : 3–11. Pitman. London, England.

KISSEN, D. M. 1965. Possible contribution of the psychosomatic approach to prevention of lung cancer. Medical Officer **114:** 343–345.

KISSEN, D. M. 1966a. The significance of personality in lung cancer in men. Ann. N. Y. Acad. Sci. **125**(3): 820–826.

KISSEN, D. M. 1966b. The value of a psychosomatic approach to cancer. Ann. N. Y. Acad. Sci. **125**(3): 777–779.

KISSEN, D. M. 1966c. Psychosocial factors, personality and prevention in lung cancer. Medical Officer **116:** 135–138.

KISSEN, D. M. & L. G. S. RAO. 1968. Steroid excretion patterns and personality in lung cancer. This monograph.

KOWAL, S. J. 1955. Emotions as a cause of cancer: Eighteenth and nineteenth century contributions. Psychoanal. Rev. **42:** 217–227.

LANGNER, T. S. & S. T. MICHAEL. 1963. Life Stress and Mental Health. Vol. II. The Free Press of Glencoe, MacMillan Co. New York, N. Y.

LESHAN, L. L. & R. E. WORTHINGTON. 1956a. Some recurrent life history patterns observed in patients with malignant disease. J. Nerv. Ment. Dis. **124:** 460–465.

LESHAN, L. L. & R. E. WORTHINGTON. 1956b. Personality as a factor in the pathogenesis of cancer. Brit. J. Med. Psychol. **29:** 49–56.

LESHAN, L. L. & M. REZNIKOFF. 1960. A psychological factor apparently associated with neoplastic disease. J. Abnorm. Soc. Psychol. **60:** 439–440.

LESHAN, L. L. 1966. An emotional life-history pattern associated with neoplastic disease. Ann. N. Y. Acad. Sci. **125**(3): 780–793.

MEERLOO, J. A. M. 1954. Psychologic implications of cancer. Geriatrics **9:** 154–156.

RENNEKER, R. 1965. (Unpublished observations.)

SCHMALE, A. H., JR. 1958. Relation of separation and depression to disease. I. A report on a hospitalized medical population. Psychosom. Med. **20:** 259–277.

SCHMALE, A. H., JR. & H. P. IKER. 1964. The affect of hopelessness in the development of cancer. I. The prediction of uterine cervical cancer in women with atypical cytology. Psychosom. Med. **26:** 634–635.

SCHMALE, A. H., JR. & H. P. IKER. 1966. The psychological setting of uterine cervical cancer. Ann. N. Y. Acad. Sci. **125**(3): 807–813.

SROLE, L., T. S. LANGNER, S. T. MICHAEL, M. K. OPLER & T. A. C. RENNIE. 1961. Mental Health in the Metropolis. Vol. I. McGraw-Hill. New York, N. Y.

DISCUSSION OF THE PAPER

DR. SOLOMON: I should like to comment that the work from the Kissen and Bahnson groups is very complementary. I should also like to comment on the finding of relative lack of projection and increased repression, which I also consider evidence not only of repression (in the sense that these negative views of the world are not being projected, or remain unconscious), but also of conscious suppression in terms of reporting such feelings.

Repression may not be specific for cancer itself, and this would raise some questions about being able to extrapolate the concept of repression on the somatic and psychological levels, in that your findings are parallel to those of ours in patients with the autoimmune diseases.

One of the most striking things in our patients, for example, is the way in which they describe their spouses. Patients with autoimmune diseases describe their spouses in either of two ways. One is in such idealized terms that such an individual really has not existed for the last 1968 years. The other is to make elaborate excuses and justifications for remarkably sadistic and brutal behaviors, describing it, again, in a rather idealized way. I do not believe that this is true of all psychosomatic patients, since our comparison group of hypertensive patients shows a great deal of hostility and projection.

Therefore, I wonder whether this particular pattern is not related to some propensity of this function of the immunologic system. I particularly think that this occurs in the presence of decompensation of these particular methods of coping, and these characterological defenses, which would tie in with the other papers you mentioned in terms of loss, depression, and so on. If these methods were really working for the patients, they might be disease-free. These are, I think, particularly fragile defenses, very brittle ones, and cannot stand too much confrontation with a reality that is very contradictory to their wishes or expectations.

I certainly agree that there is strong evidence for this particular pattern, but I question whether it is related to somatic regression, or, rather, more related to some basic physiological dysfunction that effects various disease states.

DR. GREENE: I am very much impressed with this study; I am a little bit amazed by it. I should like to say something about what came up after the last presentation about accuracy of data. I think that what one gets in terms of data to some extent has to do with how one goes at the patient in terms of the data that is wanted.

For instance, in terms of smoking, I am sure you would have different responses if the interviewer was smoking a cigarette, compared to if he was not. I think my main question is: How were you able to do these tests on a sample of patients with cancer? And I should like to know something about what the patients were told was the purpose of this, and to what extent were these a very select group of patients with cancer, on whom you were able to do these tests?

DR. SHANDS: I was a little troubled by what seems to me to be an oversimplification in your basic assumption. That assumption is that people are as similar to each other as inbred rats; the assumption is not stated, but it is implicit in the notion of "control groups."

I have been preoccupied for 20 years with the problems of "suitability" for psychotherapy—with how certain human beings differ from others without obvious external difference. My conclusion is that suitability is highly correlated with what can be called "cognitive competence," which may parallel "immunological competence" at a much lower level.

From the words you use in connection with the cancer patients, I can conclude that they are less cognitively competent than controls. In other words, I should guess that they would be less suitable for psychotherapy. The further conclusion is that the problem they present is far more complicated than would be suggested by a "diagnosis" of "simple depression."

DR. MARJORIE BAHNSON: Regarding Dr. Solomon's points, we are very much aware that the utilization of projection and regression that we describe in cancer patients may not be solely characteristic of cancer patients. As a matter of fact, we are extending our analyses to include sick controls. We find that there probably is a substratum of diminished projection, at least on some of the dimensions, as compared to well controls. In this respect, some other somatically sick patients seem to resemble cancer patients. The sick controls appear to fall between the cancer and well subjects, depending on which categories of illness and which age groups are being compared. To date, two sick groups, one a hemophilic group, the other a coronary heart-disease group, have been compared with the cancer and well groups. We are finding different patterns of projective defense and significant differences on other dimensions among these various subject groups. We are not prepared to summarize this material at this time. However, we realized that the state of being sick itself, whether by reason of immunological disability or whatever, probably does direct the psychological defensive apparatus to a certain level of projection or denial on some dimensions of emotion.

Also, we find, as we enlarge our samples, that we must be aware of differences in quality and extent of ego defenses that may appear in relation to age-grouping, both in well and sick subjects. There may very well be differences to be found between or among cancer subjects, differences that are partly a function of their ages; i.e , whether they develop cancer early or late in life. Our most recent analyses suggest, especially on the dimension of Hedonic Level and Social Interaction, that there are differences in projection among the young and old normal subjects. However, with the size of the sample we have employed, these differences were not reliable enough to override the analyses we are making.

With respect to Dr. Solomon's last point (that the repression pattern we have found may be related to an underlying physiological dysfunction, but not to "somatic regression"), I am at a loss in grasping the difference between these two formulations. Are they not simply two different ways of expressing similar thoughts, physiologic dysfunction emphasizing the mechanism, regression emphasizing the physiological end result?

With regard to Dr. Greene's point, it is difficult to collect information on cancer patients; it is difficult to collect reliable data on any patient group. One must be prepared to invest some time with each patient to let him know that one is genuinely interested in his situation. On the other hand, most cancer patients are eager to talk. Many of them are in a ward situation; many of them have come into the hospital to receive some type of treatment, often sitting in waiting areas, perhaps feeling rejected and dejected because of the busy hospital routine. Characteristically, we have invested two, three, even four and five hours in various patients with different interview and test procedures in order to provide an atmosphere, a sincere situation with them, to let them know that we are interested in their thoughts and feelings. Insofar as we can gauge, these patients were not aware that we were investigating their psychology in relation to their illnesses. Usually, we have led them to believe that we are interested in studying their attitudes toward the hospital, the routine going on, and their treatment program. This they have apparently accepted. Obviously, we think that the information we have obtained from these patients comprises valid data. Our cancer patients were unselected insofar as all patients entering the hospital and being unaware of their diagnoses, irrespective of site of malignancy, were included in the sample. Patients who were consciously aware of their diagnoses were not included.

In partial answer to Dr. Shands, in other papers, where there is more opportunity for presentation, we have tried to formulate an explicit argument for our definition of repression and projection and their relationship to depression. One of our main points has been that cancer patients are not "simply depressed" people, but that they are characterized by ego-defensive functioning which makes use of denial and repression, and which makes these persons appear as less insightful, "bland," and prosaic. If by "cognitive incompetence" Dr. Shands means that the kind and extent of ego-functioning that we have found to characterize cancer patients (i.e., denial and repression) provide an aspect of the cognitive functioning that makes a person unsuitable for psychotherapy, then we are in agreement. This is a point we may carry on in discussion at a later time.

REGRESSION AS AN INTERVENING MECHANISM: A SYSTEM-THEORETICAL APPROACH

Árpád Mezei and György Németh
Korányi National Institute for Tuberculosis, Budapest, Hungary, and National Health Service, Hungary

Problems Bearing on the Anality of Cancer Patients' Characters

All that has been assumed so far concerning psychosomatic-effect mechanisms is that chronic or fatal illness must be related in some way to the structure and life history of the personality in which it occurs. Of course, a more precise definition of this interrelation is no easy task. Neumann and Morgenstern (1947) have shown that the concepts and inferences drawn from the humanities, including those of sociology and psychology, are so vague that they do not lend themselves to scientific treatment. Concerning our field of investigation, Grinker (1965) holds the same position, and as to particular issues, Brown (1965), commenting on the theory of Booth (1964), states that while it is a highly interesting theory, it is based on an arbitrary interpretation of records, lacks experimental and statistical validation, and even goes beyond the data furnished by the records.

In such circumstances, we should be better off if we succeeded in reducing intuitive theories to their provable cores. The essence of Booth's theory is that cancer patients are anally fixated persons (Booth, 1964a). The concept of anality dates back to Freud, who observed that experiences associated with digestive-organ functions, though playing an important part in every type of personality, will become dominant in some way in particular subjects (e.g. if educational conditions and toilet training have been too strict). The anal person is, in addition to his coprophilia, thrifty or even miserly, wilful, obstinate, and pedantic. These findings were later confirmed by Ferenczy (1913) and Abraham (1923), and were refined by several others, so that by now not only anal experiences are thought of as bearing on personality, but the existence and mechanism of the anal character as an entity is assumed to be a psychiatrically accepted concept.

In accordance with the task we have set ourselves, that of reducing the concept to its provable core, we accept for the moment only the existence of anal experience, and wish to examine whether its presence and importance can be demonstrated in the case of cancer patients. For this purpose we adopted a procedure based on the following considerations.

The occurrence of the responses "anus" or "caudal bone" is a very clear manifestation of the anal drive in the Rorschach record. Another, though less explicit, sign of anality is the animal response "rats" or "mice," since these animals are of an anal type. Animals have a symbolic meaning to man, and the kind of animal and testee will see in the blots is bound to be characteristic of him (Phillips and Smith, 1953; Rychlak, 1959).

Accordingly, we have counted the occurrence of these responses in a random sample of 50 cancer subjects and 50 controls matched for age, sex, and education. We have found, as shown in TABLE 1 that the occurrence of these anal responses was higher in the experimental group: while only 12% of the normal subjects produced them, they occurred in 42% of the cancer subjects which is significant on the 0.03 level.

This fact seems to suggest that cancer patients are more anally oriented. We are now going to investigate this problem more closely.

TABLE 1

PREDOMINANTLY ANAL RESPONSES IN THE RORSCHACH RECORDS OF CANCER Ss COMPARED WITH NORMAL CONTROLS*

Specification of Anal Response	Cancer Ss N = 50	Normal Ss N = 50
Anus, Caudal Bone	8	2
Rats, Mice	13	9
Percentage of Ss Producing the Response	42	22

* Significance: $p = 0.03$.

In addition to the character traits already mentioned, the anal person may manifest, as a reaction formation against his love for dirt, excessive preoccupation with cleanliness. Should the anality of cancer patients show itself predominantly in such traits, their behavior would approximate that of normals. However, if we are to find out something more about the relation of anality to cancer, we must look beneath this facade and deal with the developmental aspect of these traits.

Anal experiences have been shown to arise at different stages of the ontogenetic development; thus, a given anal fixation may derive from different developmental phases. Then there are developmental phases preceding those at which anal experiences and fixations occur. These are even more archaic and primitive and regression to these archaic phases may be responsible for increasingly severe pathology. Miserliness, obstinacy, and constricted preoccupation with cleanliness, if kept within reasonable bounds, are normal character traits. But when they derive from earlier fixations, the motivating anal drives are more vehement, and therefore the ego has to defend against them. This is the way obsessional neuroses develop, the anal origin of which has been recognized by Abraham (1923). Anal origin, however, is likewise valid of melancholia (Freud, 1917), a component factor of the cyclic psychoses (Katan, 1940), and particularly of paranoia, in which the anal drive assumes such dimensions that personality will be destroyed (Freud, 1911). The anal nature of melancholia and paranoia was examined later, largely by Klein (1932). Of these findings, the following bear on our investigations.

The melancholic regresses to such an early phase of personality development that the distinction between self and the external world is yet uncertain, and the paranoid patient regresses even further: to a phase where not even the unity of personality has yet developed. At this stage—in early infancy—self and nonself are still unintegrated, the mother's breast has not become an integral part of a being that is nonself. At this age, feces is for the infant an aggressive, dangerous, living something. This experience has been observed by us even beyond the period of infancy in some oversensitive, not quite adequately educated children, and its presence in psychotics can frequently be demonstrated. One of our patients suffering from rectal carcinoma (now deceased) reported a dream in which he found a large amount of feces in the toilet that first turned into bread and then into a bear that started to chase him.

Accordingly, if we assume that the anality of the cancer patients bears on the development of a cancer-prone personality, we must state definitely which of the anality forms enumerated are prevalent in a given case of cancer.

According to Booth (1964a, 1964b), cancer is associated with anal personality features; i.e., with a form of anality that does not go far beyond what might be accepted as normal. Dunbar's (1954) cancer personality functions in a seemingly conflictfree manner, although highly scrupulous and governed by the defenses of denial and reaction formation. Obsessional neurosis, which is more intimately linked up with anality, has not often been associated with cancer so far; but melancholic depression is considered to be a cancer equivalent by Immerman (1917), and paranoia, constituting the most severe regression in terms of anal organization, was assumed to be a cancer equivalent by Lewis (1936). The profile described by LeShan (1965) seems to be a synthesis of reaction formation and melancholic depression arising on an anal basis.

Thus it appears possible to match the cancer personality profiles given by various authors with one or several of the manifestations of anal drive; i.e., with the anal character traits, depression, paranoia, and others. Anality, being a common factor in the theories proposed by various authors, may constitute a suitable basis for integrating apparently conflicting theories.

The Problem of the Intervening Mechanism

Several authors have held the position that the anal personality structure predisposes to somatic illness, beyond the anality-cancer association. Zauner (1964) affirms that obsessional neurosis is usually accompanied by definite somatic pathology. Associations of this kind, however, are established on a statistical plane without involving the intervening mechanism.

With regard to this mechanism, the initial difficulty is to conceptualize the transition from the level of psychic processes to the level of physical events. Authors generally believe that the course of events, when described in a psychological frame of reference, can be followed only in the area of psychology. Thus, Kütemeyer (1965) states that, as a consequence of anal regression, great amounts of hostility and ambivalent emotion are accumulated in the patient. Others, going beyond this, state that the chances of somatic involvement grow with the severity of regression. Bahnson's theory (1964) is an elaboration of this principle. However, clarification of the intervening mechanism was not attempted.

In order to establish a conceptual link between the psychic and physical levels, we suggest conceptualizing normality and the different stages of regression in the personality as states of equilibrium maintained at different levels. The ideally complex form of this state is the one found in the normal personality; a personality with dominantly anal character traits would then represent the reduction of such an ideal form. Different forms or types of personality all represent different forms of equilibria maintained at identical or different levels of complexity. The fact that all organic, living structures are forms of equilibria–more precisely, flux equilibria–has been pointed out by several authors since the middle of the last century, but the absence of a more exact definition leaves this statement without implications. The problem that has prevailed throughout is that the relation between the known forms of equilibria could not be demonstrated, and the introduction of assumed new and complex forms served only to increase the uncertainty in this respect. According to Lalande (1928), the common factor in physical and chemical equilibria is only their denomination. This must have led Cannon (1939) to use the new term "homeostasis" to describe the structure of living beings, although intuitively it was certainly clear to him that homeostasis is nothing else than one of several complex forms of a basic equilibrium.

The introduction of the thermodynamic approach has made it possible to reduce the number of problems that have arisen in this field. Within this frame of reference, the interrelations of physical and chemical equilibria become clearly visible. The real world has been shown to be composed of a series of more complex and more simple equilibrium structures, and now there is no reason why we might not assume the existence of hypercomplex forms characterizing living beings. These forms are on a higher level of complexity than those known so far, and are still amenable to mathematical treatment. Such forms, owing to their greater complexity, deviate from the known forms, but this difference is only secondary. Therefore, the theory of Bauer (1935), according to whom living organisms do not constitute equilibria but are structures remaining steadily at a certain distance from the states of equilibria, does not represent the rejection of the equilibrium concept, but only the widening thereof. Later theories, e.g. those of von Bertalanffy (1956) and his followers, take into account that systems performing work cannot be in perfect equilibrium; accordingly, they classify living structures as open steady systems, i.e. flux equilibria.

Based on the above consideration, we may assume that the psychic system likewise constitutes an equilibrium system in which the different levels of the variable factors will always add up to an approximately balanced overall system. The idea that forms of personality constitute forms of equilibria has already emerged in the literature by representatives of general systems theory (Kretch, 1956). The psychoanalytically oriented Alexander (1950) referred in an earlier work to neuroses as reduced forms of equilibria as compared with the normal state. Some of these authors use the term only as an analogy, while others (Kretch, 1956) apply the scientific concept of equilibrium, but only for the purpose of description. The concept and its scope of application has not been defined to such a degree that it might become a basis for further inferences. Our position is that such a definition is possible and may enable us to make some statements concerning the intervening mechanism between psychic and physical entities.

To begin with, some general rules governing the series of equilibria must be formulated. The first of these is the apparently valid rule that *within a given system a definite ratio of the variable and invariable factors is being maintained.* It is involved in Cannon's statement, according to which the admirable constancy of certain parameters in the organism is achieved by means of considerable variability. On the basis of this principle, the rank order of the various forms of equilibrium may be established. In the case of psychic functioning, the variability encountered is of such a high degree that the separation of the various dimensions of change constitutes an unsurmountable difficulty. It can be well perceived that the psychic system strives at preserving its identity with all its might, but identity represents an entity that cannot be broken down into its component parts, not even to such an extent that the physiological functioning of the organism can be shown to be made up of equilibria like blood-sugar levels or oxygen levels.

Another, somewhat simpler rule concerning the structure of serial systems of equilibria may be formulated as follows: Succeeding forms of equilibria may be conceived as series of surface levels in a continuous field. *For the elaboration of a higher level form, a greater amount of energy is needed,* similarly to the fact that the higher a physical body is to be raised in the gravitational field, the more energy is required. The energy of the complex structures is accumulated within these as potential energy. When, for some reason, the complex form falls back to a lower level (i.e., is transformed to a simpler form), *the potential energy of the system will be transformed into kinetic energy.* In the case of simpler systems, such kinetic energy simply leaves the system, as in the form of radiation when radioactive substances are broken down. In the case of psychosomatic systems, the situation is more complicated.

Implications for the Psychic Subsystem

When the potential energy of the human psychosomatic system has been turned into kinetic energy owing to a regressive event, the change produced in the psychic subsystem appears in the form of strong aggressive drives. Since the psychic subsystem is autoregulative, it will record the intensity grade of functions occurring in it. Increased aggression will be fed back to the governing center of the subsystem and perceived as anxiety. Normally, anxiety is the signal for being menaced by hostile interference from without. But when regression has gone as far as the early stages, where undifferentiated forms prevail, the capacity for differentiating between self and nonself, between external and inner reality, begins to disappear. Accordingly, in such cases the increased aggression may be turned both ways, against the self or against the world. The frequency of suicide in melancholia will illustrate this point. The signaling of free aggression as anxiety is therefore justified.

The course of aggression produced by the release of kinetic energy in the psychic subsystem may be followed, to a certain limit, with the help of psychological tests. In the Rorschach, it is expressed by interpreting the blots as bodies that are mutilated, damaged and so on. We have shown in previous studies (Mezei & Németh, 1963, 1965; Németh & Mezei, 1964) that chronically ill subjects interpret the blots with the help of the normal body image: by projecting the organs of the head and chest into the upper and those of the abdomen into the lower parts of the cards. The cancer patient will also make an attempt at following this course, but does not succeed: he is unable to identify the organs looked for with the corresponding part of the blot. This attempt at and failure in utilizing the body-image in the interpretation of the blots constitutes the characteristic feature in the Rorschach records of subjects suffering from cancer or other kind of malignant disease, and it is on the basis of these signs that malignant disease and particularly cancer may be diagnosed from the Rorschach protocols with a certain amount of confidence. In addition, these records include the verbalizations of self-depreciation, and appeal for help, since these subjects make themselves responsible for their failures and emphasize their own ignorance and helplessness. Numeric data of the occurrence of these signs computed for 50 cancer subjects and 50 controls matched for sex, age and education are shown in TABLE 2.

This falling to pieces (or dissolution) of the cancer subject's body image, being a destruction of the body, must be looked upon as a result of self-aggression; i.e., aggression turned toward the self because of lack in differentiation between self and nonself.

Implications for the Somatic Subsystem

The lowering of the equilibrium level by way of regression that takes place in the psychosomatic system will lead to an increase of kinetic energy in the somatic subsystem, as well. It is a change in which a psychic event degenerates partly into physical energy. The biophysical-biochemical process that is assumed to arise at this stage may be said to bear on the kinetic-potential energy balance of the organism. The increase of kinetic energy is evidently proportional to the extent of regression, and on this basis the theory of Bahnson and Bahnson (1964, 1965) and others may be considered valid.

TABLE 2

FREQUENCY OF MAIN MALIGNITY RORSCHACH SIGNS IN 50 CANCER Ss COMPARED WITH 50 NORMAL CONTROLS*

Specification of Malignity Score	Frequency		Percentage of Total Frequency	
	Cc Ss N = 50	Controls N = 50	Cc Ss N = 50	Controls N = 50
Dissolution forms (organ or body part not found–not in the right place, withdrawn, etc.)	48	7	87	13
Emphasizing ignorance or incompetence (rejection of percept or whole card, excessive "I don't know" s)	191	78	71	29
Self-depreciation	8	2	80	20
Experience of being menaced ("terrible," "frightening," etc.)	27	7	80	20
Asking for help	13	5	72	28
Total	287	99	74	26

* A preliminary draft of the detailed malignity-sign list may be obtained on request from A Mezei, Korányi, National Institute for Tuberculosis, Budapest, XII, Pihenö u.l. (Hungary).

Accordingly, the intervening psychic mechanism causes an increase of the kinetic energy in the system, with ensuing imbalance due to the excess of energy.

Ways of Binding Excess of Kinetic Energy

It has been observed that when a cancer patient produces intensive paranoid symptoms, the progression of the neoplastic growth is slowed down. This appears to indicate that paranoia is one of the ways of utilizing and binding the excess of kinetic energy, just as is the proliferation of tumor cells.

Another way of influencing the course of the malignant process is by turning aggression toward the external objects. This has already been stated in our earlier papers (Németh & Mezei, 1964, 1967) and by Renneker and co-workers (1963).

Some further clinical observations, also reported earlier (Németh & Mezei, 1967), will fit into this frame of reference. It has been found that tumor subjects who change their symptoms more frequently tend to have a better prognosis. Apparently, symptoms are changed before self-aggression can take root within one pathological process, and the change seems to enter into the service of self-preservation.

Another clinical observation (Németh & Mezei, 1967) is that subjects with malignant tumors tend to delay turning to the physician. This delay, or even lack of call, may be attributed to the inability of the subjects to interfere with their self-destructive drives; it just shows their passive giving up, the participation of the ego by noninterference with the destruction of the self.

Conclusion

Summing up, we believe that the problem of the mechanism by which psychic experience bears on somatic events can be solved if psyche is conceived as a complex energetical system and not as an absolutely separate entity, and if we assume that, when such a system degenerates, by way of regression, a considerable amount of kinetic energy is released.

References

ABRAHAM, K. 1923. Ergänzungen zur Lehre vom Analcharacter. Int. Z. Psychoanal. **9:** 27–47.

ALEXANDER, F. 1950. Psychosomatic Medicine. W. W. Norton & Co., Inc. New York, N. Y.

BAHNSON, C. B. & M. B. BAHNSON. 1964. Cancer as an alternative to psychosis: a theoretical model of somatic and psychological regression. *In* Psychosomatic Aspects of Neoplastic Diseases. D. M. Kissen & L. LeShan, Eds. : 184–202. J. P. Lippincott Co. New York, N. Y.

BAHNSON, C. B. & M. B. BAHNSON. 1965. Role of the ego defenses: denial and repression in the etiology of malignant neoplasm. Ann. N. Y. Acad. Sci. **125:** 827–845.

BALTRUSCH, H. J., K. AUSTERHEIM & E. BALTRUSCH. 1964. Psyche – Nervensystem – neoplastischer Prozess: Ein altes Problem. Z. Psychosomat. Med. **10:** 157–168.

BAUER, E. 1935. Inhalt und Methode der theoretischen Biologie. *In* Probleme der theoretischen Biologie. B. P. Tokin, Ed. : 333–346. INRA Verlag. Moskau-Leningrad.

BERTALANFFY, L. VON. 1956. General system theory. General Systems **1:** 1–10.

BOOTH, G. 1964a. Cancer and humanism. *In* Psychosomatic Aspects of Neoplastic Disease. D. M. Kissen & L. LeShan, Eds. : 159–169. J. P. Lippincott Co. New York, N. Y.

BOOTH, G. 1964b. Krebs und Tuberkulose im Rorschachschen Formdeutversuch. Z. Psychosomat. Med. **10:** 176–188.

BROWN, F. 1965. Relationship between cancer and personality. Ann. N. Y. Acad. Sci. **125:** 865–873.

CANNON, W. B. 1939. The Wisdom of the Body. W. W. Norton & Co. New York, N. Y.

DUNBAR, F. 1954. Emotions and Bodily Changes. Columbia University Press. New York, N. Y.

FERENCZY, S. 1913. Stages in the development of the sense of reality. Contributions to Psycho-Analysis. Badger. Boston, Mass.

FREUD, S. 1911. Psycho-analytic notes on an autobiographical account of a case of paranoia (dementia paranoides). *In* The Standard Edition of the Complete Psychological Works of Sigmund Freud. **12:** 9–82 (1958). Hogarth Press. London.

FREUD, S. 1917. Mourning and melancholia. *In* Collected Papers. **4:** 152–170 (1959). Basic Books. New York, N. Y.

GRINKER, R. R. 1965. Psychosomatic aspects of the cancer problem. Ann. N. Y. Acad. Sci. **125:** 876–882.

IMMERMANN, S. L. 1917. Manic depressive psychosis associated with malignant conditions. N. Y. Med. J. **106:** 828. (Quoted by BALTRUSCH.)

KATAN, M. 1940. Die Rolle des Wortes in der Schizophrenie und Manie. Int. Z. Psychoanal. **25:** 2.

KLEIN, M. 1932. Die Psychoanalyse des Kindes. Int. Psa. Verlag. Vienna, Austria.

KRETCH, D. 1956. Dynamic systems as open neurological systems. General Systems **1:** 144–155.

KÜTEMEYER, W. 1965. Psychosocial aspects of cancer. 4th Int. Conference on Psychosomatic Aspects of Neoplastic Disease. Torino. (In press.)

LALANDE, A. 1928. Vocabulaire Philosophique. Felix Alcan. Paris.

LESHAN, L. 1965. An emotional life-history pattern associated with neoplastic disease. Ann. N. Y. Acad. Sci. **125:** 780–793.

LEWIS, N. D. C. 1936. Research in dimentia precox. Nat. Committee for Mental Hygene. (Quoted by BALTRUSCH.)

MEZEI, A. & G. NÉMETH. 1963. Untersuchungen zur Psychosomatik maligner Tumoren mit Hilfe des Rorschach-Tests. Z. Psychosomat. Med. **9:** 265–270.

MEZEI, A. & G. NÉMETH. 1965. The specific nature of malignity in cancer: a tentative psychodiagnostic approach. 4th Int. Conference on Psychosomatic Aspects of Neoplastic Disease. Torino. Mimeographed ms. (Obtainable from Authors.)

NÉMETH, G. & A. MEZEI. 1964. Personality traits of cancer patients compared with benign tumor patients on the basis of the Rorschach test. *In* Psychosomatic Aspects of Neoplastic Disease. D. M. Kissen & L. LeShan, Eds. : 12–17. J. P. Lippincott Co. New York, N. Y.

NÉMETH, G. & A. MEZEI. 1967. Clinical and psychological data bearing on prognosis in cancer. Int. Psychosomatic Week. Rome. (In press.)

NEUMANN, J. VON & D. MORGENSTERN. 1947. The Theory of Games and Economic Behavior. Princeton University Press. Princeton, N. J.

PHILLIPS, I. & J. S. SMITH. 1953. Rorschach Interpretation: Advanced Technique. Grune and Stratton. New York, N. Y.

RENNEKER, R. E., R. CUTLER, J. HORA, C. BACON, G. BRADLEY, J. KEARNEY & M. CUTLER. 1963. Psychoanalytical explorations of emotional correlates of cancer of the breast. Psychosomat. Med. **25:** 106–123.
RYCHLAK, J. F. 1959. Forced associations, symbolism and Rorschach constructs. J. Consult. Psychol. **23:** 455–460.
ZAUNER, J. 1964. Zwangsstruktur und Organsymptomatik. Z. Psychomat. Med. **10:** 169–175.

DISCUSSION OF THE PAPER

DR. BAHNSON: I think we will have an opportunity later to discuss some of the concepts introduced in this paper. However, I do want to commend Dr. Mezei and Dr. Nemeth. Of course, there are sometimes problems of communication, challenging problems with symbols and language, and I think that some of the terminology presented in this paper appears somewhat alien to us. Just the same, I think that it is very important to notice that Dr. Mezei is making an impressive attempt to tie together a somatic system process with what he has been working with for many years: a dynamic symbolic process. He attempts to relate phenomena on a psychological behavioral level to a systemic level that we have been talking about in quite different terms over the last days. He is as bold as few of us have dared to be in terms of relating different systems to each other, and I think we should be thankful for this and ponder his concept of anality, which certainly may be related to defensive systems and to perception of the environment, when we discuss these systems in greater detail.

GENERAL AND ORGANIC-SPECIFIC OBJECT RELATIONSHIPS IN CANCER

Gotthard Booth

New York, N. Y.

The nature of the object relationships of cancer patients was studied against the background of the object relationships found in tuberculosis patients. The biological rationale of this approach is provided by the epidemiological fact that cancer has replaced tuberculosis as the major disease liability of a genetic subgroup of the Caucasian populations of Australia, Europe, New Zealand, and North America. Cherry (1924, 1925) demonstrated that in all these countries the sum of tuberculosis and cancer deaths in the adult populations has remained, since the middle of the last century, a stable 20% of the total mortality due to diseases. In 1960, Berkson demonstrated specifically that the combined tuberculosis and lung cancer death rates since 1930 show the same reciprocal relationship between the two diseases in spite of the rapid rise of lung cancer. At the conference on which this monograph is based, Margolin pointed out that there is no cancer among the Ute Indians, an inbred population that lost its genetically tuberculosis-prone members after the tribe had lost its freedom in the last century. Furthermore, at the same conference, there was a demonstration of the existence of a specific immunological relationship between cancer and tuberculosis.

In view of the great difference between the somatic disease processes of cancer and of tuberculosis, it was assumed that a change of object relationships had taken place not only on the cellular, but also on the psychobiological, levels. This hypothesis was investigated by comparing the reactions of these patients to ten identical objects: the ten nonrepresentational inkblots that Rorschach (1942) designed 50 years ago for the purpose of psychodiagnostic experimentation. As I demonstrated previously (1946), the differentiation of somatic groups required methods of perceptanalysis different from those used in the study of psychiatric conditions, in the narrower sense of the term.

It proved possible to establish that cancer and tuberculosis patients, respectively, do respond differently to the specific psychological demands represented by the ten inkblot pictures. Twenty-nine pairs of contrasting gestalt tendencies could be defined (Booth, 1964b, 1965). Two criteria of significance were used: 1. The specific gestalt tendency occurred at least twice as often in one clinical group as in the other, and vice versa. 2. The individual members of each group responded to more Rorschach pictures according to clinical diagnosis than according to the type established for the contrasting clinical group.

FIGURE 1 illustrates the relative frequencies of the two types of gestalt tendencies in the two clinical groups as they occurred in response to the ten inkblot pictures; TABLE 1 sums up the degree of correspondence between clinical diagnosis and Rorschach diagnosis. Recently, 12 more Rorschach records of cancer patients were obtained. With the exception of two skin cancers, one case of leukemia, and one breast cancer, the records fitted into the predicted type.

The gestalt tendencies were discovered in the Rorschach records of 15 still undiagnosed lung cancer patients, and of 82 tuberculosis patients who had served Korkes and Lewis (1955) in their study of the psychological patterns related to the prognosis of tuberculosis. Subsequently, I found that the lung cancer criteria

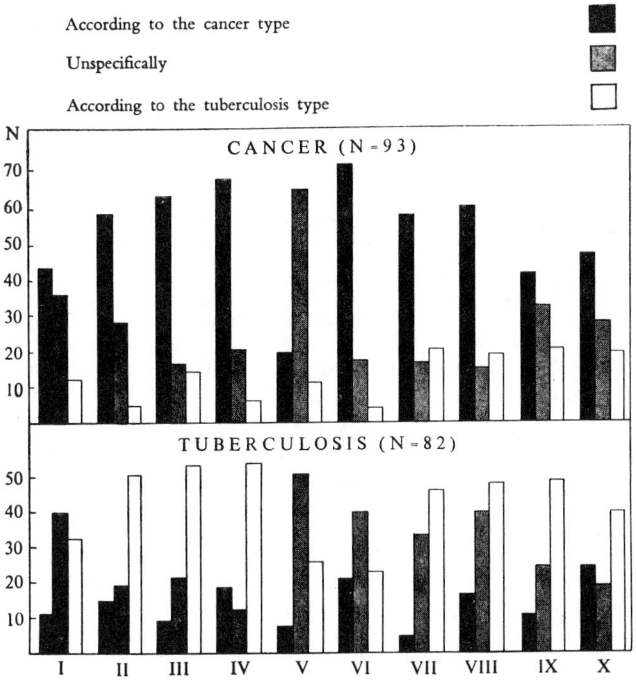

FIGURE 1. Number of patients with cancer and with tuberculosis, respectively, who responded to the individual Rorschach inkblot pictures according to the cancer type of perception, unspecifically, and according to the tuberculosis type of perception. (Reproduced from "Irrational Complications of the Cancer Problem," [Booth, 1965] in the *American Journal of Psychoanalysis,* **25**(1): 41–55, with the permission of the Editor, Harold Kelman, M.D.)

applied also to other cancer sites. Fifty of these additional records had been originally obtained by Shrifte (1962) for her study of psychological patterns related to the prognosis of cancer.

The perceptual tendencies of the cancer group were definitely unrelated to the presence or absence of disease: 13 records had been obtained by me up to 25 years before there had been any symptoms of disease, 46 patients were sick at the time of testing, and 35 had been operated successfully. In the tuberculosis group, the characteristic perceptual tendencies obtained equally in 41 cases with bad prognosis and in 41 cases that were pronounced either cured or having a favorable prognosis. The conclusion, therefore, appears justified that the different gestalt tendencies of the two clinical groups express constitutional differences between the two groups with respect to their object relationships.

The psychological interpretation of the prevailing gestalt tendencies led to the following formulations:

1. Tuberculosis-prone individuals are characterized by the prevalence of the need for reaching out toward others for mutual relationships analogous to the mutuality of male and female. In psychoanalytical terms, they are predominantly genital types. These patients are symbiotic personalities dependent on sharing life with others, and flexible in the pursuit of this objective.

TABLE 1
CORRESPONDENCE BETWEEN CLINICAL AND RORSCHACH DIAGNOSIS*

Clinical Diagnosis	Rorschach Diagnosis	Cases	%
Lung Cancer (n = 26)	Cancer	26	100
Other Cancers (n = 67)	Cancer	64	95½
	Tuberculosis	3	4½
Tuberculosis (n = 82)	Tuberculosis	74	90.3
	Cancer	6	7.3
	Neutral	2	2.4

* Lung cancer = experimental group.

2. Cancer-prone individuals are characterized by the prevalence of the need for establishing unilateral control over certain chosen objects. In psychoanalytical terms, they are predominantly anal types. These patients strive for autonomy and depend on their power for maintaining the object relationships originally chosen. This need leads to rigidity and makes it difficult to replace lost objects.

The preceding conclusions from the Rorschach records agree with the clinical observations of independent observers:

Tuberculosis patients, according to Wittkower (1949) and Kissen (1958), have an "inordinate need for affection" that makes "the break of a love bond" a typical trauma preceding the disease. In the light of the psychodynamics of this group, I interpret the infectious process as the regressive compensation for the frustrated symbiotic needs. This regression, however, tends to be reversible under favorable circumstances, because tuberculosis patients are animated by a strong need for adequate, mutual object relationship. They are flexible in this pursuit. Their "inordinate need for affection" accounts for their "eternal hopefulness"; the *spes phthisica* is the subjective aspect of the tendency toward changeable and often reckless symbiotic involvements found in this group.

Cancer patients are very different. They too have experienced the loss of an important object, but the relationship had not been characterized by affectionate mutuality, nor have they maintained an attitude of "eternal hopefulness". LeShan & Worthington (1956) found that cancer patients have been dominated since childhood by a feeling that their opportunities for satisfactory object relationships were very limited. By great effort, in spite of their basic pessimism, they had succeeded in creating a meaningful way of life for themselves. Once they had lost the hope for maintaining their individual ways of life, they fell prey to despair. They became depressed. Freud (1917) described the psychodynamics of depression as a turning of part of the self into the lost object. In cancer, the depressive process is somatized: part of the body is turned into the lost object by way of the neoplastic process, specifically the organ involved biologically or symbolically in the lost object relationship. The "object" being firmly implanted inside the body, the patient no longer reaches out toward external objects for satisfaction of his frustrated psychobiological needs. He does not "project" as much as noncancer patients, in terms of Bahnson & Bahnson (1968).

As mentioned in the beginning, epidemiological and immunological data strongly suggest that the contemporary cancer-prone population had developed in the 20% of the total population that died of tuberculosis in the middle of the last century. In view of the different psychodynamics of cancer and tuberculosis, it must be assumed that a new environmental factor brought about the radical change of personality development in members of the same gene pool. Under the conditions prevailing in the middle of the last century, the vast majority of subjects became personalities characterized by their need for affectionate, symbiotic relationships, and by their sanguine, optimistic temperament in sickness. Under present-day conditions, the vast majority of the same genetic group has become characterized by a need for autonomy and object control, and by an irreversible depression reaction to a loss of object control.

A profound psychological personality transformation such as the one described can take place only during the first year of life. The research of René Spitz (1965), now also supported by Harlow's (1965) experiments with monkey babies, has made it clear that the tuberculosis type of affectionate, symbiotic character can develop only in the beginning of life from the affectionate interplay between baby and mother. Breast-feeding, in most cases, provides the most favorable conditions for this outcome. Bottle-feeding leads to the same results, if the infant receives an adequate amount of physical affection. Otherwise, the personality development of the subject is stunted in the ways described as characteristic of the cancer group.

Now it is a well-established fact that the advance of cancer in the middle of the last century began at the time when more and more people reached cancer age who had been artificially fed. This had been the result of the industrial revolution, which forced working mothers to leave the "dry-feeding" of their babies in the hands of grandmothers, maiden aunts, and other siblings. At first the infant mortality was very high, but gradually the methods improved, and bottle-feeding became widely accepted by mothers and physicians even when neither economic nor physical conditions made it necessary. The change from physiological nursing to milkbottle, formula, and sterilizing procedures obviously involved distraction from the direct mother-child interaction in breast-feeding. As mentioned above, bottle-feeding is as healthy as breast-feeding if it is done with an adequate amount of affection. The risk for the bottle-fed infant is created by the fact that it can be done in a completely mechanical way, and all display of affection is the result of either instinct or of conscious intention. Not so long ago, the prevailing medical attitude even deliberately discouraged the cuddling of babies as "unhygienic," or as bad for the development of a sound character.

What makes the risk of frustrating the affectionate needs of babies even more serious is the fact that the stunting of their psychosexual development tends to be cumulative in their descendants. There is a striking similarity between Harlow's (1965) heterosexually incompetent monkeys and their baby-battering female descendants on the one side and the contemporary human scene on the other. The recent survey of Newton & Newton (1967) indicates a worldwide decline of the capacity for breast-feeding and its circular relationship with heterosexual incompetence. That the predisposition for cancer results partly from modern child-rearing practices is most strongly suggested by the fact that, within the last 25 years, childhood cancer, formerly a rare event, has become the second-ranking cause of death in childhood (Ariel & Pack, 1960). Greene (1958, 1959) has given convincing descriptions of the mothers of leukemia children.

Unquestionably, the adequate amount of affection necessary for normal infant development varies. As mentioned above, in the genetically tuberculosis-prone 20% of the population, the innate need for affection is particularly high. It follows that their likelihood to suffer frustration as a result of depersonalized nursing is greater than that of other genetic groups. This would account for the fact that it was the tuberculosis-prone segment of the population that was so profoundly affected by the introduction of artificial feeding. The genetic influence on the effect of identical infantile experience on adult behavior has been demonstrated experimentally by Ginsburg (1967). Four inbred strains of mice were subjected to handling; weekly weighings and cage transfers were carried out by picking up the mice by the tails with a forceps, instead of permitting them to walk. One strain developed more, another strain less, aggressive adult behavior than the unhandled controls. Two other strains developed the same adult behavior, whether they had been handled or not.

The change from tuberculosis to cancer in the same genetic human population can be traced to the introduction of artificial infant feeding and the implicit overemphasis on the physical needs of babies at the expense of the psychological needs. Whereas under the conditions of old-fashioned breast-feeding infants with great need for affection developed symbiotic adult object relationships and the "basic trust" (Erikson, 1963), making them responsive to therapy, the same genetic type of children has become subjected increasingly to the frustrations contingent on bottle-feeding. As a result, they became depression-prone, and experienced object losses as irretrievable. They developed cancers as internalized substitute objects, and became resistant to therapeutic measures.

The Localization of Cancer

Epidemiological studies indicate that the primary tumor develops in the organ that is specifically related to the frustrated psychophysiological object relationship. Such frustrations occur as the result of two psychodynamic conditions: 1. An intolerable conflict develops between the basic striving for an autonomous object relationship on the one hand, and the demands of a symbiotically motivated organ function on the other. The genital organs and the female breast provide typical occasions for this internal pathogenic constellation. 2. An external object is lost as the result of either environmental contingencies or the decreasing vitality of the aging individual. Often, both external and internal factors are involved.

The following examples may illustrate the first eventuality of object loss due to conflict between autonomic needs and symbiotic demands of a psychobiological function:

Cervical cancer occurs most frequently in women who are highly motivated for sexual activity, but who are prevented from achieving orgastic satisfaction by their need for autonomy (Rotkin, 1962; Rotkin *et al.*, 1965; Stephenson & Grace, 1954). Nuns, clearly representative of women with low low sexual motivation, hardly ever develop this form of cancer (Gagnon, 1950).

Prostate cancer is particularly frequent in those cultural groups in which men frequently engage in love-making short of coitus (Marcial, 1960; Quisenberry, 1960).

Breast cancer is related to frustration of the nursing function (Adair & Bagg, 1925; Macdonald, 1942; Quisenberry, 1960; Marcial, 1960). Even in a population of genetically unselected mice, 15% develop mammary cancer if they are prevented from nursing their litters (Bagg, 1936). Cancer-prone women are liable to repress a strong genetic motivation for nursing because their autonomous needs inhibit them in carrying out the mutual intimate interaction of nursing as well as of sexual intercourse (Newton & Newton, 1967). In addition to the inner conflicts, which cause frustration of the nursing function, the prevailing professional attitudes of physician and hospital nurses, as well as socioeconomic conditions, often discourage mothers from breast-feeding, even though they may be intellectually well motivated. The preceding observations on the influence of somatic frustration of the nursing function should be extended also to the cancerogenic effect of frustrated psychological nursing motivations. My own observations are in agreement with the very detailed psychoanalytical account that Inman (1961) gave of the life history of an unmarried nurse with breast cancer. Although this anecdotal material does not prove anything, it serves as a reminder that the dynamics of cancer are best understood by those who obtain full information from these generally reticent patients.

Forms of cancer related mainly to environmental frustrations may be illustrated by two examples:

Lung cancer has, as secondary genetic determinant, a general predisposition toward lung disease (Tokuhata & Lilienfeld, 1963). Many epidemiological observations on tuberculosis (Dubos & Dubos, 1952) and on lung cancer (Report of the Surgeon General, 1964) have established that these respiratory diseases are highly correlated with migration, urbanization, and socioeconomic deprivation. In other words, the "respiratory type" is strongly motivated for seeking satisfactory object relationships away from his native environment. Members of this group become sick when they encounter hopeless frustration in the city or the foreign country where they had expected to find fulfillment of their needs. The role of the lungs as expressing a need for independent mobility is readily understandable. Phylogenetically, the emergence of the lungs allowed animal life to migrate from the ocean to existence on land. Ontogenetically, our individual existence begins with the first breath after nine months of aquatic existence in the womb. Even as adults we inhale deeply when we have escaped, or hope to escape, from a confining situation.

The epidemiology of lung cancer is consistent with the concept that frustration of strong needs for change of milieu is related to the occurrence of lung cancer. For instance, among all nations the British people have by far the highest incidence of this disease. They are presently confined to their densely populated island after demonstrating, during 300 years of Empire building, that they are most highly endowed for establishing themselves in foreign regions of the world. In the countries with a large Anglo-Saxon population, but offering greater freedom of social and geographic mobility (Australia, Canada, New Zealand, and the United States), the lung cancer rate is less than half that of Great Britain (Doll, 1955).

Another suggestive example of the relationship between lung cancer and a frustrated desire for independent mobility is provided by the contrast between West Berlin and Japan. In 1962 West Berlin had the highest incidence in the world, 111.0 male deaths/100,000 population, while Japan had the lowest of all industrialized nations, 9.3/100,000 population (World Health Organization, 1965). The rigidly authoritarian culture maintained in the latter country until 23 years ago was hardly favorable for the breeding of a high contingent of individuals striving for independent mobility.

Stomach cancer also appears clearly related to the frustration of a psychophysiological organ function. The disease is definitely related to poverty (Surgeon General's Report, 1964). Since the depression year 1930, the incidence of stomach cancer has fallen to less than one-half (Berkson, 1960). In 1960, the United States had the lowest rate among the industrialized nations, and Japan, the highest.

The Clinical Importance of Object Relationships in Cancer

Understanding the nature of object relationships of the individual cancer patient has considerable practical importance. After the neoplasia has been removed physically, the prognosis depends on the psychophysiological rehabilitation of the patient (Evans, 1926; Pendergrass, 1961; Booth, 1965). This means that a new object relationship must be found to replace the pathogenic loss. Some patients do so unaided; others benefit from professional help in understanding their needs (Meerloo, 1954; Booth, 1965, 1966). Cancer, like suicidal attempts, is often a social signal. Unless the message is heeded, possible prophylactic measures against a recurrence may be neglected.

In order to improve the results of cancer therapy, much more knowledge must be acquired about the specific object relationships involved. Such additional knowledge can be acquired if, in the future, the psychological history of the individual patients will arouse the interest of many more physicians and psychologists. That the prevailing concern of the medical profession is still far from this interest is documented by Everson & Cole's (1966) recent monograph on spontaneous regression of cancer. Although a number of highly suggestive case histories are given, neither the text nor the index touch on the psychophysiological implications of the clinical reports. While waiting for a more favorable climate of medical opinion, we must help those physicians and patients who understand cancer as a personal reaction to a personal loss, and not as a demonic, impersonal invader of the body. I agree with the statement of Bahnson & Bahnson (1966) that unconsciously "the creation of a tumor may be as important and meaningful to the cancer patient . . . as the creation of a plastic form to the sculptor." Psychophysiological therapy demands that, after physical removal of the tumor, we lead the patient from his unconsciously created substitute object back to an object with which he can relate consciously.

Summary

The psychodynamics of the object relationships of cancer patients can be differentiated from those of tuberculosis patients by means of Rorschach's inkblot pictures.

Cancer-prone individuals belong to the segment of the population that is, like tuberculosis-prone individuals, genetically motivated for a high degree of symbiotic, affectionate object relationships.

Infants belonging to this genetic group are particularly liable to be traumatized by the depersonalized nursing methods introduced under the influence of the industrial revolution. Medical science has made artificial nursing physically successful, but, until recently, has overemphasized the physical needs of infants at the expense of their needs for symbiotic, affectionate interaction with their mothers.

Inadequate symbiotic experience with the mother profoundly affects the subsequent object relationships of the genetically predisposed baby. Instead of the flexibility and mutuality of tuberculosis patients, the cancer-prone individuals depend anxiously on unilateral, rigid control of their objects.

Loss of an important object relationship is experienced by cancer-prone subjects as irretrievable, and leads to conscious or unconscious depression. The depression is somatized in the form of neoplasia. The tumor represents an inalienable substitute for the lost external object.

The neoplasia is localized in the organ involved psychophysiologically in the frustrated object relationship.

Understanding of the pathogenic object loss is important for the rehabilitation of the patient.

References

ADAIR, F. E. & H. J. BAGG. 1925. Breast stasis as the cause of mammary cancer. Int. Clin. **4:** 19.

ARIEL, I. M. & G. T. PACK. 1960. Cancer in infancy and childhood. N. Y. J. Med. **60:** 409.

BAGG, H. J. 1936. Functional activity and mammary cancer in mice. Amer. J. Cancer **27:** 542.

BAHNSON, C. B. & M .B. BAHNSON. 1966. The role of ego defenses: denial and repression in the etiology of malignant neoplasm. Ann. N. Y. Acad. Sci. **125**(3): 827.

BAHNSON, M. B. Ego defenses in cancer patients. This monograph.

BERKSON, J. 1960. Smoking and cancer of the lungs. Proc. Staff Meet. Mayo Clin. **35:** 367.

BOOTH, G. 1946. Organ function and form perception. Psychosom. Med. **8:** 367.

BOOTH, G. 1964a. Cancer and humanism (Psychosomatic aspects of evolution). *In* Psychosomatic Aspects of Neoplastic Disease. D. Kissen & L. LeShan, Eds. J. P. Lippincott Co. New York, N. Y.

BOOTH, G. 1964b. Krebs und Tuberkulose im Rorschachschen Formdeuteversuch. Ztschr. Psycho-Somat. Med. **19:** 176.

BOOTH, G. 1965. Irrational complications of the cancer problem. Amer. J. Psychoanal. **25:** 41.

BOOTH, G. 1966. The cancer patient and the minister. Pastoral Psychology (Feb.) **17:** 15.

CHERRY, T. 1924, 1925. Cancer and acquired resistance to tuberculosis. Med. J. Aust. **2:** 372, **1:** 582.

DOLL, R. 1955. Etiology of lung cancer. Advances Canc. Res. **3:** 1.

DUBOS, R. & J. DUBOS. 1952. The White Plague (Tuberculosis, Man and Society). Little, Brown and Co. Boston, Mass.

ERIKSON, E. H. 1963. Childhood and Society. 2nd edit. W. W. Norton & Co. New York, N. Y.

EVANS, E. 1926. A Psychological Study of Cancer. Longmans, Green. New York, N. Y.

EVERSON, T. C. & W. H. COLE. 1966. Spontaneous Regression of Cancer. W. B. Saunders. Philadelphia, Pa.

FREUD, S. 1917. Mourning and melancholia. Coll. Papers. **4:** 152. Hogarth. London.

GAGNON, F. 1950. Contributions to the study of the etiology and prevention of cancer of the cervix of the uterus. Amer. J. Obstet. Gynec. **60:** 516.

GINSBURG, B. 1967. Genetic parameters in behavior research. *In* Behavior-Genetic Analysis. J. Hirsch, Ed. McGraw-Hill Book Co. New York, N. Y.

GREENE, W. A. & G. MILLER. 1958. Psychological factors and reticulo-endothelial diseases. Psychosom. Med. **20:** 124.

GREENE, W. A. 1958, 1959. Role of a vicarious object in the adaptation to object loss. Psychosom. Med. **20:** 344, **21:** 438.

HARLOW, H. F. & M. K. HARLOW. 1965. The affectional systems. *In* Behavior of Nonhuman Primates. A. M. Schrier, H. F. Harlow & F. Stollnitz, Eds. Academic Press. New York, N. Y.

INMAN, W. S. 1961. Can a blow cause cancer? Brit. J. Med. Psychol. **34:** 271.

KISSEN, D. M. 1958. Emotional Factors in Pulmonary Tuberculosis. Tavistock. London.

KORKES, L. L. & N. D. C. LEWIS. 1955. An analysis of the relationship between psychological patterns and outcome of pulmonary tuberculosis. J. Nerv. Ment. Dis. **122:** 524.

LESHAN, L. L. & R. E. WORTHINGTON. 1956. Some recurrent life history patterns observed in patients with malignant diseases. J. Nerv. Ment. Dis. **124:** 469.

MACDONALD, I. 1942. Mammary carcinoma, review of 2636 cases. Surg. Gynec. Obstet. **74:** 75.

MARCIAL, V. A. 1960. Socioeconomic aspects of the incidence of cancer in Puerto Rico. Ann. N. Y. Acad. Sci. **84**(17): 981.

MARGOLIN, S. This monograph.

MEERLOO, J. A. M. 1954. Psychological implications of malignant growth. Brit. J. Med. Psychol. **27:** 210.

NEWTON, N. & M. NEWTON. 1967. Psychological aspects of lactation. New Eng. J. Med. **277:** 1179.

PENDERGRASS, E. P. 1961. Host resistance and other intangibles in the treatment of cancer. Roentg., Radium Ther., Nucl. Med. **85:** 891.

QUISENBERRY, W. B. 1960. Sociological factors in cancer in Hawaii. Ann. N. Y. Acad. Sci. **84**(17): 795.

RORSCHACH, H. 1942. Psychodiagnostics. Grune & Stratton. New York, N. Y.

ROTKIN, I. D. 1962. Relation of adolescent coitus to cervical cancer disk. JAMA **179:** 486.

ROTKIN, I. D., N. QUENK & M. COUCHMAN. 1965. Psychosexual factors and cervical cancer. Arch. Gen. Psychiat. (Chicago) **13:** 532.

SHRIFTE, M. 1962. Toward identification of a psychological variable in host resistance to cancer. Psychosom. Med. **24:** 390.

SPITZ, R. A. 1965. The Frst Year of Life. Int. Univs. Press. New York, N. Y.

STEPHENSON, H. & W. J. GRACE. 1954. Life stress and cancer of the cervix. Psychosom. Med. **16:** 287.

SURGEON GENERAL'S REPORT ON SMOKING AND HEALTH. 1964. U. S. Public Health Service. Washington, D. C.

TOKUHATA, G. K. & A. M. LILIENFELD. 1963. Familial aggregation of lung cancer in humans. J. Nat. Cancer Inst. **30:** 289.

WITTKOWER, E. 1949. A Psychiatrist Looks at Tuberculosis. Nat. Assoc. Prev. Tuberc. London.

WORLD HEALTH ORGANIZATION. 1965. Epidemiological and vital statistics report. Mortality from malignant neoplasm of larynx and of trachea, bronchus and lung, 1950–1963. **18:** 316.

DISCUSSION OF THE PAPER

DR. BENNETTE: I think Dr. Booth's observations are very rich, with respect to the possibilities of interpreting some of the psychosocial and epidemiologic factors, and I hope it may be possible to design some experiments to see whether one can in fact establish correlations between what Laing calls invalidation of contact and feeling-exchange between parents and their children and the subsequent manifestation of illness.

There is one question, specifically, and that may be answerable. Did Harlow's autistic monkeys in fact develop neoplastic diseases?

DR. BOOTH: No. I asked Harlow, specifically, and he said that they had no observations so far, but the monkeys, for some reason, were very uncooperative about producing diseases.

DR. WILFRED ABSE (*University of Virginia Hospital, Charlottesville, Va.*): I was very much interested in your notions about the phylogenetic basis of cancer of the lung, for example. In hysterical disease, of course, elucidation of pathoplastic fantasies are very important; pseudocyesis with fantasies of pregnancy, to give a very simple one. But in general, with cancer patients it is very difficult to elucidate fantasies.

I understand from what you say that you feel that these belong to the phylogenetic realm, rather than to the individual realm of experience.

DR. BOOTH: I feel that phylogenesis provides a general basis, but it is just the basis of the pathoplastic experience, like the basis of a pyramid. Its apex is the very specific individual manifestation. For example, last week I heard from a man that he had been castrated because of a cancer of the prostate. Nine years ago I had taken his Rorschach because he was involved with one of my patients. In the tenth Rorschach card, he saw what happens to the testicles of the bull after the Spanish bull fight: the ladies get it. The man was truly a victim of the ladies. He had observed blood in his urine for a whole year, but had seen a physician only when he became handicapped by a metastasis in the hipbone.

DR. SALK: I am not sure precisely what I want to say, so I will start to say something and see what comes out. The reason for this is that I am in the very anomalous position of being both a member of the audience and a participant. And one of the observations that you made, followed by an interpretation, prompts me to make some comments upon the relationship between observation and interpretation.

You made some observations about cervical carcinoma and proceeded to offer an explanation for the observations. In other circles, cervical carcinoma is believed to be a venereal disease. Under these circumstances, it is hardly a wonder that very few nuns get cervical carcinoma.

DR. BOOTH: Yes, but some have become nuns after having had many children.

DR. SALK: In view of the statement that you made about the relationship between cervical carcinoma and orgasm, I don't know that that answers the question implied.

DR. BOOTH: I am aware of the virus theory of cervical cancer, but this has no bearing on orgasms. Herpes simplex involves a latent virus that often becomes manifest under emotional stress.

DR. SALK: But this does help clarify what I am about to say. After the first session, Dr. Solomon asked why I was being so objective, and why I didn't speculate, as he knows I am prone to do under other circumstances. I guess I have not done so partly because I try to let the data speak for themselves. There are different styles of dealing with observations that are objectively describable.

This morning I heard a great deal, not of the data speaking for themselves, but you speaking about the data and offering many dynamic or process explanations for a set of observations: for example, the differences you noted between patients with tuberculosis and patients with cancer. I think that many of the observations that you make are very sound, but it would be very interesting to consider alternative explanations just for comparison sometime, to see how different people look at the same set of data. I have illustrated this by an alternative explanation for the cervical carcinoma story.

I could do the same thing for the tuberculosis-cancer story and bring to bear a number of hypotheses and suggestions, but it would be incumbent upon me, of course, to prove that any of these hypotheses or suggestions were valid.

This would necessitate the construction of a series of controls and a great deal of detailed examinations, testing, and analysis to arrive at valid conclusions. I make this comment at this point simply to say that it is worthwhile to have a conference made of persons who come from different disciplines, not merely to hear what each other is saying, but also to observe how the individuals from different disciplines and different backgrounds think.

DR. BOOTH: My paper presented in very aphoristic form personal observations and pertinent publications of others. Over the last 15 years I have studied this material for other hypotheses that would account consistently for the many facets of the epidemic development of cancer, but I have not found any other satisfactory explanation. A fuller account of my work will demonstrate that my hypothesis agrees with the findings of many other observers who had approached cancer from a purely somatic point of view. Today's paper summarized the main points of all this material, not to prove anything, but to illustrate my method of investigating the psychophysiological aspects of cancer.

INTEGRATION, DISCIPLINE, AND THE CONCEPT OF SHAPE

Harley C. Shands

Department of Psychiatry
Roosevelt Hospital
and
College of Physicians and Surgeons
Columbia University
New York, N. Y.

Reviewing published opinions of the past half-century reveals a gradual change in basic frame of reference in the broad field of investigation, especially in the subfield of investigation of human problems. It has become increasingly clear that the scientific approach to problems so successfully based upon causal analysis (assuming a linear progression in a deterministic framework, and using precise statistical methods for evaluation) has not been nearly so useful in helping us understand the human condition and the problems that differentially affect human beings. To say this another way, it is obvious that the standard scientific approach has not given us hoped-for results in psychiatry, whatever its benefits in basic sciences.

Beginning at a point that can, for many purposes, be localized at the half-century mark, a new development has increasingly asserted its influence. Basically, this approach selects as its primary "object" not a thing, but a system, or an organization. Instead of causal analysis, we turn to a communication analysis, utilizing notions of feedback loops, of organization, integration, discipline, and the like with reference to the system of interest. A basic difference is the assumption that we have to begin with an on-going system, already in action; observation then orients itself to differences rather than to new, or newly caused, events.

Investigations leading us to this new theoretical position are easy to find; many have been familiar as works of genius for decades. Names coming readily to mind include Bernard, Cannon, and Sherrington in physiology, Whitehead in philosophy, and many others. Specific contributors to the new mode include Bertalanffy and Bentley in midcentury. Communications theorists e.g. Wiener and Shannon have familiarized us with new formal methods and with mathematical statements applicable to these newly restated problems. Most astonishing of all, the still quite new fields of molecular biology and immunology in the contemporary scene depend almost exclusively upon these ideas. (Lwoff, 1966)

From ideas associated with this new point of view in active fields of research, we find it possible, by making certain alterations in the terms we use, to describe processes across previously unbreachable barriers. Ideas about organization in the broadest sense have a direct bearing upon the ancient problem of "mind" and "body," more elegantly put as the psychophysiological relation. In this monograph we are considering the larger problem with specific reference to cancer.

When it was first suggested that "mental" events could cause cancer, the notion appeared ridiculous to many. Ideas and feelings appear to exist in a universe totally different from that of neoplasms and viruses. How could the one cause the other, or the other be an effect of the one? The resolution of this kind of problem has been taken a great leap forward by recourse to description at a different level of abstraction, using a different method of conception.

André Lwoff, the molecular biologist, gives a clear statement of general principles in saying, "An organism is an integrated system of interdependent structures and functions. An organism is constituted of cells, and a cell consists of molecules which must work in harmony. Each molecule must know what the others are doing. Each one must be capable of receiving messages and must be sufficiently disciplined to obey. . . An organism is a molecular society, and biological order is a kind of social order. Social order is opposed to revolution, which is an abrupt change of order, and to anarchy, which is the absence of order."

From his special field, Lwoff points out that viruses are found often in latent states, "repressed" in symbiotic condition amounting to a stand-off: the virus is not hurting its host, nor the host its "guest." When a traumatic event occurs, derepression may ensue, and when it does, the virus-guest rudely takes over the crucial functions of the host in assuming control of the cellular system in which it has been living. The traumatic events are multiple and varied; they include ultraviolet radiation, hormone treatment, menstruation, and "emotion," among others. The result of the proliferation of the virus may be a viral infection, as in the common appearance of herpes simplex in a person sick for some other reason.

The point I want to make is simply put when we consider the virus in such a case as a set of instructions, functioning somewhat as the sealed orders carried by a ship's captain on a secret mission. At a given signal, the captain opens the letter in which the instructions are concealed, and then, under ancient compulsions in which he has been thoroughly disciplined, undertakes to change his course according to the orders to which he now newly finds himself subject. A properly disciplined captain is prepared to sacrifice himself and his crew in response to his orders. I suggest that many of the catastrophes to which men find themselves subject may similarly be occasions in which inherent instructions quite suddenly gain control because of untoward events acting as signals or precipitants. Depending then upon circumstances, the result may be 1) a pitched battle in which the new instructions are eventually canceled or 2) a revolutionary takeover resulting in a victory for the invader (often a Pyrrhic victory, since the invader can live only as long as does the host), or 3) an anarchic state in which the manifestations of malignant neoplasia may be the principal occurrences.

In this general hypothesis, it is no longer necessary to speculate on "how the mental affects the physical." It is enough to realize that human organization requires multilevel integration. The human being can be so traumatized by the loss of a relative that he may go into a decline and die without much "being wrong" with him. The human being, convinced of having been cursed with an infallible curse, often proceeds to die. The human infant separated from its mother exhibits severe retardation in its development, as the studies of Spitz (1965) show. The list is endless. Even rats show the phenomenon of sudden death under conditions of severe stress, as Richter's studies (1957) indicate.

When we examine these lines of evidence, taken from many studies and pertaining to many different species of animals as well as to man, we find it possible to say that the "lesion" occurring is a loss of integration, a decrease in the level of organization in the system including both individual and his systematic context. "Man does not live by bread alone," which is to say that nonmaterial and personal relations are at least as important in the general scheme as are adequate supplies of food and water. To maintain a high level of organization requires a high level of supply of orderliness, or negentropy, to use Schrödinger's (1945) term. In dependable, regular relations, the organism "obeys" predictable instructions—but when the whole is altered, the organism becomes subject to instructions otherwise quite alien.

We need not look far to find clear examples of such changes, from quite different situations. The young male coming into adolescence finds himself "listening to a different drummer"; he becomes quite abruptly responsive to different "orders," especially those having sexual connotations. He finds himself a "different person"; in the case of one psychotic young man, the patient could not think himself "the same" when sexually aroused and when not so aroused. In a different context, we are all familiar with the striking changes taking place in mobs and crowds. There a "normal human being" may find himself vigorously participating in a riot or a lynching, impervious to the usually effective system of instructions we call "conscience."

We can go further and point out that these altered sensitivities to instructions are valued differently in different situations. Unless the young male responds to different instructions, the species will not be reproduced. Unless the crowd can change individual orientations, human beings cannot be converted; they will not evolve into various social organizations or conquer new territories, terrestrial or ideological. On the other hand, if instructions change, the result can be chaos, anarchy, or malignant neoplastic growth. Plasticity, flexibility, the capacity to change are ways in which we describe a two-edged blade, usable as a surgical scalpel or as a murder weapon. The general problem is the manner in which complex systems are organized to obey instructions in the interest of regularity—and the ways in which such complex organizations break down into disorderliness, temporary or protracted.

My own interest in the general problem of disorderliness stems from a study done about the time we first became interested in the psychological aspects of the cancer problem. We began with an interest in cancer as a disorganizing factor in human lives (Shands *et al.* 1951), coming then to the conclusion reviewed in the first of these conferences, to the effect that a personality is most accurately described as an informational system that must be kept in a state of orderliness through the receipt of general, predictable messages. At about the same time we studied a group of schizophrenic patients undergoing insulin coma therapy (Shands & Menzer, 1953). We had available at that time only crude measures of lymphocyte and eosinophil numbers to estimate the degree of stress involved.

Insulin coma is an extreme physiological emergency; the patient literally is at the point of death for periods of several minutes to an hour. We found that the repetition of this trauma led to a startling randomization or disorderliness in eosinophil numbers. In control studies, all patients exhibited a ceiling eosinophil count of 300 cells/cu mm; after a number of comas, the upper level (quite unpredictably) reached 8,000 in some, but not all, patients.

One interesting correlation was that patients who seemed better integrated in their premorbid state showed far less randomization. After the "therapy," the patients were quite uniformly far less difficult to deal with—but they were, as well, flat, in the psychiatric sense: unemotional, and very much less human and interesting than before. When we tested their responses to stress by measuring the drop in eosinophil numbers that had been very consistent in control experiments prior to the study, a similar complete loss of integration could be found. When we took this a step further by using ACTH, we found, on the contrary, that the specifically physiological response was quite normal. The conclusion we reached then, and it is a conclusion repeatedly reinforced since that time, is that overwhelming trauma, often repeated, may well make human beings more manageable and less difficult to care for. The "therapeutic" effect seemed to be somewhat like that of a fuse, separating a previously integrated organization into noncommunicating parts. From this beginning, the intervening years have been a period of continuous preoccupation with questions of organization and communication in a formulation general enough to include both psychological and physiological as special cases.

In the first of these conferences, personality was described as an informational system (Shands, 1966). Here I want to follow out some consequences of a further generalization of this idea, based upon a suggestion made by Schrödinger (1945) that life can be defined as a continuous extraction of negentropy for use in a continuously maintained system. This central idea is consonant with system theory (von Bertalanffy, 1950) and with information theory as well (Wiener, 1948; Shannon, 1948). With this idea, information, organization, regularity, and orderliness are seen as nearly identical with the negative of entropy. Both physiological and psychological processes are characterized by organization; therefore, if one considers organization as the primary abstraction, then a theory of organization becomes the general case of which physiological organization and psychological organization are special cases (Shands, 1968c).

In a brief review of the conceptual evolution of the past hundred years, we can begin with Bernard's (1865) formulation of an internal milieu as a rather concrete way of describing the orderliness of the cellular environment in the buffer systems. Cannon's (1932) suggestion of the broader term, *homeostasis,* and Sherrington's (1906) term, *integrative action,* both refer to organization in specific contexts of investigation of neural mechanisms. The general case is discussed by Piaget in terms of *homeomorphisms* (or *isomorphisms*) discernable in parallel forms to be found at the level of perceptual mechanisms, of sensory-motor intelligence, and at the highest level of abstract operations. Other aspects of shape, pattern, and form are discussed by D'Arcy Thompson (1961) and by those concerned with the development of artificial intelligence (Selfridge & Neisser, 1960). When we consider all living subsystems as primarily concerned with maintaining the same shape through organizing processes of input and output, it becomes apparent then that the notion of *identity* (Erikson, 1964) is another special case.

Whenever we seek theoretical solutions, we operate in the broad area of homeomorphism. All we can know we learn by transferring a pattern from a context in which it is familiar to a context in which it is unfamiliar. The discoveries of mankind are based upon analogies previously unsuspected, or metaphors previously not applied to the situation under investigation.

The propositions I want to advance here rest upon a very simple notion; namely, that we can, in relation to living systems, usefully substitute the term *instruction* (Shands, 1968b) for familiar terms such as stimulus, input, or even cause. Any significant input carries information, which means by definition that it "makes a difference," and in accordance with the principle of homeostasis-homeomorphism, the system must, if it is to maintain its shape within tolerable limits, act to reestablish the regularity disturbed by the input of the information. Food "instructs" the chewing apparatus to chew and the digestive apparatus to churn and mix and to secrete its characteristic juices. Each phase of digestion ends when the processed substrate no longer issues appropriate instructions. The fact that we generally construe such sequences attributing agency (and consciousness) to the other party is alternative (and complementary) to this view.

Adopting this different convention, traditional distinctions disappear. When we use the term *instruction* in this very broad sense, we understand behavior as a continuous ongoing process, continuously shaped and reshaped by myriad instructions. As the organism lives and learns, it deals with instructions in more predictive terms, so that as it becomes more sophisticated in both phylogenetic and ontogenetic context, the organism is characterized by an enhanced ability to anticipate instructions. Shaping characteristically also involves retrospective instructions in positive or negative feedback. Sequences of behavior are retrospectively facilitated or inhibited by contingencies of reinforcement, and the retrospective assessment operates as a predictive influence on the next exhibition of the behavior in question.

I have elsewhere explored the reasons for suggesting forcibly that what we ordinarily call "conscious" behavior boils down to behavior susceptible to description, and thus to the basic idea of verbal behavior (Shands, 1968a). Here I want simply to point out that starting from the top level of the behavioral armamentarium of the human being and proceeding to lower levels, instead of starting at the bottom and proceeding toward the more sophisticated levels, appears to be the procedure of choice in the formation of theories as well as (in Freud's prescription) the rule for the application of a psychotherapeutic point of view.

Human affairs feature the idiosyncratic use of symbolic method using verbal tokens. But when we examine a host of recent findings in genetics, immunology, and virology, we find unsuspected analogues to the process of abstraction, hitherto considered simply a function of symbolic process. Abstraction rests upon the biological capacity for a shape to be used to instruct a living system to reproduce the same shape, a basic pattern widespread in nature. When we understand that one of the possible consequences of this method is endless replication, we find a model for at least some forms of neurosis and cancer.

The immediate impact of our cancer study was to obliterate many distinctions often made between the "imaginary" and the "real." We found, to what now seems my naïve astonishment, that the disturbances of "real" trauma were very similar to those of "neurotic" trauma. The disturbance to the informational economy involved centers around the input of novelty (Shands, 1967), and in turn the novel can be circularly defined as the unexpected or unexpectable.

Taking the next step, we can then say that "personality" has an important family resemblance to a program (Shands, 1963), as the term is used in computer technology, and to grammar as this term is used in relation to symbolic-linguistic systems. In all three cases we deal with what might be called, perhaps tautologically, *structures of instructions.* In all three cases the entity is primarily one having a shape differentiating it from its surround. I would suggest here that the appropriate term for that surround is *context* rather than *environment:* when we say an organism lives in an environment, we suggest that the two are fundamentally different, but when we say that something exists in a context, we more easily think of system and subsystem, mutually or transactionally interdependent. Using this model, we see that when the context is "natural," the system responds to "natural" instructions; when in a human context, instructions may be as well "artificial," "symbolic," or "conscious."

Personalities, programs, and grammars are internally structured in ways usually so regular as to have a high degree of redundancy. The subsystem "expects" (Cantril, 1950) a continuous series of instructions, and in the normal case each such instruction sets off a train of inner programmed instructions affecting the subsystem. Learning, in the broadest sense, is a process of establishing a stable system of inner communication related to the instructions received from the larger system. We can speak of the internal processing of information and the setting up of stable sets of internal instructions as *discipline*. After a period of learning, a disciplined subsystem predictively relates itself to its context, and the stability of its own internal discipline predictively discounts a wide range of novelty in the relation of system and subsystem.

In the human context, processing instructions at more and more general levels allows the subsystem to become so disciplined that it can tolerate amounts of novelty that are unbearable (traumatic) to less sophisticated systems. Many transient relationships – as between parent and child, perceptor and novice – buffer the latter during a developmental period: these relationships "temper the wind to the [naked] lamb." Premature rupture of such a relationship may expose the unsophisticated member to traumatic injury.

Human beings have to develop programs oriented both (1) to the social context, and (2) to the nonhuman and inanimate context. This amounts to a dual adaptation. Both system and subsystem in either context are continuously involved in sending and receiving instructions, and in obeying, ignoring, or defying instructions received. Much of learning involves experimenting with the limits of tolerance. Through modern science and technology, human beings have achieved an astonishing capacity for instructing the inanimate context to "obey"–in mines, factories, smelters, and the other manifestations of man's grasp of scienific law. The obvious, corresponding failure to maintain appropriate discipline in social systems stands in sharp contrast to this remarkable success; a measure of the failure is that, as human beings, we obviously do not know what kinds of discipline are socially appropriate, and each cultural subsystem tends to set up its territorial claims in opposition to other subsystems.

When we consider the vicissitudes of growing and learning in a developmental context, we understand the different outcomes of programs of instructions more comprehensively. The obsessive-compulsive person is one in whom symbolic instructions have attached exceptional ("magical") potency; he is over-disciplined in many obvious ways. When we study such a person, however, we find him under-disciplined in his capacity to follow human instructions. His counterpart, the delinquent, is inadequately responsive to symbolic instructions, but delinquent behavior is too ready an obedience to instructions conveyed by the context of the moment..

During the second world war, Bartlett (1947) investigated highly skilled activities. "Skill" is a term used primarily in relation to muscular activities; it is appropriate here because "highly skilled" is a term close to "disciplined" in its connotations. The skilled person demonstrates a high degree of integration in relating instructions received from the context and from inside himself. Every skilled movement integrates the demands of the context with the movement sequence from which the response to the outer demands takes origin. Bartlett points out that there are two thresholds of significance with relation to highly skilled work. The lower threshold is that of indifference, the upper that of tolerance; certain instructions are too weak to be known, and certain tasks remain beyond the capacity of even the skilled person.

These two thresholds change in temporal sequence; repeated learning, with drill and repetition, results in changing the level of both thresholds. The skilled person ignores many cues distracting to the unskilled person, while at the same time he is acutely sensitive to nuances he has come to understand as significant. The skilled performer is more efficient and more tolerant of performance, husbanding his resources by performing only the essential activity. With practice, the skilled performer is able to carry on for much longer periods of time. In the opposite direction, prolonged activity eventuates in evidence of impairment and of fatigue. These tend to be associated with changes in the two thresholds: the tired person is less sensitive both to significant cues and to his own deteriorating performance. When tired, he has to work harder than when fresh, for the same result.

This general description covers a variety of skilled performances. Skills include speaking and writing, as well as directing an aircraft or motor car; the physiological activity of the body fits the scheme as well. Cannon points to the importance of realizing that the infant "learns" homeostasis through training autonomic activity, and contemporary investigators more and more present immunological theories in terms of prior "instruction" by an attack of the pathogenic agent or through the "laboratory" of vaccination. We can consider evolutionary progress in species as the manifestation of learning "by the species," through the selection of mutations aiding skillful adaptation to the environment.

Application of these ideas to problems of disease requires that we first consider the analogies that dictate our theories. Descartes' pervasive influence has mostly led us to understand the animal body as a machine, responsive to instructions of a causal nature. This notion is easy to follow when we consider that a machine has to be turned on in some manner, from a previous state of passive inactivity. When we then turn the machine off, we do not have to consider issuing "Stop!" instructions – it is included in the loss of power supply. The animal organism, on the other hand, is categorically different, since it runs (necessarily and unavoidably) without pause from conception to death. To turn off some ongoing pattern of behavior in the living organism often requires a specific "Stop!" instruction. We have paid far too little attention to this problem, although (cf. obsessions and compulsions) it is obviously of importance when we take it into account.

A recently clarified case in point is the problem of obesity. A number of studies now present strongly suggestive evidence that obesity is not so much caused, as by too large an appetite or by disorders of metabolism, as it is a function of a disordered susceptibility to the cessation instruction. The fat person, to say it simply, does not know when to quit eating; it is not that he is hungry so much as it is that he is responsive to the food's implicit instruction, "Eat Me," like Alice confronted by the little cake in Wonderland.

In various kinds of learning, we can ignore the problem of the cessation instruction simply because human beings are limitedly docile. They tend to issue the cessation instruction to themselves. In many deviant conditions, however, we find that this is no longer the case. In a psychosomatic context, I have mentioned the problem of obesity. In a psychiatric context, we find the cessation problem uppermost in phobias, "crystallized conflicts" (Shands, 1968b), and obsessional and compulsive disorders. At the immunological level, allergic disorders are primarily acute inflammations that do not follow the ordinary path of cessation through resolution; hay fever, for instance, is a protracted rhinitis and conjunctivitis. We find a striking parallel in myth in the story of the sorcerer's apprentice who learned how to turn on the broom but could not turn it off, and in the addictions we find a very similar pattern. In all these we can understand an organization with a usually predictable shape becoming deranged by a loss of the terminal boundary. The boundary that limits the extent of the organized process is ruptured, and the process becomes perseverative, like a broken record.

The principal characteristic of neoplastic tissue is that it responds to instructions saying "Grow!" without being then obedient to the ordinary instructions that say "Now stop!" This lack of terminal obedience is often associated with the activity of filterable viruses, and when we turn our attention to these part-organisms, we find the pattern typical. An active virus enters a cell and diverts the physiological processes of that cell to its own use, thereby initially establishing something of an analogy to the cuckoo that lays its eggs in the nest of another bird after pushing the appropriate eggs out of the nest. The special feature of the virus molecule's activity is that under favorable conditions, it tends to replicate itself endlessly. It requires an active process of cutoff to suspend the activity of the virus; the virologists speak of "repression" in this connection, with "derepression" when some traumatic event affects the capacity of the cell to resist takeover by the virus (Lwoff, 1966).

The repressed virus becomes a part of a situation, imbedded in that situation in a manner making it impossible to differentiate part from whole. The part retains its potential autonomy, and it appears again in an autonomous state when derepressed. Then the liberated virion is freed to scan its surround to find a suitable host for the subsequent takeover. Whitehead (1925), in his "philosophy of organism," points out that the part is an aspect of the environment for the whole. In the case of the virus, the part takes command of the whole.

The aspect of this transaction to which I want to call special attention is that a virion can be considered an instruction. In its basic activity, it is like any "to whom it may concern" instruction, moving freely until it encounters its appropriate second party. In the ordinary bodily economy, as Wiener has noted, hormones, (chemical messengers) have such a function, as does the aversive message of the skunk's odor. Through the circulating humoral instruction, the pituitary gland as a central source of master messages controls the activity of endocrine glands throughout the body.

The message carried by the virus has one major difference from the message carried by the hormone; namely, that since its goal is to replicate itself, it is potentially infinite in its activity. No humoral message can so transcend its goal; the destiny of the humoral message is to terminate at its target origin. When we see this difference, we grasp that the virus in its own peculiar character is analogous to the symbolic message, rather than to the chemical message. The message carried by the symbol, or by the symbolic system as a whole, is highly similar to that carried by the virus, in that the symbolic system has as a primary goal the replication of itself in other hosts. Since the symbolic message as pure shape (Schrödinger, 1951) is never used up, it is potentially infinite in its dissemination; its only limitation is in the number of potential hosts.

Internalizing a symbolic system is like internalizing a virus: no matter how inapparent the difference, the host is never again the same. Under appropriate circumstances of susceptibility, the host can become the victim of the internalized instruction; I see disaster of this sort as the core problem of neurosis in the symbolic context, as the consequence with a de-repressed virus may be a spreading infection.

The extraordinary homeomorphism then evident is that the relation of cell and virus reveals the basic structure of abstraction. In both instances, the part comes to gain control of the whole in functioning as an instruction oriented toward its own replication. For this reason, the part operates autonomously and without natural termination. The feedback system comes to be positive, rather than negative, and success breeds further success – while we must always then remember that from the other point of view, failure breeds further failure. What is success from the point of view of the part is failure from the point of view of the whole.

The point of central significance is that we have been fundamentally in error in likening living systems to inanimate objects and physical systems. The inanimate system cannot learn, whereas the living system has to learn if it is to come to the full deployment of its potential for adaptation. The developmental history is as crucial an aspect of the living system as are its component molecules. We must always bear in mind that there are many different explanatory ideas about disorder of any kind in a living system. In relatively simple situations, a cause-and-effect explanation may yield significant insight for effective methods of understanding, but in many others, linear formulation is misleading.

An organism progressively learns to dispense with preceptorial buffering as it internalizes preceptorial methods in a gradual increment of discipline. The process described by Cannon at the level of automatic learning is homeomorphic with processes of cognitive learning. Disorder is to be understood in terms of integrative function, with the clear implication that integration is learned progressively. In the course of learning, temporary crises occur in which the input of novelty may be for the moment partially disabling; in many of these instances the need for buffering by a preceptor reappears temporarily. When the crisis is successfully weathered, the result is an increment of integrative capacity. If the crisis is inadequately met, if temporary buffering is not available, there may be a further worsening of the adaptive state because trauma impairs adaptive mechanisms, through positive feedback.

Viruses are like ideological patterns existing for extended periods in some kind of fragile equilibrium, inducing a morbid state when trauma allows rerelease of the dangerous pattern and its spread among previously uninvolved aspects of the system. Hoffer (1951) points out in his studies of the mass movements of the twentieth century that alien ideologies tend to affect the frustrated and the disadvantaged. We scarcely need remind ourselves of the relevance of his predictive comments in the present state of affairs in our universities, our country, and in the world. It need scarcely be noted, either, that when we say "alien ideology" we speak in relativistic terms, since the nature of human cultures is such that any imported ideology tends to be alien. Since the incident at the Tower of Babel, man's condition has been that of enmity toward his conspecific fellow of a different persuasion.

The thought I want to present, then, can be restated in terms of the subject matter of this monograph. It is that the disorder of physiological function seen in, say, hay fever, is analogous to the disorder of cognitive function seen in obsessions and in phobic states. At a different pair of levels of function, the disorder of loss of terminal control is that seen in neoplastic illness and that metaphorically evident in the myth of the sorcerer's apprentice who could turn on but not turn off. In the broadest context, the process is that of abstraction, the use of a part to instruct the whole; and inherent in abstraction are the potentialities of neurosis. When we see the extensive homeomorphisms from level to level in this model, then the interrelation of emotional and neoplastic disorder appears theoretically inescapable; we have already seen in many different contexts that the empirical relation is readily observable.

References

BARTLETT, F. C. 1947. Measurement of Human Skill. Brit. Med. J. **1:** 835, 877.

BENTLEY, A. F. 1950. Kennetic Inquiry. Science **112:** 775–183.

BERNARD, C. 1865. An Introduction to the Study of Experimental Medicine. Macmillan Co. 1927. New York, N. Y.

CANNON, W. B. 1932. The Wisdom of the Body. W. W. Norton & Co., Inc. New York, N. Y.

CANTRIL, H. 1950. The "Why" of Man's Experience. Macmillan Co. New York, N. Y.
ERIKSON, E. 1964. Insight and Responsibility. W. W. Norton & Co., Inc. New York, N. Y.
HOFFER, E. 1951. The True Believer. Harper & Row. New York, N. Y.
LWOFF, A. 1966. Interaction among virus, cell and organism. Science **152:** 1216-1220.
RICHTER, C. P. 1957. On the Phenomenon of Sudden Death in Animals and Man. Psychosom. Med. **19:** 191–198.
SCHRÖDINGER, ERWIN. 1945. What Is Life? Cambridge University Press. Cambridge, England.
SCHRÖDINGER, ERWIN. 1951. Science and Humanism. Cambridge University Press. Cambridge, England.
SELFRIDGE, O. P. & U. NEISSER. 1960. Pattern recognition by machine. Sci. Amer. **203:** 60.
SHANDS, H. C. & J. E. FINESINGER. 1948. Lymphocytes in the psychoneuroses. Amer. J. Psychiat. **105:** 277–285.
SHANDS, H. C., J. E. FINESINGER, S. COBB & R. ABRAMS. 1951. Psychological mechanisms in patients with cancer. Cancer **4:** 1159–1170.
SHANDS, H. C. & D. MENZER. 1953. Eosinophil variation in the course of insulin coma therapy. Amer. J. Psychiat. **109:** 757–766.
SHANDS, H. C. 1963. Conservation of the self. Arch. of Gen. Psychiat. **9:** 311–323.
SHANDS, H. C. 1966. The informational impact of cancer on the structure of the human personality. N. Y. Acad. Sci. **125**(3): 883–889.
SHANDS, H. C. 1967. Novelty as object. Arch. Gen. Psychiat. **17:** 1.
SHANDS, H. C. 1968a. Psychoanalysis and the twentieth century revolution in communication. *In* Modern Psychoanalysis. Judd Marmor, Ed. Basic Books. New York, N. Y.
SHANDS, H. C. 1968b. Crystallized conflict. M.S. thesis delivered at Speech Communication Center, Univ. Wis. at Milwaukee. Feb. (To be published.)
SHANDS, H. C. 1968c. "Coping with Novelty." (Unpublished.)
SHANNON, C. E. 1948. A Mathematical Theory of Communication. Bell System Tech. J. **27:** 379–423.
SHERRINGTON, SIR CHARLES S. 1906. The Integrative Action of the Nervous System. Yale Univ. Press. New Haven, Conn. 1948
SPITZ, R. A. with W. G. COBLINER. 1965. The First Year of Life: A Psychoanalytic Study of Normal and Deviant Development of Object Relations. Chapter **XIV:** 267–284.
THOMPSON, D'ARCY. 1961. On Growth and Form. Abridged edit. Cambridge University Press. Cambridge, England.
VON BRETALANFFY, L. 1950. The theory of open systems in physics and biology. Science **111:** 23–28.
WHITEHEAD, A. N. 1925. Science and the Modern World. Mentor Books. New York, N. Y. 1960.
WIENER, N. 1948. Cybernetics. John Wiley & Sons, Inc. New York, N. Y.

DISCUSSION OF THE PAPER

DR. SALK: I found this to be a very fascinating discussion, and had the impulse to want to break in at a number of points along the way. Dr. Lwoff spent about six months at our institute this past year, and he is a most extraordinary scientist, a highly intuitive person—I used the word poet two days ago—and he is one of the rare people who can describe the field in which he has worked in the terms in which you have interpreted them.

He is basically an artist and his work is magnificent, and, as you all know, he shared the Nobel prize with two other remarkable people about two years ago. He is fundamentally a molecular biologist, but he sees the gestalt of what he is doing, and it is for this reason that he made so significant a contribution. He spent time trying to understand the shut-off mechanism, at the molecular level. If you look at the organization, or the order in a cell that becomes neoplastic, it is equally clear that the regulatory mechanism has somehow been jammed in the on-position rather than the off-position. Molecular biologists are applying themselves to try to understand precisely the structural nature of the process that is involved. And they are trying to define precisely the chemical elements responsible for neoplasia.

Now, earlier you talked about linguistics, and said that language was uniquely human. Other forms of communication between animals are merely communication. Human language is a specialized form of communication. You then jumped to the molecular level, and I was glad that you did that, because there are parallels in that both express forms of communication. The code needs to be translated, and what we tend to do with abstraction is to code them, and then they have to be decoded again.

We have a strange institute because Roman Jacobsen, the linguist at Harvard and MIT, has spent several months of each of the last several years with us, working with Dr. Bronowski, who gave a lecture the other day on magic and science. What has been going through my mind during this conference, in part, has been about the nature of the evolution of thought processes in attempting to explain natural phenomena. There was a time when magic was a way in which we could explain things. Now we use science as a way of explaining things. Perhaps I can tie the two periods together by using the phrase that Bronowski used when he talked about the difference being between black magic and white magic.

I suppose I could characterize some of the discussions that I have been listening to as gray magic. An attempt is made to take an observable fact and offer an explanation that is almost magical in its quality. What we are really trying to do is to understand nature. What are nature's explanations of the phenomena that we observe? And that, perhaps, is the difference in the approach that I hear from the two different sets of minds that are both addressing themselves to this very interesting and complicated problem.

Dr. Shands: It seems to me that the most important problem that we are now confronting is whether or not the frame of reference in science that has existed triumphantly for over two hundred years is now appropriate to the requirements of this era.

It is my own opinion that traditional science is obsolete. What is succeeding it is a much broader field, concerned primarily with communication and organization, of which science forms a special case.

Dr. Abse: What I was going to talk about has become distracted by the dialogue between Dr. Salk and Dr. Shands. I certainly do not agree with you, Harley, that we depart from science. However, I feel that your discussion is relevant.

Many years ago, actually in 1885, there was a book called *The Life of Speech*, by Wegener, who was a German linguist. It is a very remarkable book, in that he shows that language evolves in the child through a process on the one hand of orderly emandation, (I cannot go into all the aspects of this), but on the other hand, what is very important for the evolution of discursive language is the metaphor. And in the work, as you know, of Suzanne Langer, this business of symbolic transformation acquires a great deal of importance. In fact, it is through metaphor—the evolution of live and dead metaphor—that discursive language evolves, and it is fundamentally posited upon physical impressions that we have to use for semantic movement in order to encompass novelties. And in this way, we acquire a basis for an orderly view of the universe.

When somebody has a psychosomatic disorder, in general, there is regression in one part of the mental apparatus. I think that this part, however, gets dissociated from another part. There is still orderliness. There is orderliness in one sector, there is organization in one sector, but there is another sector that is disorderly, in which there is regression; there is regression in the symbolic transformation, so that you get back to the fundamental physical processes. I think that what we are dealing with is a certain loss of shape in one aspect of the ego, the body ego part of the total mental ego.

DR. SHANDS: When one says "organization," it presupposes that there are many different lower-level organizations, any one or any number of which can be in good working order, or in fair working order, except that something is interfering with the total integration. It would seem to me that it is entirely logical that if something catastrophically disturbing happens at the symbolic level, in terms of the discovery of some terrible event or the receipt of some dreadful news, it is quite likely that the whole organization will be temporarily disorganized while preparing itself for reconstitution.

PART VI. THEORETICAL PSYCHOPHYSIOLOGICAL CONSIDERATIONS

GENERAL DISCUSSION

Claus Bahne Bahnson,* *Moderator*

Department of Psychiatry
Jefferson Medical College, Philadelphia, Pa.

When we planned this conference, there were several of the members of the conference committee who thought we should have a chance to sit down as informally as we possibly could and discuss some of the main concepts and issues that might have arisen during the first half of the conference, before we enter the last day of the conference, when we will try to integrate some of the ideas that were presented. There is no agenda at all for this session, but in order to make it a little easier for all of us, I suggest that we might talk about one of several things. We could talk about the general theoretical problem of this conference, the relationship between experience and physiological function as it pertains to malignancies. Several of the participants have alluded to this; certainly, Dr. Salk brought it up on the first day, and several others have been struggling with relevant concepts. We have been wondering how one might conceptualize the role played by psychodynamic or experiential processes, and about the way they may interact with endocrinological, immunological, and other processes.

There have been different opinions about this. Some participants have operated in terms of more reductionistic formulations, approaching the malignancy problem as a multifactorial situation. These formulations assume that one must consider several factors, but that these in a way all are independent processes with a common target. There have been other formulations, like that of Bennette, framed in existential terms, conceptualizing existence not so much as a physiological process, but as some kind of experiential expanse that may be manifested on different levels.

Many of us have been struggling with the whole problem of what one can call psychosomatic relationships and the complementarity of interaction between different system levels. Since we think differently about this, some of us may raise, discuss, and amplify this problem.

Another possibility for this meeting, I think, is to take off from the greater biological refinement that has been introduced in the conference with the consideration of different types of immune responses and different mediators of this response. Dr. Salk, Dr. Weiss, and Dr. Klein introduced the discussion of the immune response on the cellular and the humoral levels as two complementary and perhaps interacting systems, and pointed out that one cannot consider immune responses as a simple one-track process, but must deal with it as a differentiated and very complex subject matter. The phylogenetic implications of the time table for "invention" of the different branches of the immune response certainly seems relevant at this point.

I am impressed by the recommendations of Dr. Klein that we should think of devising experiments–equations–that can elucidate the exact relationship between well-depicted experiential or psychologic states and specific immunological reactions, whether they be on the cellular or humoral levels. Here is a whole area that could be taken up in discussion.

* Present address: Eastern Pennsylvania Psychiatric Instiute, Institute of Pennsylvania Hospital, Philadelphia, Pa., and University of Connecticut, Storrs, Conn.

A third area that comes to mind, as a free association, is the problem that Dr. Margolin presented yesterday, the problem of "open systems," originally introduced by Grinker, the relationship between social psychological and sociological variables (for example, in the Ute Indians) and psychodynamics processes such as the interaction between a social system and the specific handling of aggression that may involve both the particular depressive matrix and the defensive solution of it. Here, I also think of ego defense in terms of Kissen's and my own emphasis of defense against certain affective potentials.

These, then, are three possible starting points. Why do we not, any of us, on this basis, raise whatever idea or train of thought that comes to mind? I think we should then be on our way.

DR. MARGOLIN: I am most interested in the references to a possible phylogenesis of cancer. It seems to me that logic would compel us to postulate an equally plausible biogenetic origin of the mechanisms of immunity, especially in relation to the incidence of malignancy in the lower vertebrates. Among such organisms, it is suggested or implicitly stated that there are no malignancies, only regenerative processes. That is to say, an animal whose limb is removed will regenerate that limb.

There are many tissues in the human body that continuously or episodically regenerate without undergoing neoplastic changes. Hence, the phenomenon of tissue constancy is not necessarily unique. I was also interested in the suggestion that the immune process develops phylogenetically in higher vertebrates as a way of coping with lethal neoplasms.

I should like to suggest a counter hypothesis, namely, that in all vertebrates below the amphibia, tissue growth is regulated by a hyperimmune state that inhibits neoplasms. Subsequent phylogenetic evolution, especially of organisms with internalized regulatory systems, led to some lessening of the immune state and increase of the neoplasms. I think that this broadly stated hypothesis is as plausible as the one it opposes.

At the same time, however, I do not think it is a better statement than the one that was proposed. I merely wish to emphasize that because we are all very facile, we run the risk of misleading each other with our impressive and ingenious explanatory statements.

DR. SOLOMON: May I add something to that problem, so that you can respond to that, too. I was visting a friend who was working on the phylogeny of the immune response, at Stanford's Hopkins Marine Station. Apparently, there is some evidence of quasiimmunologic memory of a primitive sort in the echinoderms, which are probably closer to the vertebrate line than any other invertebrate phylum. Foreign material to which there was previous exposure is more rapidly phagocytized. In discussing this matter with the director of the Hopkins Marine Station, he raised the question whether or not memory develops simultaneously phylogenetically in the nervous system and in the immune system, since these animals can learn simple avoidance tasks and can undergo simple conditioning. I believe there is no evidence of immunologic memory in flatworms, and I think the evidence for behavioral learning is pretty weak in flatworms. I am not very good at this, but the question was once raised and discussed whether a possible reason that the immune system and the central nervous system may have some relationships and tie-ins is that both systems learn by experience and that it is conceivable that the molecular basis of memory by means of RNA-coding is similar in both. I wonder if you, Dr. Salk, would comment on this, in view of Dr. Margolin's question, possibly from both the phylogenetic and the theoretical points of view.

DR. SALK: These are both very good questions, and I think they provide an excellent basis upon which to enter into a discussion of the question of the association between psychological factors and neoplasia.

In the instance that you mentioned, the question is whether there is a cause-and-effect relationship or whether it depends only on an association. The two events may happen to occur at about the same time, phylogenetically.

DR. MARGOLIN: Implying that they are neither causes nor effects of each other?

DR. SALK: They simply are parallel phylogenetic phenomena. That is, phenomena that occur independently at essentially the same points of time in evolution.

DR. MARGOLIN: Nevertheless, they can be necessary or sufficient without being cause and effect.

DR. SALK: Necessary, but not necessarily related. The immunologic system, without a doubt, when it was invented, contributed enormously to survival, under circumstances in which survival would otherwise have been impossible. There must have been some forerunner of the immunologic system that may have served a similar function or similar purpose. If not, the integrity of the organism could not have been maintained. Parasitism would have prevailed. I think this is self-evident.

The organizational integrity of the organism in relation to its external environment is preserved and protected by the immunologic system, or whatever was the forerunner of the immunologic system. I do not know the nature of the ordering mechanism that preceded this. The immunologic system is the kind of ordering mechanism that preserves the integrity of the organism against being disordered. This has enormous survival value.

The same thing would be true of the internal environment, as in mammals or other multicellular organisms. The immunologic system has to adapt to the recognition of self versus not self. And it is clear that some cleansing mechanism was necessary; hence, the phagocytic system and the immunologic system clearly have a relationship to each other. I am reasonably certain that, phylogenetically, parts of it are really quite old and other parts are only newly developed, in the same way that you have the old and the new parts of the nervous system. These have developed with time.

I do like to think of the immunologic systems and the nervous system in parallel. I remember thinking this way and talking about it rather early. Perhaps more than a dozen years ago I had occasion to give a talk to a psychiatric group in Chicago. I talked of the immunologic systems as having the same relationship to the external environment as does the nervous system in providing a sensing mechanism, a recognition mechanism, and a responding mechanism. I think of the immunologic system and the nervous system as being parts of the somatic system, by contrast with the genetic system; the environment does not have a direct effect on the genetic system. The two systems that are necessary for maintaining the integrity of the organism in relation to the external environment are the nervous system and the immunologic system.

We can carry this discussion further, speculatively, and say that as life became more complicated, both systems became increasingly complex. All of the structures that were developed, developed because of a need. Our problem now, is to try to understand structure-function relationships. Even when we measure a structure called antibody, this says nothing about the functional nature of that particular antibody. About 1950, we studied antibody response over a period of a year, taking weekly bleedings from monkeys given a single injection of antigen and testing the serum by three different methods. Subtraction curves developed from the results of the different methods of measurement did not give a straight line, but yielded curves, which indicated that there were different molecular species that rose and declined at different rates. At that time, one measurement was regarded as equivalent to another, and without respect for what is the functional meaning of these molecules.

DR. MARGOLIN: Dr. Salk, I wonder if, in addition to the general theory you have been outlining for us, we might respond to your questions, namely: "How does the psychological aspect become coherent with this molecular and neural system?" You have described a provocative formulation in which the complexities of the immune systems and of the central nervous system were evolutionary inventions in the service of a more general immunological and molecular system. In such a system, many lawful relationships would operate. For example, the law of mass action would make antigen-antibody reactions predictable and measurable. In psychophysiological or ethological terms, the organism can learn or become conditioned in order to reduce the concentration of molecular factors that are determinants of the immune responses. Thus, the central nervous system, together with its mental functions, can influence the immune process by altering the internal and external conditions of the organism. In this concept, the aim of the mental apparatus would not be to interfere with the lawful relationships and the principles that govern these biological mechanisms, but rather, to modify internal and external situations that attenuate their influences.

If behavior is not realistically and teleologically adapted to the biological processes, the maladaptive biological effects can be enhanced. It would appear, therefore, that the principles of adaptation are not intended to reduce the immune processes, but to influence their effects.

DR. MARC LAPPE (*Institute for Cancer Research, Philadelphia, Pa.*): I have difficulty following the discussion. I think we are taking off from somewhere and ending up somewhere else. I should like to add some ballast to these flights of fancy. Perhaps this is the least useful thing to do, but I cannot help trying to get some hard facts into the discussion, for one thing, I think, hard facts about evolution and antibody production. It is a pretty hard fact that the cellular response, which is supposedly the response that first appeared and which is functional in rejection of neoplasms, appeared, as far as we can tell, at the same time as the humoral response was established. The lowest animal in which both responses are found is the hank fish, and correct me if I am wrong. Therefore, if the humoral response really is not functional in rejection, and the cellular response is the response for which the immune system was "created," these two responses should not have appeared at the same time. Of course, we are talking of a scale of millions of years, and it is possible that if you went to the proper species (which we may not be able to define), the cellular response may appear earlier.

As far as the conditions of hyperimmune responses in lower animals is concerned, I think that when you talk about immune responses, you ought to make clear that in our terms of reference these are adaptive immune responses, not the general immune responses of the system. Adaptive immune responses have been searched for in lower species as far as immune responses go, and Ben Campbell, for example, had lobsters around for a year or so that he immunized. He reported that he looked very extensively for either antibody reactions or what he thought might be something like an anaphylactic reaction, and could not find either.

Others have exposed snails to albumin, radioactively tagged, and found that they sequestered it and stored it under the shell for a long time, for years in fact, which seems rather difficult to understand, not knowing much about the zoology of the snail.

The question is, why would the system go to the very extreme length of having an animal go into anaphylaxis, if the purpose is really just to serve as a warning? How much of a warning do you need, and at what point does a warning become useless?

DR. BENNETTE: You ask the question, "What do we understand by immune response?" It seems to me that we have been concentrating throughout this meeting solely on the immunological reactivity aimed at retaining the integrity of the cell against invasion by mutant clones of cells, or by microorganisms, or by foreign substances. No attention has been paid to the morphostatic possibilities of activity in the immune system.

If, as Burnet believes, the immune system is concerned not only with the surveillance mechanism that keeps the cell in an organized state, but is actually concerned with the control of differentiation in a morphostatic system (and this is a big "if"), then we have here the possibility of considering the effects of immunity in a much broader sense, involving the control of differentiation in some fashion. The question then arises as to what extent we should consider the cancer process as being a defect of growth and differentiation. According to the model of Smithers, who has presented the other side of the picture to the somatic mutation theory, the idea is that the cancer cell is not a diseased cell, but a cell which is behaving abnormally as a result of the buildup of differentiational abnormalities. May I mention here the following observation: If you have a traffic jam, there is no great sense in studying the internal combustion engines of the individual automobiles. What you need is something to untangle the jam. When you have a jam in the differentiational controlling mechanisms, whatever these morphostatic mechanisms may be, it could well be that behavioral changes promote genetic changes, antigenetic changes and all kinds of other inducing mechanisms that produce the autonomous malignant cell. Therefore, could we perhaps look at the immune system in this broader light as a possible morphostatic system?

DR. SALK: I think it would be good to put the immunologic system aside for the moment and concentrate on the point that you have just raised, about the origin of the cell that just multiplies without respect to the order within the organism itself, and becomes neoplastic. Those who are interested in the mechanism whereby this occurs have tackled the problem in a variety of ways. One of the most elegant of which I am aware is the one that Dulbecco is using. He is studying temperature-sensitive mutants of the polyoma virus to try to determine which genome of the virus, of which there are only six or eight, in contrast to about a million within the cell itself, gives rise to the neoplastic condition. One of the expressions of neoplasia in the system that they are using is the loss of contact-inhibition. This means that when the normal nonneoplastic cells are allowed to grow on tissue culture, they grow in a monolayer. And when the cells come in contact with each other, they stop growing and do not form in multilayers, but stop multiplying.

On the other hand, when cells have become neoplastic, there is a loss of contact-inhibition, and the cells simply pile up, one on top of the other. That is a very simple marker for recognizing the existence of neoplasia. And this is something that can be induced *in vitro*. I do not want to go into more detail other than to say that with a simple, elegant system such as this, it is possible to show that the introduction of viral material into the cell is all that is necessary to bring about this alteration in state. In the intact animal, the immunologic system enters and plays a role in defense of the organism itself.

Those who are interested in the problem of the origin of neoplasia are also beginning to think about the problem of differentiation, as well. Differentiated cells are beginning to be studied; an attempt is being made to make them neoplastic and have them remain in their differentiated state. The very fascinating problem that developmental biologists are attacking is the question of the mechanism that is involved in the turning-on and turning-off of genes after the first cell division: the second, third, fourth, and so on. This then eventually results in the cell's becoming a differentiated cell, still with the same genetic load that was present in the beginning. The expression of the different functions is the result of the turning-off of genes that were active or potentially active originally, so that the multipotential cell, which is the single cell, then becomes more narrowly defined by the turning-off of genes. Therefore, when neoplasia occurs, the cell does not necessarily have the same function characteristics, although it may have them. It may become anaplastic; it may regress to an earlier form. The neoplastic cell now has become an entirely different animal, in the sense that it is now independent of the controlling mechanisms of the organism as a whole. Now the immunologic system responds to it as if it were foreign material, depending on the sensitivity of the recognition system or the degree of difference that is revealed to the immunologic system by the changes that have occurred in the neoplastic cell.

Dr. Bennette: The question of differentiation should be thought of as being an inducer mechanism that turns genetic information on and off. This seems to be very important when it comes to the question of the possibility of spontaneous remission with maturation. Research has shown that in the mouse one may take one tumor cell that is anaplastic and apparently fully differentiated and produce from this cell a tumor mass that contains fully differentiated tissue. One cannot regard the original cell as being genetically committed to its neoplastic condition, but it is rather subject to complex controlling mechanisms that must in some way, it would seem to me, modify the induction and repression mechanisms of the genetic information.

Could this be the mechanism of morphostasis, and if it is, is it operated through immunocytes? If it is operated through immunocytes, then we need to look at the immunological system as a system that, by reason of its extraordinary capacity of evolution and mobilization in response to all sorts of different situations, may itself be a psychobiological system. I have the poetic picture of a man whose bones and muscles and organs have been removed, and all he has left is lymphoid tissue. You have a ghost of a man and loads of lymphoid tissue, and you have dispersed lymphoid tissue, and you have dispersed lymphoid cells moving around and responding to stimuli, responding to the needs of the situation, as Burnet put it. The possibility of the heterogeneity of the immune system as a whole, coupled with this capacity for its quite extraordinary ability to respond appropriately to the situation, seems to me to imply that the immune system has a meaning, that it is a meaningfully operating system, functioning at levels of organizational control that may contain some leakage with psychic mechanisms, if one uses the word "psychic" as to include the concept of the unconscious.

Dr. Salk: Let me say that the immunologic system is what it is largely because of its reaction to the external environment, in the same sense that the nervous system is what it is, to a very great extent, by virtue of what it learns, by virtue of its experience with the external environment. I will try to tighten up this analogy by saying that in a germ-free animal there is very little lymphoid tissue, as we all know. If you wait long enough in the course of development, before exposing the animal to antigens, you lose the capacity for the animal to learn, so to speak, to develop immunologically competent cells, not unlike the autistic child, or animals that have been blinded for a period of time and then are exposed to light later; they have lost the capacity for sight to develop.

In this sense, I think antigens are equivalent to experiences. I look upon ideas, in a way, as equivalent to antigens, and I therefore see the two systems working very much alike, and separate, in a sense, from the rest of the organism, in that each owes a great deal of its structure to the nature of the experiences that it has had in the course of development.

DR. SOLOMON: There is some new experimental evidence that I think may bear on this problem of the relationship of experience to the reactivity of the immune system. In a complex and intriguing way, these observations provide a hint of the way in which central nervous events may play a role in self-surveillance and autoimmunity. I refer to Michison's work, which the Nossal and Burnet group feel is among the most significant work that has come out recently in regard to the concept of tolerance. It used to be thought that tolerance could be induced only by exposure to massive amounts of antigen that paralyze the system. Therefore, the reason that tolerance can be induced in the young animal more readily is that the relative amount of immune system versus the amount of antigen is different. But Michison has shown that specific tolerance can be induced not only by vast amounts of antigen, but also by very minute amounts of antigen. Somehow, the continual exposure of the system to very small amounts, almost a few molecules, of antigenic material keeps the system from reacting against it.

DR. BENNETTE: This is what is known as a globulin interaction, to some extent, is it not?

DR. SOLOMON: No, I do not think it is. Now, Michison's findings are quite intriguing to me from the point of view of autoimmunity, but they may also relate to cancer. One concept has been that the immune system does not react against some tissues because their antigens are "sequestered" and do not come into contact with the immune system, for example, because of thyroglobulin. If some inflammatory lesion or injury occurs, the immune system may "see" the antigen for the first time and react against it.

In the case of the thyroid, new work has shown that if one cannulizes the thyroid vein, it can be demonstrated that thyroglobulin comes out into the circulation. Thus, thyroglobulin is not novel to the immune system. Moreover, recent work has shown that the amount of thyroglobulin that is secreted is related to stress events. Therefore, it is quite conceivable to me, for example, that some central nervous system-mediated event could increase or even shut off the exposure to some antigen to which the immune system is being kept tolerant by minute stimulation. On the other hand, tolerance could be induced by changing the degree of exposure. In this regard, various concepts in relationship to membrane permeability might be important. Antibodies themselves may affect membrane permeability. Abnormal antibodies and autoantibodies or release products of their intereaction with antigens, such as histamine and serotonin, might effect membrane permeability in such a way as to alter the exposure of certain tissues to the immune system. Thus, one can envisage a very complex system.

Although I have reservations about his work, at the recent APA meeting Heath claimed that the antibrain globulin he calls "toraxein" alters the permeability of a very specific region in the septal area of the brain, allowing IgG to deposit inoligoderdroglia. Heath stated that if one gives this substance, which he derives from schizophrenic sera, after tagging it with fersitin, it can be picked up in these cells. If one gives the toraxein first and then gives normal gammaglobulin, which is tagged, the normal gammaglobulin can be found in these cells, because their permeability has been altered.

Once again, I consider most intriguing the concept that the exposure of the immunologic system to either tiny amounts or larger amounts of antigen may determine whether the system is tolerant or reactive. This degree of exposure, in turn, might be altered by nervous events, possibly by means of endocrine mediation.

DR. STERN: As a nonimmunologist and as a person who asked the question of one of the immunologists, whether or not immune mechanisms were of concern in the initiation or induction stage of cancer, I wonder if the way these mechanisms affect the genetic endowment of the cell can be explained.

DR. SALK: The immune mechanism?

DR. STERN: Yes. This is one thing that would have to be involved by definition.

DR. SALK: It need not influence the genetic mechanism in the cell. It simply has to affect the membrane of the cell.

DR. STERN: Is this to be concerned with the initiation of the tumor?

DR. SALK: I believe that anyone that may have answered that question may have had the following in mind: The tumor had formed.

DR. STERN: I am aware that immune mechanisms are involved in the control of cancer. But I was concerned as to whether or not they were involved in the induction or initiation of cancer.

DR. SALK: I cannot imagine how they could be involved in the induction or initiation.

DR. SOLOMON: They can be, if some viral or some other carcinogenic agent, which is ordinarily reacted to immunologically, is not prevented from reaching its target.

DR. SALK: But that is stretching it. I do not think you want to do that, do you?

DR. LAPPE: This is H. M. Green's theory of carcinogenesis. There is no evidence supporting it, but I would refer you to his work.

DR. SALK: I think you can accept the answer that the immune mechanism is not responsible for the initiation of neoplasia, unless there is someone here who thinks otherwise.

DR. AMKRAUT: I do not know. We have been dealing in analogies. There is one analogy in bacteriology. You can convert a smooth colony to a rough colony of bacteria, and this is genetically controlled by producing antibodies, by providing antibodies to the capsule.

DR. SALK: I have trouble with both the question and the answer, simply because I think I know what you have in mind.

DR. STERN: If you are talking about the control of cancer, it is quite clear to me that immunomechanisms could be involved, but if you are talking about the induction of cancer, that is different.

DR. SALK: I also think that is quite different. There is one thing that I would like to say, and that has to do with the induced enzyme synthesis in bacteria. This also has something to do with learning, in a sense.

All of you are familiar, I am sure, with the experiments done by Monod and Jacob, in which it was demonstrated that bacteria with a certain enzyme expressed the capacity to form this enzyme only when the substrate was put in medium. They could distinguish the organism that was genetically programmed to form this enzyme from those that were not capable of forming this enzyme. The point of interest is that the enzyme is not formed unless induced by the presence of the substrate. This is a beautiful and highly efficient system.

Now, the same thing happens in the learning in the nervous system, which has an enormous capacity. The same thing is true of the immunologic system. It has an enormous capacity that has to be turned on, by a stimulus that in a way is equivalent to the substrate for the enzyme. Therefore, we see at different levels of phylogenetic development similar processes, similar patterns of relationship between the organism and its environment. And if you now want to extend this to the relationship between the immunologic system and the nervous system, we said earlier that we think of each of these as separate systems, and when the systems get together within the organism, it is hard to believe that they do not have some cross-relationship in which each affects the other.

Now, this could happen easily by means of hormonal influences, and now I speak of chemical mediators of communication, rather than direct nervous connection, of molecular connections in the form of bits of information that are transmitted between the two systems.

DR. SOLOMON: Do you think of RNA information transmission between the two systems?

DR. SALK: That's going too far. When Dr. Klein put on the board the antibody response of young and old animals to passively transferred cells, you recall that the older animals' reaction was weaker than that of the younger animals.

Before the discussion is closed, I thought that I should refer to some work that has not yet been published, done by Carlo Baroni, now in my lab, who has done recent work at the University of Pavia, Italy, where he showed that thyroxine and growth hormone were both necessary for normal antibody formation in the dwarf mouse. This mouse is essentially nonresponsive immunologically, but the injection of growth hormone and thyroxine are together capable of making this a normal animal so far as its immune response is concerned. This raises the very important question as to whether or not growth hormone and thyroxine are essential for immune response. This would be an example of a hormone that connects these two systems. This is an example of a chemical mediator of information, not specific information in the sense of antigen-antibody information.

DR. WEINER: The studies around the world that look at the distribution of the polio virus, particularly in the poorer elements of the world population, showed higher titer levels to the polio viruses. For a virologist, these titers are of great interest. However, a cardiologist studying the same population would observe low serum cholesterol levels and relatively low occurrence of heart disease. A cancer investigator would observe little occurrence of cancer. A psychologist may observe little evidence of alienation, and so on. Depending upon the investigator, the same population is examined with a specific set of measurements. Now, as a biostatistician, I find myself raising the question: Do you in fact want to integrate your measurements so that in this case the psychologist, the virologist, and the cancer epidemiologist can pursue intelligently the common problem, namely, human cancer?

I think there is a tremendous need for integration of the results, so that a relationship may be described as a psychophysiologic phenomenon. The specialists must integrate their thinking, as well as their results. The immunologist must, for example, admit the existence of an endocrine system. The point is that the purpose of this conference is not completely being met, in the sense that each of us is still pursuing our own separate paths. The problem at this conference, as I understand it, was to integrate this work so that we could develop a series of new studies using measurements from immunology, measurements from endocrinology, measurements from psychology—all devoted to the common laboratory animal or the common human being.

DR. SALK: I think you would have no difficulty if a clear question were formulated and put to you, and you then would help design the studies that would be necessary to show whether there is significance or not, to give you a valid "yes" or "no."

DR. WEINER: I think there is more to it than just the number of subjects or the particular design. I think the statistician has to involve himself, if he is going to be of real value. He must involve himself in the choice of the measurements that are most meaningful. As I listened to the various papers presented, I heard many indications of defects and problems in terms of measuring from the immunological point of view, as well as in measuring from the endocrinologic point of view. And I am sure tomorrow the psychologists will tell us of the difficulties in measurement from the psychological point of view. Therefore, I do not think that it is quite as simple as trying to keep the statistician outside.

DR. SALK: He must understand the concept. He must open himself to understanding the concept without trying to worry about statistics at the moment. A much more beautiful experiment must be designed.

DR. WEINER: That is what I am trying to point to. It is my impression that the concepts are being weighted inappropriately at the present time, with too much emphasis given to immunologic factors. Indeed, what mechanism "controls" this system?

DR. LESHAN: I wonder if one of the problems is not a communications block we see here. You speak of a correlation between two things. I think you mean something quite different. We are dealing with a general pattern in a total organism and how this pattern, that we might label "cancer," shows itself on various arbitrarily conceptualized levels, and how these levels relate to each other. This is not, it seems to me, a problem that will be solved by attempting to correlate two things together. What we need to do is to start to follow the purpose of the conference, to consider what happens on each of these various hierarchical levels and what the total pattern is. This is what we are trying to get at here. What is the total situation of this organism-in-an-environment, the total situation we have labeled "neoplastic disease?"

DR. BAHNSON: I think we all must be a little more humble and patient with each other. It seems that there are several of us who have tried, maybe in a naïve way, at least to keep an open mind in terms of exploring a possible interaction between different systems of approach and different psychobiological levels of function. I think it takes a very long time before it becomes possible, without being too superficial and without pushing too much, to communicate about the isomorphism between different observational and conceptual systems. I think, however, that some starting points already have been introduced, and I should be very pleased if we could go back to some of these main points that Dr. Salk, particularly, mentioned. I think that the discussion of these points already has brought us close to the interdisciplinary issues. The similarities between the function, or role, or the conditions of invention, of the nervous system (and, may I add, of the experiential system, which is another aspect of the nervous system) on the one hand, and the immune system on the other, already provides us with working blocks for a model. Before saying a few more things about it, allow me just for a moment to be very naïve.

We have heard much about a postinvader relationship between antibodies and antigens. This seems to me to be an archaic and misleading statement. I think that we should rather consider that we are "hosts" to all the cells that constitute our physical being, normal and neoplastic. The way in which we have heard a neoplastic state described by Dr. Klein, Dr. Weiss, and Dr. Salk makes it quite clear that it is not really a sudden invader. It is, rather, a complex development of some of the conglomeration of cellular matter that constitutes our bodies. Dr. Bennette's formulation has been in line with this thinking.

I think this is an important consideration, because if you approach the problem this way, then you can more readily apply parallelism or isomorphism in the conceptual integration of the psychological organization of the person (or the nervous system, if you so prefer) and the immune system in the same person. In other words, if we conceptualize the psychobiological system as one that demands control—and control, of course, is a metaphor, a concept that we impose on observations we make of the well-functioning organism—we can then describe a breakdown of control in terms of dysfunction of antibodies, disturbance in the balance of endocrines, or inadequacy of symbolic ego functions. What I am trying to say is that we are not really dealing with an invader, but with a breakdown of control resulting in changes in certain cells, for reasons that are very complex.

If we allow ourselves to think not only about the psychological or nervous system and the immune system, but also about the similarity, communication, and complementarity between the two systems, then it may become possible to translate events from one system to the other, or at least to find links of importance. If we use such a model, and give ourselves a little margin here, in terms of translating from one system to the other, then I think that many promising avenues will present themselves. One of them was proposed by Dr. Prehn today, when he referred to development from amputative to immune reaction, when moving from the lower vertebrae to higher forms. Similar formulations have been presented previously by Dr. Lang Stevenson and Dr. Adolphe Jonas, and Dr. Margolin also has addressed himself to this very intriguing point. In addition there may be several other approaches that can be used in an attempt to translate between the nervous and the immune systems, both of which monitor interactions with the environment.

DR. RIFFENBURGH: It would seem that there is a basic idea that has not been brought up; that would tie together the frayed points of this discussion of the last half hour; we will continue talking at cross-purpose without it. That is the role of DNA in memory. Take the DNA spiral from a neural cell; it is about six feet long and can accept a vast encoding; for example, several volumes of the *Encyclopedia Britannica*. There is no reason why this DNA can not be coded to react conditionally. If you will forgive a neophyte's mode of expression, it might be viewed as follows: Given a certain type of electrical and chemical stimulus to the neural cell, the DNA instructs the RNA, which then instructs response. However, given some other frequency and amplitude of electrical stimulus and another type of chemical bath, say, a different sodium-potassium rate of exchange, an entirely different type of response might be instructed by the DNA that would completely explain the slime mold's behavior that Dr. Bennette brought up.

Let us examine memory with this kind of thinking. The genetic structure of the DNA is passed on not only when the whole organism is reproduced, but also when individual neural cells are reproduced. Think of short-term memory as being a difference in graded potential of the cell. Continued stimulation and, therefore, retention of this graded potential for a long enough time affects the RNA amount, which then affects the DNA in the nucleus. You will note that the more material memorized, the greater is the amount of nonnuclear, cellular RNA in the RNA/DNA ratio; so you can see a change occurring with increased memory.

The control of differentiated cells is quite understandable; the problem arises in the dedifferentiation. There is apparently an erroneous instruction or a bar preventing the interchange of instructions between the DNA and nuclear or even nonnuclear RNA. About how this would happen, I can do nothing but conjecture. Once a response arises from a cell with an erroneous instruction or no instruction at all, the dedifferentiation process seems understandable. How the instruction comes in is what is crucial in all this discussion. I have probably not expressed these ideas well because I am more of a general modeler than a specialist in this area, but the ideas do seem relevant.

DR. SALK: Let me go back for a moment to the ideas that Dr. Bahnson put forth. Let us say that we have the nervous system. Separate from it, we have the immunologic system. And let us say we have the system that makes hormones. We agree now that these three are important elements in our discussion. And finally, we have the neoplastic cell. How did that cell become neoplastic? This is the important question that we are asking. Before we consider the other questions, let us talk about that for a moment.

Now, let us consider all other conceivable possibilities. One obvious one is viral invasion. That is something that comes from the outside. Another could be irradiation. Again, it is an effect that is introduced from outside, and affecting, let us say, the DNA, or possibly even RNA, but nevertheless producing a damage to the hereditary information, or to the information that is then translated into proteins in the decoding process.

Now, what is viral invasion or x-ray? Essentially the same mechanism is involved, because it affects the protein design-function, which in turn disrupts the control or regulatory mechanism within the cell, so that you now no longer have a cell that is regulated as are the other cells. These are two external influences. But then the same thing could happen also merely as a result of a copying error. That is an internally arising change.

The mode of action of chemicals (for example, methylcholanthrene or other such substances, or sunlight in the formation of skin cancer), in one way or another have some effect upon the information within the cell that in turn is translated in a way that produces what, for the normal cell, is a copying error. You either have copying errors or you have a disruption in the organization of the information-containing system within the cell.

DR. SOLOMON: You need only one copying error. After that you may copy the erroneously copied cell.

DR. SALK: That is what I mean. When I say "error," I am talking about a transmittable copying error, which is what the virus produces. It produces a change, and once that change is introduced, it is maintained. You then have what I refer to as an essentially independent organism, because it has not arisen as a result of differentiation, through what you might call normal evolutionary development, and does not necessarily have survival value. When this occurs after the period of maturation, then it could be a cause of death, but would not necessarily be lethal for the species as a whole.

The question that I suppose we are now asking is, "What is the relationship of the nervous system, the immunologic system, and the endocrinologic system to the system I have just described?"

DR. STERN: I should like to add one possible mechanism, and that is the mechanism of gene control by hormone action. The genetic endowment of cells is capable of an entire repertoire of activity–the expression of which may be initiated by hormones.

DR. SALK: Yes, I did not mean to exclude it, and you are quite right. There are very likely other influences as well. They all have such an effect.

The mode of action of hormones is one of the darkest areas of biology. And this is an area that is going to become elucidated by the molecular biologists in the next few years, I am sure. Some hormones produce an effect by action on the cell membrane, some have effects on RNA, some have effects on DNA. And the classification of hormones in this respect is still an area of darkness.

DR. STERN: It is true that it is quite dark. However, in human cancer, for example, virus has not yet been proved to play a role, so that the possible role of hormones is quite important to consider, even though it is an area of darkness at the moment.

DR. SALK: I do not question that they do play a role with their control of self-replication. And where the copying error comes in, I do not know. For example, it has been shown that animals that are hyperimmunized are more likely to get lymphatic leukemia than are unimmunized animals. Here you are forcing cell replication and increasing the probability of a copying error.

DR. SHANDS: The title of this conference said something about "psycho-physiological," but we bog down here repeatedly in the biological-physiological stratum–over and over again. I think this is because it is easier to manage. But human beings are not concerned only with an endocrine system, with an immunological system, and with a nervous system, but also with a symbolic system. The symbolic system really is the central system in which we all live. And it is very easy to ignore it completely, as I think we are doing.

When we say that memory exists in DNA-RNA, that is true of nonverbal animals. Verbal animals have memories that are coded in words, a conscious memory. If anybody can find a conscious memory that is not a verbal memory, I should like to see it.

DR. SALK: All right, then, how are you going to get that symbolic system to make cancer?

DR. SHANDS: Isn't that just the point?

DR. SALK: Yes, but you are the one who raised that question, not me. Now that you raised it, I should like to hear some discussion.

DR. SACERDOTE (*Mt. Vernon, N.Y.*): I agree with you, Dr. Shands about the fact that we have not been talking about what is really the title of this conference, especially from the point of view of a clinician dealing with cancer, advanced or less advanced. For me, the problem is this: I think there is fairly general agreement among all the participants that in all probability, immunological factors have something to do with eliciting or regulating or inhibiting growth. Very well. I think there is general agreement on this other point at least, about the so-called hypothalamic-pituitary-adrenal axis having either specific effects on the cells as you, Dr. Stern, are suggesting, or at least on how fast the tumor mass is growing or not growing.

I think one point that we have not considered at all, and I don't know whether I could suggest any experiment on human beings or lower animals to prove or disprove it, is that there may be a possible direct effect from the central nervous system, by the highest centers of the central nervous system, specifically upon individual cells or groups of cells. I do not think we have discussed this part at all tonight.

I think it would be very interesting to think, at least, of the possibility of some laboratory experiment or clinical experiment to prove or disprove that there is some direct relation between, let us say, a symbolization that our cortex can create, whatever its actual chemical mechanism at the DNA or RNA level, and its effect on a breast cancer, for instance, because this is the practical angle, as raised in the paper by Dr. Katz today, of trying to see if different ways for the individual to react to stress or to cope with emotional factors will have a certain measurable effect on the mortality or the length of survival of the patient who has the cancer. Is there another possible action, besides the generally accepted mechanism of stress acting on the pituitary gland, and indirectly on the adrenal glands, that may alter the level of the cortisone or of the androgens, as compared with the level of the estrogens in the case of breast cancer? Is that the only mechanism, or is there the possibility of the existence of some particular nervous mechanism that, in a particular woman who is prepared to–and accepting of the fact that she is going to die from cancer, will prevent control of the existing or of the beginning of a new cancer, or of a metastatic one? Is there any specific mechanism anybody can think of that can be tested through laboratory or clinical experiment in this direction?

DR. SOLOMON: I should wonder in that regard about direct nervous influence. There has been some work in this area in relation to experimental arthritis, for example. There is a clinical observation that patients who develop arthritis after a hemiplegia do not get the disease in the paralyzed limb. Kuzell did an experiment denervating limbs in animals and inducing arthritis by administration of adjuvant, and the arthritis did not occur in denervated limbs. On the other hand, if the peripheral nerve is stimulated electrically, there was an increase in arthritis. I wonder if there is any work that anyone is aware of, regarding tumor transplantation or the use of chemical carcinogens in denervated limbs.

DR. SARCERDOTE: I do not think – if I may interrupt – this is pertinent, because, if you have something like denervation of the tissues of the gastrocnemius muscle, or of another muscle (that was presented today), there is always the possibility that there may exist many other factors: alterations in circulation, alterations in activity because the muscle becomes inactive, and so on. And I do not think it applies to something much more refined; that is, to a specific effect on individual cells or groups of cells, rather than the massive effect of cutting off the complete nervous supply.

DR. BAHNSON: Are you saying that we should not think of the intervening mechanisms, but think of some other pathways, other than through the systems we are talking about? I would be concerned about that, because I think that we mind-oriented people must bend over as far as we possibly can, in order to communicate with the biological workers, and not only talk about psychological conditions that we then cannot transmit, or cannot get any handle on, in terms of the physical process. I think we all know that there are relationships between experiential states and cancer. I think that is why we are in this business, that is why we are talking. But I also think it is our duty to try to see what the possible mediating mechanisms are, and this is why we are getting into the immune and hormone fields and whatever other fields exist.

DR. SACERDOTE: I agree completely with what you say. I think that we are all accepting these interrelationships. I am all in favor of having this wonderful selection of experts in the fields of immunology and biochemistry and endocrinology. I am just suggesting one additional area that I think should be studied, too. I am not saying that it is unimportant, even from the viewpoint of the psychophysiological aspects of cancer, to study the relationship between the nervous system and the immunological system, or between the nervous system and the endocrine system. I am all in favor of studying them. I believe that they are all important in the genesis, the development, the permanence of cancer. But I think that there is still another area that can be studied. This area may be more apparent to the clinician, especially to one who has been in both fields, in internal medicine and in psychiatry, besides having been in biochemistry years ago. As clinicians, we are aware of the fact that in certain individual cases there might be a selective effect of the highest centers of the nervous system upon some particular group of cells or tumors. We definitely cannot say—we do not know—whether these cells become differentiated again after they have become undifferentiated or whether the undifferentiated cells die away and the normal ones redevelop. I have the impression that there is at least a theoretical possibility of a direct effect of individual groups of neurons reaching individual cells.

DR. SOLOMON: I think, as does Dr. Bahnson, that perhaps what you are trying to do now, is back away from this more specific systems-orientation to a more global and encompassing view of the problem. Perhaps this conference has served to illustrate that already, at this point, there are some specific things that we do know in a very modest way about the means by which environmental and mental events influence the onset and course of cancer. I was asked today, "Well, what does all this mean? What does this have to do with the treatment or prevention of cancer?" That rather brought me up short. I have also found myself, especially this evening, having a kind of identity crisis and thinking, "I am a psychiatrist, and look what am I talking about here."

When I tried to answer the inquirer, I made several points based essentially on some things that have come up today. One was with regard to the patient already with cancer. I said that a sensitive clinician should be aware whether or not the patient is struggling with strong emotions about his situation while unable to express his feelings and deal with them. In this case, some opportunity for ventilation, expression of these emotions, would be very helpful, in order to discharge some of the affect. On the other hand, if the individual is using strong mechanisms of denial and repression, perhaps successfully, questioning him about it or confronting him with the issue would be maladaptive in terms of his psyche and physiology.

My questioner then said, "Well, how is the clinician supposed to know what he is dealing with, whether this is a denial, whether it is a repression, or whether it is really just a suppression and the patient is conscious of his situation and in great turmoil?" I replied: "In addition to his perception and intuition, why doesn't the clinician obtain 24-hour corticosteroid excretion levels? This information would provide some indication of the integrity of the psychologic defenses and perhaps provide a guide as to whether the physician should explore issues with the patient or let sleeping dogs lie."

As a physician, I am basically concerned with prevention. If we are aware that certain psychological parameters, the social situation, personality predispositions, and stress events all may relate to oncogenesis as well as to other physiological as well as psychological decompensations, perhaps we can be aware of what constellations of factors might provide a high risk in the statistical sense. Such psychiatric techniques as crisis intervention, particularly around important losses, may be very important when we realize that loss, depression, or situations that are not adequately coped with have such important physiological consequences.

I do hope we try to extrapolate the knowledge that we have, even at this very primitive stage, to real human beings in clinical situations, using our admittedly meager knowledge to help people.

DR. STERN: May I make a suggestion, Dr. Bahnson? As I see it, Dr. Salk has started us off on the right foot when he defined what a cancer cell is. And in my view, if you are going to discuss the psychological or the cultural or the external factors with regard to cancer, you may have more success if you talk about the end result—cancer—at two levels; that is, the cancer as it exists, an existing cancer, and the initiation of cancer; and with regard to the two levels, the psychological factors may differ for initiation and for control. I think that it is very obvious that immunological factors are very important in the control, as are also, probably, hormonal factors.

But I think that linking those factors in control with some psychological or behavioral concepts will be easier to do if we divide these two concepts: initiation and control of cancer. I think they will probably come out to be quite different, and yet there may be psychological factors in both.

DR. SOLOMON: Evidence that Dr. Weiss presented makes it seem that initiation and progression are not that different. Thus, the differentiation you are making seems somewhat artificial.

DR. LAPPE: From the point of view of cancer biology, the best place to start from is the idea that all of the potential tumor cells may have initiated at the time of birth; from prenatal exposure, carcinogens are vertically transmitted viruses; subsequently, all you are doing is controlling the cells. And indeed, this is the only information we have from immunology, and we know very little about what kinds of controls are operating at the very early stages.

May I, since I have the floor, throw out a radical idea that may fuse some of the concepts we have been discussing. This is a concept that makes us (that is, Dr. Prehn and the people in his laboratory) interested in these focal points in phylogeny when there seems to be a flipover, when you start getting tumors and start losing regenerative capacities, because it is at this point in phylogeny that we think we see the abrogation of the higher nervous system control turning over to a lymphoid system control.

It is a platitude to tell you that there is a centrepolization of the peripheral nerves that goes on with phylogeny, and one of Singer's greatest discoveries in regeneration, I think, is that the number of peripheral nerves that are still left determines whether or not regeneration can occur. And as these nerves become centrepolatally retracted to achieve our higher functions, which is what is happening at the level of the enphystoma, we are left with regenerative capacities in the peripheral limbs. In these peripheral limbs, tumors apparently can be controlled. When, at a higher level in the reptiles, say the frog, just after metamorphosis, we have retracted these nerves and do not have the ability to regenerate, we do get tumors. I think there is experimental evidence that tells us that the lymphoid system may be replacing the nervous system and controlling what the Germans call "morphogenetic fields." One of the most obscure experiments is the one that has shown the tremendous influx of nerves that occurs within a few days after exposure to a carcinogen. This is why we are concerned with immunology, perhaps more correctly than with the higher nervous system, because we feel the higher nervous system has abrogated control of cells to this lymphoid system.

DR. SALK: I think the point that was made is a good one. We tended to spend much of the time discussing mechanisms, simply because we were goaded into doing so. I think we ought to hear from those who are more familiar with the evidence for the relationship between psychological events and the neoplastic process. We do not for one moment disregard the fact that the neoplastic process is occurring in a whole organism.

As you were speaking a moment ago, there came to mind the occurrence of the herpes simplex lesion. All of us have had the experience of having reactivation of this lesion, not only under the influence of sunlight or wind or infections, but under the influence of psychological factors of which we are not unaware.

Now let us for the moment forget about the question of mechanism that is involved either in that process or in the initiation of the neoplastic process or in the control of neoplasia, and listen for a few moments to something about the phenomenon itself, of the relationship between psychological factors and the neoplastic process as an expression of some symbolism.

DR. SHANDS: I want to call attention to a conviction that apparently, I share with very few other people, which is that the symbolic system is as real and solid and regular a system as is the immunological system or the nervous system.

DR. SALK: You talk about the nervous system and the immunologic system. Can you talk about the symbolic system in the same way?

DR. SHANDS: No, you cannot. That is the interesting thing. You can measure many aspects of it, but if you want to know where it resides, it resides "in consensus," which is a curiously unsatisfactory answer, I am sure. Like the immunological system, unless the symbolic system is internalized, unless a person is trained appropriately in the symbolic system, he becomes unable to learn. Bruner's data indicates that an unschooled child beyond the age of nine is incapable of any further cognitive development.

Most of us actually live primarily in symbolic systems, sharing consensually symbolic values. It is the impalpable but completely regular quality that is so baffling about symbolic systems.

DR. SALK: Can you imagine how that brings about neoplasia?

DR. SHANDS: No, but I think that is the question that we are concerned with, at least from the title of this conference.

DR. SOLOMON: Do you feel that symbolic events play a role? For example, may breast cancer be more likely to occur in a woman who has conflict about mothering?

DR. SHANDS: That is too hopelessly simple.

DR. SOLOMON: I have a resistance to analogizing on the hysterical model in psychosomatic disease.

DR. SHANDS: The classic case that is always quoted in this matter is that of the man who was violently allergic to roses, who started sneezing when someone brought in a paper rose. The fact is that the shape does assume prepotency.

DR. SOLOMON: But he did not have antigen-antibody reactions. Experimentally conditioned asthma evokes wheezing behavior in the absence of antigen-antibody reaction.

DR. SACERDOTE: The clinical picture is the same: The patient is just as uncomfortable and the breathing capacity is just as totally reduced whether that is caused by a symbolic rose or by one made out of paper, or a natural one to which he has developed antibodies. I can go one step further, which might have some relationship to the symbolic concept. We are distinguishing, certainly in the human being and the lower mammals, the so-called autonomic nervous system. Actually, it is not so autonomic as we conceived it to be, as we studied it in medical school. For instance, we take as an example of autonomic nervous system response the pupillary response to light; this is supposed to be an autonomic response that we are not controlling. It has already been proved that a number of individuals can be trained to control the pupillary reflex.

Let us look at all the reactions, for instance, of the gastrointestinal tract to stress that may be effected through the sympathetic nervous system, or, more often, through excessive stimulation of the vagus nerve. It has been proved definitely that certain individuals, through psychological means (one of which I am familiar with–hypnosis) can learn to control selectively spasms of the gastrointestinal system that otherwise would be controlled only in a very massive way by anticholinergic drugs.

So, going off on this point, I believe some of the ability of the central nervous system to have some control, at least on the functions and perhaps also on anatomical changes of other parts of the body, may be mostly nonused and non-trained, rather than really absent, and it was from that point of view that I was thinking of the possibility of the child's having learned to sneeze and to develop asthma when seeing the artificial rose because he had learned that a rose causes that. Actually, he is not creating the asthma consciously. He responds that way.

These are not areas that are in contradiction with all that has been studied and brought to this meeting, which has been very important and very basic. But I think of other areas that certainly need elucidation; it would be a question of bringing some of the action back to the psychological areas.

DR BAHNSON: May I come back to the main concepts that we have introduced? I think that before we got off the track a bit, we discussed how to get from what we usually call experience, clinical situation, or affect and feeling, to the physical end result of cancerogenesis. I think Dr. Salk had in mind a model in which, going from antecedent to consequent, one would move from experience and affect, through the hormonal system, through the nervous system, and through the immunological system, finally arriving at the end result of the malignant cell.

DR. SALK: I think of experience as related to the nervous system. Do you?

DR. BAHNSON: Yes, I do, but, I have made reference to experience rather than to the nervous system, because our observations are in terms of self-reported and observed behavioral phenomena, and not in terms of physiological processes in the nervous system. Whether what we think and feel or what we see in a microscope is more "real" is a matter of philosophical discourse. The fact is that many behavioral and psychologic studies have shown that there is a relationship between experience and cancer, they do not specify how this experience may be mediated. This is what we have learned in several meetings over the last ten years, and I think that these correlational relationships have been sufficiently well demonstrated not to be considered hearsay any longer. They have been demonstrated on a statistical basis much beyond the usually accepted probability levels.

This is all good and well. However, the question arises: Should we, or should we not, try to elucidate the mediating process? This process may work directly via the nervous system, as Dr. Sacerdote suggested. There are several studies—I do not know how good they are, how solid they are—that have indicated that interruption or monitoring of efferent nerve paths result in changes, inhibition, or facilitation, of the development of cancer cells. Some of the work presented today by the Russian group, Kavetsky and Balitsky and their co-workers, illustrated the possibilities of this approach. They have systematically interrupted the flow of information from the central nervous system to malignant target tissues and have observed subsequent changes in the behavior of tumors. Thus, if one accepts a relationship between experience or symbolic processes and the nervous system, then nervous system alterations may provide a path. But another, and more likely path (and I think this was understood spontaneously in this conference) goes via the immune mechanisms that definitely relate to the control, if not initiation, of malignant development. The next questions then are: How can we relate experience or symbolic processes to the newly understood immune processes? How can we conceptualize this? How is it even possible to think about experience and the nervous system, on the one hand, even on a theoretical level, and about hormonal and immune systems on the other? Is there any possible way of conceptualizing potentials short-circuiting from one system to another? At that point, our discussion broke down and became diverted, and we need to understand why.

I may not have emphasized strongly enough that I and our group work most comfortably with psychological concepts, and not with immunological concepts. However, our exact purpose in this conference is to communicate with other disciplines and to understand the systems that have been developed on those levels of abstraction. And in order to do that, I think we are groping for models that will allow us to communicate.

DR. AMKRAUT: I think that the difficulties that Dr. Weiner stated very bluntly, and the difficulty that I find here, is not only one of communication, which is obvious and ought to be here, but a difficulty in recognizing the extent to which the field of each of the disciplines represented really has answers. I am beginning to wonder more and more whether, at this point in time, it is useful to try to correlate before we really go back and get more basic answers. As an immunologist, at least I am willing to concede to vast areas of ignorance. I am sure the endocrinologists will do so. I am not so sure about the behavioral scientists; perhaps they do know what there is to know. But I think, given that there are vast areas of ignorance, correlation becomes extremely difficult. I think the question one must ask from various points of view is the same question one must ask from experiments, or from any kind of setup: Is it useful? If we can have a discussion here that will lead us to set up experiments that will lead to some useful application of the information so acquired, I think, then, we should have the discussion at this point in time.

DR. SHANDS: Let me say one thing, rather in response to that. There is abundant reason for having a conference on the immunological, neural, and endocrine aspects of cancer. But if you are going to have a conference on psychophysiological correlation and leave out symbolic systems, social systems, and anthropological aspects of the thing, it seems to me that you are talking about the physiological aspects of cancer, and not the psychophysiological correlation. That is the simple point.

DR. SACERDOTE: I think the conference has been useful, even though it has been slated more in this direction. But I think if there were more mobility, so that a psychiatrist, a psychologist, a biologist could collaborate more intimately in actually working out, in studying and presenting hypotheses, and thinking together and then deciding, let us test this hypothesis with the knowledge we have, and with the help of a biostatistician (who will tell us all the mistakes we are making in trying to demonstrate our hypotheses with such an experiment), it would be even more productive. That would provide an ideal situation.

DR. RIFFENBURGH: That was a very good point about attitudes. May I make a comment regarding this concept which is strictly educational and has nothing to do with the subject matter. For 17 years I have been teaching professionals who are coming into biostatistics from other fields, and have observed that they uniformly reject the ideas at the outset. Later, when they begin to feel at home with the ideas, the difficulty disappears. This occurs in almost every field. You want to stay in your own field because that is what you know and that is the tool with which you are competent. Thus, when you get together in an interdisciplinary type of meeting, you must make a conscious effort to suppress your own field and accept those foreign to you, just to avoid blocking communication. The more foreign the fields, the more effort you must make to accept them in order to achieve any successful meeting of the minds.

DR. BAHNSON: May I just respond to Dr. Amkraut's point. I think that both Dr. Solomon and I are very much in agreement that we should come out of this conference with some suggestions about future experiments and research. However, when you talk about the heuristic aspects of thinking, I do not quite agree with you. I believe that one sometimes must also think for no good reason; one does not always have to have a pragmatic reason. But I think it would be very, very helpful if we could come out of this conference with some suggestions about what we ought to study next. We know that there is a very very crude relationship between psychological fate on the one hand, and a very crude clinical measurement of malignant development on the other. I hope that we will be able to formulate some more specific research projects that could be carried out. For example: Would it be possible, both in animals and in man, to devise experiments to study in which way particular affects and particular types of stresses are related to different aspects of the immune reaction? For example, regarding the two branches that Dr. Salk was talking about, would it be possible to study the differential effect that different emotions would have on these immune branches? Or, is it possible to classify psychological profiles as carefully as the Los Angeles group defined endocrinological profiles, and then tease out by the use of discriminant function analysis the relationships between these profiles and malignant subcategories?

I think we should be able to make some such recommendations, so that some of our behavioral science groups, instead of dealing with the very crude secondary variable, clinical cancer, can take a look at relevant aspects of some of the more refined mechanisms that we now know actually are directly related to the malignant process. I think that would be of significance.

DR. AMKRAUT: Do the psychologists or psychiatrists here feel that animal models are adequate? Do they feel there are experiments based on what they know and have heard about immunology, that one can or should carry out in man? I think this is one of the fundamental questions that confronts at least me, here.

DR. BAHNSON: I can only answer for myself and what I know from others. I think most clinicians are skeptical about animal models because there are so many differences between what you would call a stress situation in an animal and what we, as people, perceive in a very complex way. But I think that one can use both. It should be possible to start out with very crude concepts; for example, alienation and separation, as Dr. Rasmussen did when he isolated his mice. It should be possible to take crude models and use them in animals to try them out on the basic level. Then we should go on and study by the natural history method a number of people who in real life have been subjected to different types of stress conditions. During that period, as in Hamburg's model, we could study the effect on parents of the loss of a leukemic child, following at the same time exactly what was going on in terms of epinephrine and norepinephrine production. We ought to study, in the same way, the immune reactions and other physiological processes.

DR. SALK: I think this is very commendable, the moment you begin to classify certain parameters to study. And the so-called physical scientists, in a sense different from the psychological scientists, would be delighted to have the opportunity to make such correlations, because he lacks this kind of material just as the psychologists and psychiatrists lack the physiological skill. In my own laboratory, I mix up chemists and immunologists. We have the same kind of problem that has been occurring here. Every time we meet, you put up with healthy tension that gives rise to the hybridization that results in a new point of view, and eventually a new idea, and eventually a new set of experiments. So it seems to me that the conference so far has been very productive. We cannot lose our identity entirely in the discussion.

George Solomon asks why I was not speculating, and why I seem so conservative and so precise. This is what happens to me under these circumstances, whereas in my office I am likely to be very speculative and very wild. As these ideas exist and begin to work, they become more precise. It seems to me that as a result of this exposure, the psychologic scientists ought to go home with a greater feeling of confidence and a desire to make their own data more precise, to increase numbers or to make the description more exquisite, so as to segregate groups through refinement, and so that differences of a physical nature might then become evident, and perhaps to begin to do some prospective studies where profiles are established and predictions made, based on retrospective studies as to what you are likely to expect. Now, you are not making predictions but simply making observations, prospectively as well as retrospectively. This, again, can be done only if, as a naturalist, one moves in and begins to concentrate in as precise a way as possible.

DR. SOLOMON: Whether one ends up concluding that there is a direct effect between psyche and a target tissue or that there is some intermediary mechanism is relatively unimportant. The important thing is to define the problem, characterize it, and then see what the psychological and physiological correlates are.

DR. BAHNSON: I think this is the note on which to end our interdisciplinary meeting tonight.

PART VII. INTEGRATION AND EVALUATION OF CURRENT PSYCHOPHYSIOLOGICAL APPROACHES TO CANCER

PANEL DISCUSSION 1: THE NEUROENDOCRINOLOGIC APPROACH

Sydney Margolin, *Moderator*
Department of Psychiatry and Human Behavior Laboratory
University of Colorado School of Medicine
Denver, Colo.

DR. CORSON: The quintessence of all kernels of wisdom that have been presented at this session is rather difficult to summarize. So I shall choose just a few things that appear to me to be most important. One of these is the problem of philosophic orientation. I think it is important to have an appropriate philosophic orientation, if one is to do the proper scientific work. Your assumptions are extremely important ingredients of an experimental design.

I was a little perplexed by some of the philosophic papers during the last two days. And I am particularly perplexed about the discussions of the dichotomy between reductionism and what I should like to call the integrative approach in the biomedical sciences. I would be the last person to defend reductionism as the sole method of approaching science, but, certainly, it is the preliminary way of doing business in scientific research. Once having done it, one must realize that when we are discussing the physiology or the behavior of an organism as a whole, one has to think of integrative aspects. But one does not have to escape from reductionism into mysticism. Now, there are many ways of looking at the world. The scientific way is not the only one; mysticism has its place, and so do poetry and art; but one must not mix up these things. I think it is rather confusing and inhibiting of progress to attempt to use nonscientific methods in arriving at a scientific assessment of the world.

I think we all can agree that the scientific method is based on the assumption that the world exists outside of us. What we know about this world is a different story, but the assumption is that there is an objective world, and in our mind we are attempting to approach as closely as possible an understanding of the reality of this world. If this assumption is not valid, then there is no point in conducting experiments or even in making observations of natural phenomena. It would be simpler and certainly less expensive just to verbalize.

This brings me to the business of the brain-mind dichotomy. Those of us who are inclined to be in the scientific field and use the scientific method must agree on the fact that there is no mind without brain, just as there is no circulation without a cardiovascular system, and there is no urine production without a kidney, even though we may not understand completely how the kidney or the heart or the brain works. The mind must be considered an expression of the operation of the brain, and the attempt to go from one extreme of absolute reductionism to a completely mystical nonmaterial assessment of the world, I do not believe would bring any useful results.

As to what I feel would be the pressing problems that need to be attacked, I am a little bit biased, because most of my work has been in basic research. I believe that basic research is what is very sorely needed in the field of psychosomatic medicine, for a number of reasons. It would be essential, I believe, to attempt to develop what I call controlled case histories, which you can do only by long-term systematic work on animals. In attempting to study the effects of psychologic or emotional stress on cancer, I think one ought to be guided by the following considerations. Number one, one should remember that there are several kinds of psychologic stress. I think one must distinguish (and I think this is one of the major sources of confusion) between exposure to a single-stress situation (i.e., acute stress) and repeated exposure (chronic stress). I have tried to demonstrate to you that the physiologic and behavioral reactions to a single exposure to psychologic stress are quite different from those observed after repeated exposure. In fact, the major genetic differences appear only in relation to chronic stress. If you simply study a single exposure or one or two exposures of animals to psychologic stress, you may find only a few differences. Differences become particularly apparent when you expose these animals to repeated, chronic stress. That is when the genetic differences really appear.

This brings me to the second point. It is important that when one studies the effects of psychologic stress on cancer or any other possibly psychosomatic disease, one must not think of animals as "pigs is pigs." It would be advisable to conduct extensive comparative studies on different species, as well as on different genetic groups within a given species. Unless you have really seen it in the laboratory, you cannot fully appreciate how completely differently–not only quantitatively but qualitatively–animals of different genetic backgrounds respond to the same psychologic stress. If you are studying a whole group of animals and you neglect the psychophysiologic variations within the group and study the effects of psychologic stress on cancer or on other disease processes, you may find that your results are meaningless, because you are averaging many things that cannot be averaged. You are averaging horses and pigs and mice, and so on, while neglecting the qualitative differences between these individual organisms.

The other point I wanted to emphasize very strongly is the need to distinguish between avoidable and unavoidable psychologic stress. I am referring to stress in which an individual organism acquires control or feels that he acquires control, and stress during which the animal or the human subject is not capable of acquiring control–is not capable, in other words, of achieving an adaptive consummatory response. It is the pattern of physiologic and endocrine responses to psychologic stress under circumstances where the animal is not capable of achieving an appropriate consummatory adaptive response that may represent the background for the development of psychosomatic disturbances.

I tried to point out the remarkable differences between avoidable and unavoidable stress. If you take an animal with a genetic predisposition to reproduce Walter B. Cannon's "fight or flight" physiologic responses to symbols of stress, and if you take the same animal and expose him to the same conditional and unconditional stimuli in a different room and give him the opportunity to develop an avoidance response, most of these psychophysiologic responses will disappear or become markedly ameliorated. Therefore, many of the references in the literature to emotional stress, when avoidance conditioning is used, are subject to serious question, because avoidance conditioning is not much of a psychologic stress once the animal has learned how to avoid. It may be no more stressful than for a dog to become housebroken, for a child to learn how to write or to wear clothes, or go to school, or listen to a lecture. Once you have learned to perform the task, this is no longer a serious stress. It is the lack of control over psychologic situations that most likely represents the background for the development of psychosomatic disturbances.

DR. STERN: I should like to take one small page from what Dr. Corson has said, which is, of course, important and fundamental to our discussion of experimental work. That is, that within the framework of standardized experimental conditions that we all know are hardly applicable to human beings, we still must look at what we see. I think that what I am going to say is going to be in the form of a few questions from my own work, the first of which is: What can we learn about neuroendocrine factors from the use of the chemical carcinogen model? Why, for example, does the tumor localize at a point distant from its administration? The localization in the mammary gland–is this determined by some altered functional state in the cells of the mammary gland? Some support for this, I think, exists in the experimental finding that if you deliberately alter the hormonal state of the animal, you will be more likely to get tumors in the ovary, rather than in the breast of the animal.

Another question that we and other people have raised is the one that says: Is the carcinogen merely a way of accelerating tumor production? We have seen, as have others, that chemical carcinogens, and other types of carcinogens as well, have an endocrine effect. If the carcinogen acts on the brain, as we think we have indicated, and if this action is related to the later development of tumors, what does this really mean in terms of carcinogenesis?

From the experimental standpoint, what it might mean is that in carcinogenesis there may be a disturbance of regulatory mechanisms in the brain. Further experiments may indicate that the action of carcinogens is on such regulatory centers in the brain, in the anterior hypothalamus, for example, which do have something to do with the cybernetics of the neuroendocrine mechanism.

As far as what can be done in the future in the way of experiments, a number of suggestions have been made, one of them being, of course, that we would have to define exactly where the carcinogen does localize in the brain, somewhat in the manner of the work that Michaels did on the localization of estrogen. These are experiments to be done in the future.

Dr. Margolin brought up the very significant question of what we are doing to the brain in general when we manipulate it even by putting a very small-caliber needle in the brain. I think that is about all that I want to say, because I know that Dr. Margolin has some very exotic philosophical ideas that he wants to get started on.

DR. MARGOLIN: It is not true. They are exotic, but not philosophical.

DR. SOUTHAM: I think the idea behind the panel is that if you put strikingly different groups of people together on a panel it may be like knocking flint against steel: a few sparks might be produced. But all I can say so far is that I feel like a chunk of rock up here, and if anyone is good enough steel to get a spark out of me, I congratulate him.

My principal interest in the problems that have been under discussion here is how we might identify mechanisms through which psychological stresses could influence cancer. The one pathway that certainly can be suggested is through the hypothalamus, which influences the anterior pituitary and thereby controls the release of two groups of steroid hormones that do influence tumor growth.

The adrenocortical steroids influence immunological reactions and have a cytolytic effect on lymphoid cells. The steroids (estrogen, androgen, and progesterone) influence not only breast cancer, as was discussed by Dr. Stern, but also endometrial cancer.

Another lead comes from the direct investigation of urine steroid levels, as studied by Dr. Kissen and Dr. Katz and their co-workers. Those studies suggest that higher levels of the steroids of the adrenocortical type are correlated with poorer defenses against cancer. We know that high levels of adrenocortical hormone activity also correlate with poor immunologic responses, and I learned here that they also seem to correlate with a poorer psychologic response to one's disease.

I think that one of the biggest problems is finding investigative techniques that are applicable to the study of these interrelationships. We are looking at a final target, the cancer, which is several steps removed from the psychologic processes that eventually affect the target. What is the right approach? Should we attempt to study directly the influence of stress on cancer, or might we learn more by studying the influence of stress on endocrine responses, and the influence of hormones on cancer, as separate steps? Certainly the sequential approach is better for experimental control and for analysis of results, but we must recognize that this approach is useful only if we can identify potentially significant steps. I think we all are willing to admit that there may be many effects and many mechanisms of which, at present, we have no conception. It may be that the only way by which these will be revealed is by setting up the total experiment, and then, if anything happens, trying to dissect out the various steps.

Just one more point: If we do use the direct approach instead of the sequential approach, what tumor systems should we study? Studies of humans (cancer patients) are of greatest pertinence but almost impossible to control and evaluate. If we use mice or other experimental animals, we must be certain that we are truly studying cancer—not just a tissue graft. No one could find fault with a study of the carcinogenic response as reported by Dr. Stern, but, more frequently, in this type of study the investigator is tempted to implant a tumor, rather than to wait a long time for the neoplastic process to start by itself. With a transplantable tumor you can set up groups of animals, instead of dealing with individuals, and you can make mathematically satisfying measurements of tumor size, but to obtain data relevant to cancer, it is absolutely essential that a transplantable tumor be genetically identical with the host in which it is growing. Either we must study autochthonous cancer (cancer growing in its original host) or we must study syngeneic (isologous) tumor transplants. In our dissection of mechanisms we may find it useful to study homotransplanted (allogeneic) tumors, recognizing that we are studying homograft reactions that may be pertinent to cancer, but such transplants are not comparable to neoplastic disease.

Dr. Katz: It would seem to me that we are presently at something of a crossroads in clinical, as separate from animal, endocrine, and psychoendocrine considerations in cancer. We now have increasingly sophisticated tools for both psychiatric and endocrine assessments, and I stress the "both." Not only do we now have paper chromatography and double isotope techniques for endocrine assessment, but those working in the psychiatric field, I think, are aware that within the past ten years there has been a genuine push toward more reliable and valid assessment techniques for both acute "state" psychological variables and chronic "trait" psychological variables. We have also been able to establish certain correlations with increasing impressiveness, correlations between certain hormone patterns and the presence and course of certain malignancies and correlations between psychological and endocrine variables.

Nevertheless, as has been repeatedly stressed here, correlations do not, first of all, guarantee direct cause-and-effect relationships, and, second, even if causal relationships are present, they do not necessarily define the mechanisms and pathways for those relationships, although obviously they may offer hints.

It would thus seem incumbent at this point, for both endocrinologists and psychoendocrinologists to become increasingly involved in prospective, predictive, closely controlled studies, if any of these gaps are to be bridged. We are, perhaps, already beginning to get some of this in endocrinology.

For instance, there is presently a study going on in Gurnsey by the Bulbrook group, in which urines on approximately 5,000 presumedly normal women are being collected and the subjects then followed out prospectively; correlations between the urinary hormone patterns and the ultimate development and course of neoplasm are then going to be traced. Although I think some question can be raised regarding the whole concept of "premorbid normalcy" in a person going to develop cancer, I believe this is moving in the right direction.

However, in association with pure endocrine assessments, it has been very strongly suggested here that concurrent immunologic measures are going to be necessary. Psychiatric studies must now attempt to predict hormonal data, immunologic alterations, and clinical course, not just one or the other, and at the very least (and I stress "at the very least"), all of these parameters must show some correlation. Even then I would urge a word of caution. It is conceivable that certain tumors such as breast and prostate are particularly vulnerable to altered hormonal environments. But, for most malignancies, this may be a relatively minor consideration, both for the onset and the course of the illness. In other words, what we have been grappling with here, even though it has been more implicit than explicit, is really whether a psychological phenomenon can play a primary role in the etiology and/or pathogenesis of cancer.

Because of the availability of the psychic-adrenocortical relationship, it becomes highly tempting to invoke this as a pathway for an ultimate effect on immune mechanisms by psychological events. But only the first relationship in quantitatively established to any extent, and even if the second does exist, the question remains as to what degree it takes place, and whether this still might not play a relatively minor role among the various factors that play a part in the etiology and pathogenesis of cancer. While such conservatism and caution may seem strange, coming from one trained primarily as a psychiatrist, I think it is sorely needed in this particular area.

Only tightly controlled, prospective psychoendocrine studies for a variety of neoplasms will help to clarify the present obscurities. I might say, however, that I think such studies are indeed feasible and will begin to take place over the coming decade.

DR. MARGOLIN: First, I want to comment about the problem of controls and of scaling, as used in the various papers that we have heard. In practically all instances, the control situation was one in which there was a number of subjects who had cancer and a number of subjects who did not have cancer. It might properly be questioned: How does this procedure set up a legitimate and an appropriate control relationship? For example, it is perfectly conceivable that instead of setting up a binary situation of 0 cancer or of plus cancer on a scale of plus 4, why would there not have been a negative condition of cancer on a scale of minus 4? You would say, of course: How do you set up such a situation? What is cancer to a negative degree? What state of malignancy is that?

I believe that the answer to these methodological questions can be exemplified in the very fruitful contributions to this particular conference made by the endocrinologists and the immunologists. Many of their reports have emphasized that cancer is the consequence of an interacting set of varying factors whose single and combined effects would have to be evaluated or controlled. The negative scales would be used in the analyses of these factors. What class of human diseases can be scaled in this way that would be relevant to the proliferative condition of cancer?

The autoimmune diseases are characterized by alteration and/or destruction of parenchymal and interstitial tissues. Such pathological processes can be localized to one organ or disseminated to many organs. Dissemination may be equivalent to malignant metastases, in the sense that the spread of disease follows the distribution of the blood vessels within the organs. In the light of these considerations, I submit that our clinical cancer research should avoid the oversimplified cancer-no cancer statistical model. Instead, the widely accepted and valid multivariate model should be adapted whenever possible to psychophysiology of cancer data. For example, we should compare patients with cancer to patients who have autoimmune diseases.

Another factor that impressed and troubled me in our conference was the tendency to use research models as if they were explanatory. While this is occasionally possible, some inherent difficulties can be observed. For example, would they not apply to conditions that are not ordinarily regarded as neoplastic? A very good instance that has occurred to me is the condition of generalized obesity. Here we have cells that are capable of penetrating every tissue and organ of the body. We must decide whether the spread of this tissue is the result of production of new cells (as in neoplastic growth) or whether it is due to the filling up of cells that are already in existence. For many patients this disease is incorrigible–i.e., malignant. For others, as in the clinical course of some leukemias, there are relapses and remissions. In short, we have here a state of generalized metastases that is also commonly associated with neuroendocrine pathophysiology. Endocrine etiological factors have been sought in the metabolism of obesity.

Moreover, we try to treat cancer by starving it and reducing its metabolic supplies, and we interfere with the intracellular metabolism by means of drugs. We treat obesity in accordance with the same principles.

In short, the neuroendocrine model of cancer that has been ably presented to us must be less than specific if it can encompass the condition of obesity in the way that I have described. It is possible, of course, that this model is relevant, after all, if obesity can be regarded as a reversible metastatic malignancy.

More serious and more urgent is the question of whether or not we are legitimate in our choice of cancer versus no cancer as a proper control model in much of the clinical work that has been presented at this conference.

DR. ALFRED AMKRAUT (*Stanford University, Palo Alto, Calif*): It has occurred to me during these meetings, especially as a psychiatrist spoke, that perhaps in trying to produce stress models in animals, we may be looking at the wrong thing, or we may not have the proper correlate. We are looking at the input. The animal is being stressed. Should we perhaps be looking at: Is the animal coping with stress? Are there any suggestions forthcoming from the panel as to how we can do this? In other words, are controls, or some of our controls, equally under some kind of stress that we are not recognizing, and are some of them coping, and others not?

DR. BIDNER (*New York, N.Y.*): I would concur with the idea of controls other than those that have been presented. I think the confusion has been that the clinician considers as ideal the animal control model, and transposes it to the human condition. He forgets, however, that in the animal condition a control demands that all conditions except the area under study be identical. Having worked with cancer patients, as many of us have, makes me challenge the concept that a patient who has cancer or suspects that he has cancer can be compared with any other ill patient. I think this is an important consideration.

It seems to me that if one could find a similar clinical group, where a life-threatening situation would pertain, this would be helpful. I know that many studies have been done on the psychiatric aspect of patients in concentration camps and prisoner-of-war camps. Probably, that would be a good place to go to for prospective study.

DR. BRONNER-HUSZAR (*Sloan-Kettering Institute for Cancer Research, New York, N.Y.*): I wish to elaborate on just two subjects. First, I should like to comment on the question of people under an extreme stress situation that they cannot control, such as the concentration-camp situation. From what I know, it was never really established whether or not there was something added to the inmates' food to stop menses. Be that as it may, there were extremely few people who menstruated in concentration camps. For this and other obvious reasons, a hormonal imbalance somewhere along the line must logically be postulated. Therefore, I suggest that there should be a statistical investigation of those who did versus those who did not. (Ideally, if at all feasible, the latter group, too, should be screened for signs of malignant and premalignant lesions). The proportion of cancer victims in the concentration-camp-survivor population should be compared first of all with that in judiciously chosen control groups that were not exposed to stresses in any way comparable to internment in a concentration camp. I do not know of any such investigation to date, this in spite of having studied the pertinent literature and of having worked with concentration-camp survivors quite extensively.

Second, I should like to comment on the question of controls. I feel that when we investigate the importance of stress on cancer patients, we ought to set up control groups not only of the so-called normal population, but also of the diseased. Not of any diseased, either, but of patients suffering from chronic, debilitating and/or life-threatening illnesses such as, for instance, severe myocardial infarction, chronic nephritis, the collagen diseases, and multiple sclerosis, to name just a few. Pulmonary tuberculosis, fortunately, no longer seems to belong in that league, since greatly improved prophylactic and therapeutic measures have, for the most, completely altered its course and prognosis lately. Stresses inflicted by their diseases on these control groups should be, in my opinion, closely related to those imposed on the cancer patients by their illness.

DR. RAO: I appreciate that in a conference that runs only three days we cannot possibly discuss every aspect of cancer. I noticed possibly one slight omission in this discussion; that is, the problem of initiation and promotion of cancer. We talk of cancer as one process, but there is a fair amount of evidence that initiation is a process different from that of promotion, and one can have cancer for years and years and it may not spread and it may not present clinical manifestations.

If you are talking about immunological defenses, you are perhaps talking of defenses against promotion and not against initiation. I wish that some consideration would be given during this discussion to the initiation of the cancer process.

DR. STERN: I should like to answer the suggestion that Dr. Rao made, because this came up in discussion at the workshop. I do not know whether the people who are at this conference agree that there is such a difference between the initiating and promoting stages in tumorigenesis.

I think that somebody at the workshop said that there was no difference, and that this had been proved. If so, I missed the proof. I see that Dr. Rao missed it, too. Perhaps that can be brought up later. In some of my own work on cancer of the cervix, we found that the set of factors related to the early stage of cancer were different from the set of factors related to the later stages of cancer.

DR. ABSE: Can the authorities on the platform tell us something about the connections between immunologic and endocrine derangements and enzymatic derangements?

DR. MARGOLIN: The panel has a challenge.

DR. STERN: I do not think that we have come to that question, but I think that is a very pertinent question to raise at this time. It might very well give us the direction for some future meeting, where there could be some interplay between these two disciplines.

DR. WEISS: I should like to make only two brief points. Concerning the possible model of obesity, I suggest that there is an operative distinction between neoplasia and hyperplasia that should be borne in mind, and that is that hyperplasia is a response of cells capable of multiplying to a given stimulus, and that the response ceases when the stimulus is withdrawn. If the individual stops eating too much or exercises more, metastatic spread of fatty tissue is immediately arrested. Neoplasia, in contradistinction, either is maintained after withdrawal of the inciting stimulus, or the inciting stimulus remains; for example, a viral agent incorporated into the genome of the cell. So I question this model.

The only other point I wish to make at this time is that we are belaboring the question of controls. Some valid things have been said, but it should be remembered that in many experiments there is no such thing as a single satisfactory control group. One must often use eight, nine, or ten control groups for one experimental group in order to control for different aspects of that which the experimental parameters are designed to reveal; one therefore should not overemphasize the point whether this control is better than that. One needs different controls to control for different variables in total conceptual circumstance.

DR. MARGOLIN: Dr. Weiss, before you leave the microphone, may I ask if you were satisfied with your particular approach to the problem of experimental control; were you satisfied with the concept of control used in several of the individual reports to this conference? In short, are you satisfied with human cancer research based upon two classes of cases as controls of each other, one with cancer, one without cancer?

DR. WEISS: No. Satisfaction is a very broad concept and a very relative one. Psychiatrists certainly should be aware of this.

DR. MARGOLIN: Do you mean that there are several varieties of satisfaction?

DR. WEISS: Yes. If it is impossible to set up a totally satisfactory experimental circumstance, I would still settle for a limited experimental circumstance, which might at least be suggestive. I think that when one attempts to correlate psychic factors in all of their complexity to a given, extremely complex physiological process such as progressive neoplasia, it might be virtually humanly impossible for any one experiment to have all the possible controls that are needed. Hence, I would settle for several experiments in which different control groups control for different aspects of this situation. I think a very important point is that if one were to plan a prospective study, then one should incorporate many controls, or should attempt to do so. If one does a retrospective study, one might have to settle for a limited number of controls. So I am not totally satisfied. I am, however, persuaded that there is a good bit of suggestive evidence for a correlation between psychodynamic states and neoplasia. I do not think anybody is totally satisfied.

DR. STERN: May I make one comment on that? In experimental work I was very much taken with the idea that there should be the kind of a control, which I cannot conceive of myself, which would relate to something that would create a condition of chronic stress. Now, in our hypothalamic experiments we have 14 sets of animals, 14 experimental groups. But I still think that the point that Dr. Corson was making was that we do not have any real evidence of the response of the animals to chronic nonspecific stress to compare with the response of the animals to chronic experimental stress. If there is such an experimental model that anyone has in mind, I should be delighted to have it, because, I do not think that giving a vehicle to an animal as a substitute for the experimental procedure is a condition of chronic stress.

DR. MARGOLIN: Dr. Corson gave us a good example of such a stress. He pointed out that a dog can learn where he's been and received a shock. He will remember this experience for a long time, so that whenever he comes into the setting of the previous trauma, he no longer needs an external piece of apparatus to provide him with the stimulus. This is the state of chronic stress, or at least the readiness for the dog to be stressed, which appears to have already become internalized.

DR. BAHNSON: I was very much impressed by Dr. Corson's statement, because it suggests that animals also have a phenomenology, so that one cannot just deal with stress in terms of environmental parameters, but must take into consideration the particular experience that the animal has of this stress. One can describe these events in learning-theory parameters as learned adaptation to cues, but it also provides fine parallels to the human situation, in which many workers have thought of the loss or the external stress situation *per se,* without considering the individual's particular perception of the situation. Thus, Dr. Corson's comparative studies cross relate to the human phenomena that we have been talking about for quite a while.

DR. CORSON: I just want to make one remark about genetic differences, because I am not sure I really made this point strongly enough in my previous remarks. When you study genetic differences, you must consider them in relation to the genetic differences of the central nervous system. You can have black dogs or white dogs and segregate them on that basis, or on the basis of short tails or long tails. This would probably have little bearing on differences in reactions to psychologic stress. It is possible, as we have done in dogs, to segregate animals not merely on the basis of their breeds, but on the basis of their reactions to specific psychologic stimuli.

There have been some attempts in several laboratories to breed a number of generations of rats with high and low central nervous system excitability. I suggest that it would be a useful procedure to conduct such genetic-psychophysiologic-behavioral studies on higher animals, and particularly on dogs. Dogs are especially suitable for genetic-environmental-psychologic interaction studies because of the availability of a variety of pure breeds and because dogs exhibit many kinds of emotional attachments that resemble those of humans. I think it would be a worthwhile investment to do this kind of work. Psychophysiologic and psychopharmacologic data will be much more meaningful when higher animals are segregated and bred on the basis of genetic differences in the function of the central nervous system.

PANEL DISCUSSION 2: THE IMMUNOLOGIC APPROACH

Jonas Salk, *Moderator*

The Salk Institute for Biological Studies
San Diego, Calif.

DR. SALK: Our question may be expressed in the following forms. One, is there a cause and effect relationship between psychological states and neoplastic disease? It is perfectly clear from the discussions here that the matter of controls is insufficiently resolved to permit us to answer that question strongly in the affirmative.

I must at this moment comment on something that Dr. Bennette said to me, and that is that we are so polite that we have lost some of the tradition of our forebears in science who spoke out very forthrightly.

I think we really should call a spade a spade at these meetings. It sharpens our own thinking, and there is nothing impolite about saying what you really think, so long as your motive is intended to be constructive. I think it is fair to say that a direct relationship between psychologic states and neoplastic disease has not been established. We then go to the second question, which asks: If such a relationship exists, what is the mechanism whereby it is mediated?

In considering the first question regarding cause and effect in the psychopathologic pathogenesis of cancer, there seems to be two schools of thought. One school is of the opinion that there is a direct connection between the psyche and the target tissues, and another school is of the opinion that the psychic effects are mediated through such systems as the endocrinologic and/or the immunologic.

I think it is fair to say that the conference has not established any of these points as yet. It is fair to say that the conference is trying to order the questions, rather than to end with explicit answers.

Since the exact sets of causes of all of the various forms of cancer in man are not yet established, and since seemingly identical circumstances do not always produce the same effect, both schools of thought accept the idea of direct and of contributing factors. So long as the causative factors of a particular disease of man remain unknown, the field is open to all kinds of conjecture, and of this, of course, we have had ample evidence.

Until the pathogenesis of cancer is more precisely established, this field will remain one in which hypotheses will be rampant. The need, of course, is for rigorous observation, rigorous experimentation and rigorous proof. And, the purpose of this conference, in part, is to reveal where such exists and to distinguish between hard facts and soft facts, or between facts and impressions. The panel is to sum up the impressions that each of us has developed.

DR. BENNETTE: What I am going to do is to call a spade a spade, if I may. We have been looking at data, and as I see it, a datum is a given fact, and it may be a fact derived from our study of the so-called objective world or of the subjective world. And I insist that there are such things as subjective facts. I do not believe that data is the same as information. Data must be linked in order to become information, and they can be linked logically, or dialectically, or symbolically. When they are linked, you have a flow of information.

Cancer, as I see it, is a disease of the self, whatever that may mean. But, whatever it may mean, it is a mystery that is central both to immunologists and psychologists. Immunologists are forever talking about identity, recognition, self patterns, memory, learning—all these words that have very strong psychic overtones.

I think I had better try to demonstrate that I am capable of some concrete perjury, because I think we need to come down to earth from these philosophical points of view and try to establish ways of designing experiments that will bring psychologists and immunologists and others together. We have to come down to earth, and that means to say, we have to come down to the lab bench or the couch. Personally, I feel a bit happier sitting at the side of the couch, but some of my colleagues probably feel happier sitting at the bench.

What we need to ask is: What can we do together? I think we all agree that one of the things that we really must look at is the possibility for prospective human studies, recognizing that man is not just another species, but a different order of being. His difference resides in the fact that he can make history. I believe that there is a possibility here. Postoperative patients are in a situation of crisis of existence. They may know before that they have cancer, but after the operation they surely know. The surgery or the radiotherapy I see as first aid. The real crunch comes when they get metastases. And this seems to me to be the essential point of what has been called so often "the cancer problem." However, it ceases to be a problem for someone with metastases. It becomes an intense anguish of the life-death situation.

After the operation, I believe that many patients will accept psychotherapy, having been brought to the very frontiers of their existence. They not only accept it, they welcome the opportunity to explore the possible meaning of their situation. What I am suggesting is a bit of concrete poetry: the possibility that an experiment could be devised in which patients who are willing to accept psychotherapy postoperatively be given the opportunity to engage in this experience. There will be many patients who are not ready for this, who will constitute a control group. But this will be ethically acceptable, because it will not be a question for the physicians to decide, but for the patient.

Now, as I see it, psychotherapy is a process of controlled release of exactly those aspects that cancer patients, it is believed, cannot adequately discharge. I believe my colleagues here will be able to demonstrate that it is possible to make correlations between the immunological competence and the cognitive competence, as Dr. Shands called it, in the postoperative period. That is to say, it is possible to take patients in psychotherapy and study immunological profiles, and patients who are not in psychotherapy and study their immunological profiles, and patients who are in psychotherapy and who are in other fixed categories, and study their immunological profiles and so on, using as many controls as one can get. It might be possible to bring the realities of the lab and the realities of the ward together in some sort of synthesis.

Dr. Salk: Dr. Eva Klein will tell us how all this appears from her point of view, and the intention is to begin with some of the hardest information we have, which is the work in animals, and let her comment on that and give her views of the human cancer problem.

Dr. Klein: After you have been hearing all about experimental tumors and about specific antigens in animals, I suppose you think that you know terribly much about it, and that is really the case. But some of you might have wondered why we never mention the human tumors. This is because we really do not know very much about them.

We anticipate specific antigens on the basis of experimental tumors, but there is not yet one single case in which you can pinpoint the question and say that here you really find cell-free antigen. We have found a lot of suggestive evidence, and this is what I should like to point out for those cases on which we were working ourselves. There are bits of evidence that we can collect for occurrence, but what we learned from experimental tumors was to use a method that was available and that worked out.

On the basis of our experience with mouse leukemias, we turned to a tumor that occurs in Africa, the Burkett leukemia. This is a sort of lymphoma that occurs in a very well defined area, of course. Some of you, then, will think that this has some sociological importance, but I think that mosquitoes play a much greater role in this. The tumor occurs on low altitudes and in areas with a high average yearly temperature and high humidity. It is very common. It is a childhood tumor with a peak incidence of four to five years of age, and you rarely find it after 12 years of age.

It has been suggested that this is caused by a virus, and, in fact, in cultures derived from some tumors, we have found virus particles, against which, in a large number of people, antibodies were found–even in the United States, antibodies are found in about 50% of adult population, and all Burkett disease children have antibodies.

If the tumor is virus-induced, in anology with experimental mouse leukemias, we can assume that it also has a surface antigen. We therefore applied the test we used in mouse leukemia, and, in fact, we found that some Burkett patients have antibodies in the serum that reacted with this lymphoma cell. So I think we have quite good evidence that we here are considering a tumor-specific antigen.

What can we learn from that? What are the consequences? We know that this tumor responds very well to chemotherapy. Actually, this is a tumor you can cure. Now, we have cases of survival up to six years that did not recur after chemotherapy. Thus we have a good evidence that the tumor-specific antigen in this case elicits an immune response, and this helps in the therapy to eradicate the disease.

However, we know from experimental studies that we do not have much hope that we can do much to eradicate a tumor by immunological means only. So, whenever we want to look for prevention or to help prevention, what we must do is increase immunological responsiveness. I may add that in Africans, the gamma globulin level is much higher than in any Western countries, so that these children are, in fact, in a very high immunological responsiveness, in general. That is where we stand with this tumor.

The other tumor that was selected was the epipharynx cancer, again occurring in Africa. The epipharynx cancer, we were told, might be a chemical carcinogen-induced tumor. It also occurs in unusual high frequency in young adults in Africa, and is very common in people who live in huts without any outlet of smoke. These people have a fire in the middle of the hut, which is constantly kept burning to keep away insects and to warm the hut. We anticipated that the tumor has surface antigen, in this case individual antigen. And, again, by borrowing the methods from animal experimentation, we have produced some evidence that it can be the case.

DR. WEISS: I should like to begin my brief comments by attempting a reply to something that Dr. Bahnson said a little while ago and that, in a way, I believe, lies at the center of many of these discussions. This concerns the contradiction between the so-called reductionist and the so-called integrationist approach to this problem. I should like to throw out to you the obvious thought that integration and reduction are not necessarily mutually exclusive intellectual processes, when one thinks of a problem of this complexity. May I get poetic for a moment? When I look at an old painting, I attempt first of all to see the painting as a whole, but if I want to ask myself: "Is the composition good? Is the lighting adequate?", I must then attempt to reduce the entire picture into component parts and juxtapose a part here against a part there.

If I wish further to ask, "What is the makeup of the pigment?", I must actually do chemical analysis on flakes of the paint. Now, this does not mean that I look at a Rembrandt only as a chemist. It does not mean that I look at a painting only in terms of design, or light, or color, or pigment, but I look at all of these parameters, and at the same time I enjoy the painting as a whole.

I, myself, am satisfied that there is a good deal of suggestive evidence that points to some kind of correlation, and perhaps to a causal correlation, between psychodynamic states and neoplasia. I am also satisfied that the very nature of the immune response–its susceptibility to major change as a result of even relatively minor effects–makes this a very likely candidate for being one of the important matrices or pathways by which psychodynamic states translate themselves into potential susceptibility.

I also wish to throw out again the rather obvious point that some of the very best experiments in the history of science were done on the basis of hunches, on the basis of intuition, and not on the basis of any more convincing evidence than what we have available to us right now at this moment for these interactions between psychodynamic states and neoplasia. So, if the ultimate purpose of a meeting like this is to suggest better work, newer work, more extensive work, I certainly believe that the basis for such future study is present. I refuse entirely to perceive a paradox between, on the one hand, attempting to integrate into one configuration the many elements here discussed, and on the other hand, to attempt to reduce at any one point various components in this model to their own direct interaction, in order to see whether the component can be related, and from that to make an entire structure.

Now, specifically, with regard to what I think can most properly be done in the immediate future, I should like to throw out the following. I think that the hazards of any retrospective study are such that I cannot conceive of any likely retrospective study to produce the hard kind of evidence that would permit us to go beyond the area of suggestion and circumstantial evidence that is already at our disposal. I suggest that prospective experiments, prospective studies in man, are by no means impossible. There are today available in American society and certainly in many other societies very large numbers of individuals on whom fairly careful personality testing is done for one reason or another, people who are screened for certain positions in life. Many such individuals can be followed up for prolonged periods of time, so that one can do a kind of prospective study of the relationship of certain fairly well-defined psychodynamic states and eventual susceptibility to neoplasia.

If one were to introduce now an immunological parameter into such a kind of prospective study, I suggest to you the fact that one need not do heroic things. There are available to the clinicians, the epidemiologists, very common tools for getting an impression of good, bad, or intermediate degree of immunological state. The normal kinds of testing that the allergist does in order to assay whether an individual is or is not hypersensitive to a large number of environmental allergens in a large number of different kinds of immune states–these are available. A small amount of serum from a patient can give a great deal of information as to the presence of the so-called natural antibodies. The follow-up of tuberculin tests, and, again, of auxiliary reaction, provides a fairly broad degree of overview with respect to immunological states. So these things are possible.

Now, with regard to animal experiments, I again suggest the following. A great deal of information can be gained from animal experiments, provided that one is not too facile in speaking of psychological states in animals, or on the basis of very limited numbers of experiments or circumstances. I think, in closing, that perhaps the most valid experimental model in animals is not an attempt to produce in animals conditions that are simple shock circumstances, but rather, that asks the question: What kind of threat circumstances does a given species of animal experience that is a truer kind of analogy to stress in man? Perhaps the study of male animals, male rodents competing for the affection of female rodents, might be a better "natural" model of stress in animals than putting an animal onto a platform on which it receives an electric shock.

I think the point is obvious. One has to vary so-called stress conditions over a large spectrum of circumstances in order to cover the various possibilities that exist; and, similarly, one would have to ask the question of a large number of neoplastic states whether there is a correlation with different kinds of stress, and especially, stress that is within the normal experience of an animal of this species. Electric shock is not. Competition for a female is. Overcrowding is. Certain disease conditions are.

Finally, we must ask the question: What does this mean in terms of susceptibility, not only to some very artificial neoplastic circumstance, but to a naturally experienced neoplasia? What would certain stresses do to the natural leukemia incidence in a strain of mice in which leukemia is endemic? To mammary tumor incidence in a strain of mice in which mammary tumor is endemic? I especially stress the difference between different kinds of neoplasia, because one kind of immune component may be very effective against a neoplastic condition consisting of dispersed neoplastic cells, as in leukemia, and be totally ineffective against a solid tumor, and the opposite might hold true if you turn the picture around.

Animal experiments, I think, are valid provided one is not overly simplistic, and provided one varies over a large number of conditions the parameters that one is attempting to measure.

Dr. Rasmussen: I should like to continue the discussion that Dr. Weiss has introduced and to emphasize how much can and must be learned with the animal systems because, as Dr. Klein has indicated, we know very little about the pathogenesis of tumors induced either virally or by other kinds of carcinogens in man.

There is a wide variety of spontaneously occurring animal tumors in rodents that are being defined and that offer an opportunity to assess the immunologic response in relation to the pathogenesis of rodent cancer. I think it is imperative that we recognize that immunology covers a very broad category of responses that together may account for a varying degree of resistance. For example, in a virus tumor system, the specific antibody response in the form of antibody globulin either gamma A, gamma G, or gamma M, might very well be an important and even determining factor in determining whether the initial malignant conversion would occur. For instance, if the Burkett virus is transmitted by a mosquito, there can be a prompt immunologic response, and the virus infection may be arrested early. There may be no malignant conversion and no cancer. In that case, the antibody response has been very beneficial. On the other hand, the malignant conversion may occur, or the malignant conversion may have been accomplished by some other carcinogen, and this same category of antibody may have harmful impact on the progression of the tumor and may actually enhance the capacity of tumor to grow in its new host. Again, we must look at an entirely different category of immune responsiveness, cellular immunity, which is more likely to be concerned with immunity to cancer in general.

These questions are the kinds of questions which I think can be approached in experimental animals through a diversity of experimental situations, a diversity of animals with different genetic backgrounds, and a diversity of tumors.

The opportunity, I think, really to increase our knowledge in this area is enormous at this time, and since progress with small animals can be more rapid than that in the long life of human subjects, I certainly hope that this kind of effort will continue.

DR. SALK: Dr. Bennette said that he was far more comfortable sitting beside the couch. I think you can gather that there are some of us, as he already indicated, who feel more comfortable at the bench, and as we progress in this discussion we are now moving more and more toward clinical investigation from the strictly laboratory investigation.

DR. SOLOMON: I just wish to summarize the classes of evidence that emotions may affect immunity, evidence that emotions affect immunity, which in turn may affect the onset and course of cancer.

One class of evidence is that personality factors and stress events may be associated with diseases in which abnormalities of the immunologic system occur, both autoimmune diseases and diseases of hypersensitivity, though, indeed, the nature of the immunologic dysfunctions in these two types of diseases might be quite different. There is postulated immunologic deficiency of some sort, probably of the cellular or delayed hypersensitivity variety, in the case of autoimmune disease, and in the case of allergy, there is hyperreactivity or, more likely, qualitative differences in the class of antibody produced. We also have to differentiate between personality traits in terms of predisposition and effects of stress or decompensation of psychologic defenses.

The second line of evidence that emotions relate to immunity is that there are some immunologic dysfunctions in conjunction with clinical conditions of failure of psychological defenses and mental illness. The third class of evidence comprises the animal experiments on stress and immune response, about which we heard.

Next, I should like to comment on further experimentation. I agree that it is important for us to use a variety of stressful circumstances and, especially, naturally occurring situations that would be likely to be disruptive to the homeostasis of an animal population. However, we do also have a problem on the immunologic side: that of evaluating cellular immunity in a serial way. I hope the immunologists will be able ultimately to help us look better at cellular immunity in a quantitative way, in order to be able to make correlations with environmental events. This ability is crucial, because circulating antibody appears not to be the most important aspect of immunity in cancer.

With regard to human studies, I think the points made about correlation of emotional state over time with immunologic status and with ultimate onset of disease is terribly important, but I am not quite as sanguine as Dr. Weiss is about the ability to do this. We have some evidence that immunoglobulins, for example, are enormously stable in given individuals. If one checks IgG, IgA, and IgM even in the presence of intercurrent infections and major emotional upheavals, the levels are steady. Similarly, in our observations on rheumatoid arthritis, although exacerbations of the disease were correlated with the antecedent stress events, the levels of the abnormal gamma M autoantibody rheumatoid factor for any given individual remained remarkably steady.

It has been suggested by Dr. Klein that it might be useful to look at the responsivity of lymphocytes themselves after challenge by antigen. We did this kind of work in stressed animals and controls and had a great deal of difficulty in obtaining reliable results because of enormous individual differences. We have been working with lymphocyte cultures and *in vitro* stimulation in humans, looking for antibrain activity in schizophrenia. Again, we have enormous problems of individual variability, but we remain hopeful that this system may yet prove useful. Perhaps it is a bit reassuring to a psychiatrist to realize that such quantitative and testing problems exist in another field. These problems are very analogous to those we are beset with in our own field. I feel that we need a great deal more help from immunologists in order to do the kinds of longitudinal predictive studies that have been so justifiably advocated.

DR. RASMUSSEN: One important point that has, I am sure, been underneath all our discussions, although I do not believe anyone has ever said it, is that the natural history of the tumor in a rodent is really not a very good model of the natural history of tumor in a long-lived animal like man. One can talk about doing experiments in primates, other primates, but if one is going to do an experiment in a primate, a human is by far the most satisfactory and rewarding subject.

DR. SALK: The organizers of this conference were very bold indeed. To take the problem of cancer is difficult enough. To take the problem of psychological aspects of cancer is indeed heroic. These are two problems that stand so much on their own, and both are in need of so much further inquiry, that I hope you will understand when I sort it out in a somewhat shocking way in commenting, as I did. I believe that we all must feel very humble, indeed, each of us in our own little universe, feeling adequate and being able to manipulate the tools that each of us possesses, whether they be those of a psychiatrist or those of an immunologist or an enzymologist or a neurophysiologist.

Our purpose, I felt, was to define the issues, to look at the familiar from an unfamiliar point of view; that is to say, for each to look at the problem as seen by the other. In a sense, this has been a very illuminating experience for me. I think that all of us who have come here have come here with open minds and open hearts, if you will, and will have returned to our own work enriched considerably by thoughts and ideas of others.

The effect of all this, I am sure, will be to influence the kind of work that each does individually, and whether from a conference such as this there can emerge little islands of collaboration is something that only time will tell. We attempted in this presentation to indicate, as best we can, the present state of knowledge, the present state of the art. We have resisted the idea that we have any final and definitive answers to report, but wish, instead, to see the questions that need to be posed, and suggestions have been made as to how they may be posed and how they may then be approached. Unless the conference ends not merely with each person's having his own opinion reinforced, but rather with the idea that each will go back and do something differently, it will not have had as great a value as it could have had.

I want to conclude by saying that I do hope that everyone has the feeling that we are not dealing with an either/or situation, that we are dealing with both pinheads and pinpoints; we can't be both at the same moment, but we can be both in the course of time. Some of us tend to stroke the round side of the pin, and others of us do the needling. The attempt to probe for evidence is quite different from the mood in which one speculates when one nurtures hunches and intuition. But I must confess that each of us does both.

DR. MICHAEL LEVY (*New York, N. Y.*): I just wanted to say that there are islands off New Guinea and New Britain where there is a population of a million and a half covered by one physician, with limited access to hospitalization. Human beings inhabiting these islands have been seen with disease such as cancer of the cervix by the age of three or four. That means that the possibility for diagnosis prior to that does not exist. With the sophistication of current technology and laboratory possibilities, one might establish a control. At the same time, it might help or improve the health of that area. One might establish a feasible control for the etiology, the nature of the disease, and a model for investigation. This is just to comment that there are areas where such a model can be applied, where one can extend the learning from the animal to the human, if it is not possible in this area.

PANEL DISCUSSION 3: THE PSYCHOLOGICAL APPROACH

Claus Bahne Bahnson,* *Moderator*

Department of Psychiatry
Jefferson Medical College
Philadelphia, Pa.

DR. BAHNSON: The second panel, particularly, but also the first, brought up several subtle points to which I should like to address myself before we go into the panel itself. There seems to be some epistemological confusion about cause and effect. An either/or problem, whether psychological problems may or may not be related to endocrine processes, whether biochemical aspects are related to immunological aspects, and so on, has been raised. It seems to me that although there has been a general trend toward openness, many of the participants now have gotten "cold feet." I think the common "super ego" is beginning to work, with the result that more caution has been expressed in the last few hours than during the last three days. I do not welcome this development at all, but I want to emphasize the underlying point: that it is a naïve and mistaken assumption that one can talk about cause and effect at all. All we can do is organize observations over time, within different theoretical conceptual systems. We usually assign a causal antecedent effect to those events that come early in time and dependent effects to those that come later in time. Now, in our case, as Dr. Weiss so brilliantly pointed out, we have many different systems operating at the same time, with the emphasis that systems do not really exist, but are different levels of organization of processes based on our selection of methodology and theory in approaching the subject matter.

We have tried to communicate with immunologists and with endocrinologists, and have tried to listen to their language. Some of my panelists may not agree with me on this point, but I feel that they have not listened enough to our language. Dr. Bennette was correct when he said that it is perfectly legitimate to observe carefully and, in some cases, even measure experience, which is one of our most permanent companions. One should not be a reductionist to the ridiculous degree that only certain laboratory or bench observations are legitimate, and that experiences that have been obtained in a clinical setting or in a subjective or phenomenological setting become less respectable.

Of course, this is part of the pragmatic attitude in the Western world today, with its great emphasis on gadgets and meters, but we should not forget that there are other ways of assessing psychobiological phenomena.

I emphasize this point, because it seems to me that there has been a tendency to play down the respectability and the worthwhileness of studying man in terms of his experience and his psychological reactions. We have been bearing with this because we have tried to be good hosts, but there are limits, and I think that we want to stand up for the relevance of studying psychological experience.

DR. LAWRENCE LESHAN: There are many things we have learned from this conference. Perhaps one of the most important is that an individual does not just "get" the malignancy, which starts on the cellular or immunological or endocrinological or psychological level. The entire organism eventuates toward cancer. His

* Present address: Eastern Pennsylvania Psychiatric Institute, Institute of Pennsylvania Hospital, Philadelphia, Pa., and University of Connecticut, Storrs, Conn.

total biography, involving all its levels, moves in a direction leading to a total, organism-in-an-environment situation, which we term "neoplastic disease." The most dramatic aspects of this is, finally, the cellular disorganization, the inability to function on various psychobiological levels, and death. We tend to focus on the cellular level because of its very highly dramatic and visual aspects and for reasons involving the recent history of medical philosophy. Our studies point out to us very clearly, however, that "cancer" is a total organismic situation and we slice it into small parts at our peril. The different levels at which we work are clearly necessary divisions in terms of our training, our intellectual limitations, and our ability to learn. There are no more Renaissance men, unfortunately, and perhaps it is impossible today for there to be any. We need these divisions into different levels. However, we should be clear that they are myths—necessary and useful myths, but like the particle in physics, myths, nevertheless.

Henry Poincaré once said, "Modern man uses cause and effect as ancient man used the Gods, to give order to the Universe." "But," said Poincaré, "this is not because it is the most truthful system, but because it's the most convenient."

Similarly, we today in science use the concept of levels, hopefully remembering from time to time that we impose them on the data, rather than vice versa. Perhaps what we need most in this field at this time is an attempt to pull together what we know or are reasonably sure of, the hard data at each level. Each of the levels of organismic being that we have studied in cancer research has a certain amount of hard data. If we can begin to draw up a profile of these data, perhaps we can see the beginning of an overall pattern of the organismic life situation that we call "cancer."

Thus, on psychological levels, we can point to poor outlets for emotional discharge, feelings of despair and hopelessness, a strong sense of loss of relationships, and a rigid personality structure. If other specialists can add data on each level, data that they are reasonably sure of at this time, then perhaps we will be closer to the goal of this conference. It is crucial that we keep in mind that we are all specialists, and that "cancer" is a general situation; together, we may be able to understand it.

But, I must add one crucial warning about this. When we look at the data at different levels of approach, we tend to feel that the scientist working on levels other than our own are simply speculating, and not dealing in hard facts. This is because we do not know exactly what went into the background of each concept, and therefore tend to see it as verbiage resting on air. Not having done our homework at these other levels of scientific research—each level with its own logic, its own research techniques, its own history—we listen to the scientific shorthand that is given, we hear the specialists in fields other than our own talking about the data they know so well, rather than describing the data itself and seeing it as pure verbal play.

A certain amount must be taken on faith. It must be taken on faith that specialists in other scientific fields do know what they are talking about even when they disagree with each other. Unless that faith is given, we will never be able to integrate our knowledge.

Dr. Arthur H. Schmale, Jr. (*Rochester, N. Y.*): I am not sure that I have much to add to what has already been said, or to what I presented at the first cancer conference. I should like to follow up, however, on what Dr. LeShan has said, and perhaps get a little more specific in terms of the psychological setting in which cancer has its apparent onset. From our studies it is now evident that there is nothing specific about the psychological setting for the patient with cancer that differentiates him from patients who develop other diseases. Studies of medical and psychiatric patients with a wide range of diagnoses, as well as of normal health controls, grieving women, and women with cervical carcinoma have demonstrated a common pattern. Most of what has been described at this conference, as well as the previous cancer conference, can be seen as elements in this common pattern. The failure of repressions, denial, and inhibition as defenses, the loss of sources of object or self-gratification, the feelings of depression and no motivation to change things are all part of the setting in which disease, including cancer, has its onset. We have labeled this "giving up." Others have called it alienation or inability to cope. What Dr. LeShan described to us as the turning-off reaction fits with what we call giving up.

The reaction involves the thought that there is no way to achieve what one has been trying to accomplish. There is nothing the individual can do to overcome the feeling of depletion or inadequacy. Yet, the individual is unwilling to stop desiring or wishing for the unachievable goal or gratification. From our studies, we have delineated two distinct types of giving up: helplessness and hopelessness. Cancer appears to be one of the diseases that frequently makes its first appearance in a life-setting of experienced hopelessness. Data presented at the previous conference indicated that carcinoma of the cervix could be predicted in asymptomatic women who had atypical and suspicious but not diagnostic changes in their cervical cytology. The dichotomy of cancer or no cancer was based on whether the women reported before their diagnostic biopsies a reaction to a life event(s) with feelings of hopelessness within the period of six months prior to their first atypical smear.

Thus, the reaction of hopelessness may be seen as a permissive or facilitating factor that allows the cancer as well as other diseases to appear when they do. Since hopelessness has been reported prior to the onset of a number of diseases other than new growths, it must be assumed that it is a nonspecific factor that requires the known existence of a neoplastic predisposition already present within the body before a prediction of cancer can be made.

Thinking in these terms, cancer becomes a psychosomatic disease. Dr. Reiser and his group, going back some years now, with Weiner, Thaler, and Mirsky, demonstrated the relevance of such a model for predicting the onset of peptic ulcer. (The history of the individual in terms of his somatic predisposition, as well as his psychological predisposition, must be determined. With this background information, it is then possible to predict the kinds of life events that will create a reaction of psychological giving up. If and when the giving up occurs, then the somatic predisposition may, in turn, proceed to what we know as disease.)

The concept of linking what goes on at the psychological level with what goes on at the immunological, the endocrine, or the cellular level is where we are left in the dark. Dr. Bennette's idea that alienation, when it occurs, may be experienced simultaneously at cellular as well as psychic levels is a seductive one. Alienation, when defined as isolation and lack of communication, can be understood psychologically, and it also fits with the descriptions being made by those studying the activity of the cancer cell in its environment. Thus, at least the language is compatible with thinking at somatic and psychic levels simultaneously, and gets away from our previous cause-and-effect theorizing.

The psychological test data of patients already diagnosed and being treated for cancer are of limited value, in my view, for understanding the psychological factors relevant to the apparent onset of cancer or for the study of the antecedent personality configuration of the patient who develops cancer. By way of illustration, in our studies of cervical carcinoma the psychological factors found by many investigators to be present in women with cervical carcinoma were not helpful in predicting who had cancer and who did not. With our subjects, all were considered equally predisposed to cancer because of the similarity of their cytology. In fact, we found that the psychological profile said to be associated with cervical carcinoma by other investigators was present in most women of both groups—in those found to have cancer and those without cancer. From these data and the subsequent work of others, we assume that what was previously described as being associated with cervical cancer is really associated with a predisposition to cervical dysplasia. Thus, when specific psychological conflicts and biological factors considered predisposing to cancer are present in a life-setting where the psychological conflicts become or seem unresolvable, the nonspecific giving-up reaction will occur. It is in this kind of setting that cancer has its greatest chance of making its clinical appearance.

DR. BOOTH: First of all, I shall try to explain my theoretical approach, because it is different from that of the other observers. They were concerned with cause-effect chains that connect psyche and neoplasia. In this scheme, the organism is viewed as a homeostatic system that reacts to contingent environmental stimuli in predictable ways. Its inanimate model is the computer. My own psychophysiological approach is rooted in the work of Viktor Von Weizsaecker. Its central concept is the *Gestaltkreis,* the circular process of morphogenesis, an acausal process that connects subject and object. The inanimate model of *Gestaltkreis* dynamics is quantum mechanics. Their role in the neurophysiology of the brain was established by Eccles.

Von Weizsaecker demonstrated that the behavior of the organism is based on the reciprocal, simultaneous interaction between subject and object. In biological developments, subject and object are not causes of each other, but "events," as defined by Alfred N. Whitehead. They follow each other in more or less predictable sequences. Biological causality is statistical, like the causal laws of macrophysics.

The coherence of subject and environment is negatively revealed in the effects of sensory deprivation, the disintegration of the behavior of the subject if cut off from the structured object world. From this point of view, most animal experiments devoted to the psychophysiology of cancer are open to criticism because they deprive, more or less radically, the animals of their natural environments. Ethologists have taught us that animals in the laboratory do not display the purposeful behavior of which they are capable in nature. I feel that experimental cancer research would lead to more illuminating results if carcinogenic agents were applied to animals living under approximately normal conditions. Methodical variations of just one factor might make it possible to clarify further the pathogenic dynamics observed in human cancer.

The principal aim of my psychophysiological research has been to define the kind of psychosocial environment that is needed by individuals liable to develop specific diseases if their dominant needs are frustrated. The nonrepresentative Rorschach cards provide clues to the basic structural aspects of the environment that a given clinical group seeks: which formal features of a given inkblot picture are perceived, and which are ignored or neglected. The predominant gestalt tendencies of the clinical group proved to be symbolical of the relevant psychosocial structures.

Although the theory of the Gestaltkreis may appear far-fetched, its clinical application has considerable practical significance. This is immediately demonstrable in Parkinson patients. The rapid changes of the level of motor effectiveness cannot be understood in terms of anatomical lesions, but make sense if one understands the changes in terms of the changes of motivation implied in variations of the psychosocial situation. If we apply these insights, we can eventually improve the functioning and the prognosis of these patients.

The same Gestaltkreis principle applies in the case of cancer. Destruction of the tumor is only the first step of therapy. The ultimate outcome depends on the question whether the patient will find a new object to satisfy his idiosyncratic need. Some accomplish this spontaneously, but others can be helped by physicians who understand the psychophysiology of cancer.

DR. GREENE: This conference has been quite different from the last one, and I should like to comment on some things that I think have changed somewhat.

One is that there has been less concern with the questions, do or do not psychological factors play a part in the manifest development, precipitation, perpetuation, or what-have-you, of neoplasia. I think one of the most striking new developments in this conference, compared to the last, has been the rise of immunology. In spite of the fact that people say that we should not jump to questions of intervening variables, particularly in this field, it may be necessary to do so. I am reminded of the time I first did my work with leukemia patients. This was when my colleague, George Engel, said to me, "You'd better not go around saying that leukemia is a psychosomatic disease." Certain people looked at my initial data and conceptualized the relationship by making such statements as: "It has been known for years that in leukemia the white cells eat up the red cells," based on the association with an oral model in relation to depression, and so on. The only problem with this is that in leukemia it is true that the white cell's measure gets larger and the red cell measure gets smaller, but these two changes have nothing to do with each other. There is a general kind of thinking at an early stage of life when the child assumes that if one measure gets larger and another measure gets smaller, the larger one is eating up the smaller one.

At the same time, people also cast on the patients with leukemia the mourning-and-melancholia model that these patients were naturally guilty, that these patients must have been furious because they were reacting to a loss. The only problem was that in the leukemia patients, at least, there was not evidence of suppressed fury.

I think that I look forward to some increased acceptance of the possibility that psychological factors may play a part in neoplasia, because we have now not only the endocrine-mediating mechanisms as a possibility, we also now have the immunological processes as possible mediating factors. I hope and expect that there will be some fighting among the immunologists and endocrinologists over which is more important in mediating psychological factors.

I should like to say something briefly about controls. Dr. Margolin mentioned this in terms of the problem of looking at the cancer population, compared with the noncancer population. Is this sufficient? I say this, having been a person who has never used controls because I don't know where I can find a relevant population of controls. But I feel it may be important to indicate what category of patients with carcinoma one is studying. In other words, my own particular population of patients has consisted of leukemias and lymphomas, which are somewhat similar in terms of neoplasia. Dr. Kissen's populations have, by and large, been patients with carcinoma of the lung, and most of the other studies have been on groups of patients with various types of carcinoma. I think it is important to know, for instance, whether these patients were predominantly those with carcinoma of the gastrointestinal tract, which in itself may reflect, may be a function of, a particular psychological type and determine the interpretations one obtains.

I want to echo what Dr. Weiss said about possible areas of solving some of our unanswered questions by looking for and looking at persons who develop these diseases, who happen to have had psychological tests. I echo what he said because this echoes what I said at the last conference. I pointed out then that it is very difficult to get out of college these days without having had psychological tests.

I might point out that in my twins with leukemia, we have Rorschach, TAT test data on one set of the sets of twins. I don't think these data are of any significance, chiefly because the tests were done a year after the sick twin became ill. What I am doing is having a very good school psychologist take all of the data that is available from the schools on all of these sets of twins. I have told her to tease anything out of this data that she can, not knowing which twin is sick. This material goes back ten or so years on these twins before the manifest disease developed.

I also want to make a plea for looking not only at psychological variables pertaining to the development of illness in patients with neoplasia and at psychological factors that may contribute to morbidity and relapses, but also at psychological factors that may contribute to sustained remission. In particular, there has been some talk here by the immunologists about the question of spontaneous and nonspontaneous tumors in animals. There are instances of spontaneous remission of malignancies in humans. I assume that these are not spontaneous. They are related to some kind of factors. It would be important to look at these particular patients as they are available.

Dr. Bahnson: It was nice to hear again, Dr. Greene, that you do not like psychological tests, and perhaps at another conference we should talk about methodology. We have with us one panelist, Dr. Solomon, who also was on the last panel. Dr. Solomon plays this double role because he actually is both an immunologist and a psychiatrist. Dr. Solomon, please.

Dr. Solomon: I first want to mention something that really has not been brought out at this conference from the psychiatric point of view. In regard to the effect of cancer on the individual's emotions, there exists the possibility of unconscious, rather than conscious, awareness of having cancer. The cancer itself may not yet have been detected. I had two striking experiences as an intern that I should like to relate. Perhaps it is just as well to return to clinical material because I think the anecdote still does have a place, in spite of all our emphasis on research at this conference.

A board-qualified surgeon appeared at Barnes Hospital and stated: "I have a carcinoma of the colon, and I have come to this fine institution for a colectomy." How did he know it? He said, "I don't have any symptoms, I just know it." A variety of diagnostic procedures was done, and no neoplasm could be found. The patient was referred to a psychiatrist, who considered him to be an obsessive personality with a fixed somatic delusion. In view of a rather organic orientation of that psychiatry department, a unilateral prefrontal lobotomy was performed, after which the patient said, "Well, I still have my carcinoma of the colon and would like a colectomy." A lobotomy was done on the other side. I became aware of this case at a postmortem clinicopathological conference showing his disseminated metastatic carcinoma of the colon. In retrospect, the initial film taken at the time of his admission showed the carcinoma, but it had been missed.

The second case was that of a patient presented on rounds to the visiting Professor of Medicine from Oxford University. This patient had a severe mental disturbance bordering on psychosis, myasthenia (muscle weakness), and peripheral neuritis. The professor said, "Let me see his chest films, because this man obviously has carcinoma of the lung, does he not?" The answer was, "No, he doesn't." The professor looked at the chest films and asked, "What is this small shadow?" The staff said, "Those are hilar nodes." He replied, "No. There is a small primary carcinoma of the lung. These mental symptoms and the entire symptom complex are due to some humoral factor elaborated by this type of cancer." This very small and nonmetastatic cancer was removed, after which all of the man's mental symptoms disappeared. We know that the mental functioning can affect endocrine functioning and endocrine functioning can affect mental functioning. I think we're coming to know that emotions may affect immunity, and perhaps immunity may affect the central nervous system. Thus, in addition to psychological relationships to cancer, there may be important relationships between cancer and psychology, too. Perhaps we haven't emphasized the other side enough in this conference.

I really jumped at the chance to be up here with Dr. Bahnson, because I want to thank him for doing heroic work in organizing what I think has been a most stimulating and valuable conference. Dr. LeShan said before that the day of the Renaissance man is no longer, but I think Dr. Bahnson belies that. He is a musician, poet, philosopher, and scientist who is familiar with both biological and psychological concepts, and is a very generous, concerned and compassionate human being, besides. Thanks.

DR. BAHNSON: In closing, may I say that this conference could not have come about if it had not been for the very intensive help tendered by an organization committee consisting of Dr. Emerson Day, Dr. Feder, Dr. Mastrovito, and Dr. Waxenberg, as well as Dr. Solomon, who was to a high degree responsible for the invitation and involvement of the immunological participants, and for the immunological aspects of the program. I thank the organization committee for its valuable work and also extend thanks to the New York Academy of Sciences, which made this conference possible.

Printed in the United States of America